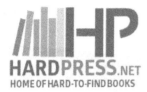

A Treatise on the Pneumatic Aspiration of Morbid Fluids
by Georges Dieulafoy

Address:
HardPress
8345 NW 66TH ST #2561
MIAMI FL 33166-2626
USA
Email: info@hardpress.net

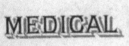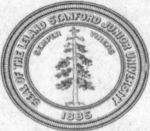

PNEUMATIC ASPIRATION.

LONDON : PRINTED BY
SPOTTISWOODE AND CO., NEW-STREET SQUARE
AND PARLIAMENT STREET

A TREATISE

ON THE

PNEUMATIC ASPIRATION

OF

MORBID FLUIDS

A Medico-Chirurgical Method of Diagnosis and Treatment

OF

CYSTS AND ABSCESSES OF THE LIVER—STRANGULATED HERNIA—
RETENTION OF URINE—PERICARDITIS—PLEURISY—
HYDARTHROSIS, &c.

BY

DR. GEORGES DIEULAFOY

GOLD MEDALLIST OF THE HOSPITALS OF PARIS

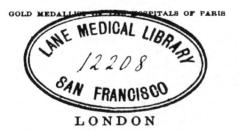
LONDON

SMITH, ELDER, & CO., 15 WATERLOO PLACE

1873

To the Memory

OF

MY ILLUSTRIOUS MASTER,

TROUSSEAU.

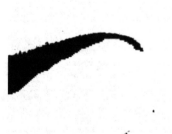

TABLE

OF

FRENCH AND ENGLISH WEIGHTS AND MEASURES.

———◆———

1 Milligramme   =   ·015 grs.

1 Centigramme   =   ·15 grs.

1 Decigramme   =   1·54 grs.

1 Gramme   =   15·43 grs.

1 Millimetre   =   ·039 inches.

1 Centimetre   =   ·39 inches.

1 Decimetre   =   3·93 inches.

1 Metre   =   39·37 inches, or 1 yd. 3·7 in.

1 Litre   =   1 pt. 15 oz. 2 drs. 111 m.

CONTENTS.

—◆—

CHAPTER IX.

PART III.

ASPIRATION OF THE SEROUS CAVITIES.

CHAPTER I.

CHAPTER II.

CHAPTER IV.

CHAPTER V.

CHAPTER VI.

PART IV.

THE TREATMENT BY ASPIRATION OF EFFUSIONS INTO THE CELLULAR TISSUE.

CHAPTER I.

CHAPTER II.

CHAPTER III.

CHAPTER IV.

PART V.

ASPIRATORS.

PLATES.

A TREATISE

ON

PNEUMATIC ASPIRATION.

GENERAL OUTLINE.

I HAVE applied the power of pneumatic aspiration which the vacuum of the air-pump supplies, to the removal of pathological fluids in the practice of medicine and surgery. The apparatus used for this purpose has received the name of aspirator, and the medico-chirurgical method itself I have called the aspiratory method. This method is applicable to the diagnosis and treatment of all fluids, and it tends to combine, under the same therapeutic unit, various methods by which the same results have hitherto been attempted. This book has for its subject the study of this method. It is divided into five parts. In the first part I give a general sketch of aspiration, and pass under review its origin, object, uses, and different applications. The second part treats of aspiration of fluids accumulated in the different organs, of cysts and tumours of the liver, of retention of urine, strangulated hernia, hydrocephalus, &c. In the third part, the aspiratory method is examined with regard to its application to the fluids of serous cavities, pericarditis, acute and chronic pleurisy, hydarthrosis, &c. The fourth part considers the application of aspiration to fluid collections in the cellular tissue, both superficial and deep, to cold abscesses, perinephritic phlegmon, iliac abscess, and blood tumours, &c. The fifth part gives an account of the different forms of the aspirator.

PART I.

PNEUMATIC ASPIRATION IN GENERAL.

CHAPTER I.

CONCERNING ASPIRATORS AND ASPIRATION.—HISTORY.—THE STATE OF SCIENCE BEFORE AND AFTER THE 2ND OF NOVEMBER, 1869.

ON the 2nd of November, 1869, Professor Gubler presented, in my name, to the Academy of Medicine, an apparatus which I had named an *aspirator*, and a paper giving a general view of a method called *aspiration*. In this paper I showed how aspiration constitutes a method of diagnosis and treatment, by means of which we can proceed with certainty and without danger in our search for pathological fluids, whatever may be their seat or their nature. Exploratory punctures, less sure and sometimes dangerous, will henceforth give place to *aspiratory* punctures, always harmless. The most delicate organs of the economy will be traversed without any bad results, and collections of fluid hidden in the depths of the tissues, will not escape our means of investigation in future. I said, in this paper, that urine could be aspirated in cases of retention, and that strangulated hernia could be reduced after the aspiration of the gas and fluids which distend the intestine.

I pointed out that the same process was applicable to hydarthrosis, pericarditis, acute and chronic pleurisy, to various kinds of cysts,—in one word, to effusions of every description, serous, hæmatic, or purulent, which can be searched for, found, and exhausted. The truly important point, which I made prominent in my communication to the Academy of Medicine, was the principle on which this method, which includes the treatment of all pathological fluids, is based; and this principle is inseparable from two conditions, namely:—(1) The use of extremely fine hollow needles; (2) the creation of a previous vacuum.

The creation of a *previous vacuum :* everything lies in this. This idea, which is so simple and of so easy an application, differentiates aspiration, at the outset, from the methods which preceded it. Since the time of Galien and his pyulcon,* surgeons of all ages have been groping about without actually discovering that which they stood in need of. Their researches, however, gave birth to various kinds of suction apparatus, such as syringes, syphons, pumps, and other instruments, which were in turn adopted and laid aside. M. Bouchut, in a learned essay,† has considered the question from an historical point of view; he has informed us of the numerous alterations and modifications made in these apparatus from the time of Galien till now, and he has shown their insufficiency. After the subject had been abandoned for a long time, the sixteenth and seventeenth centuries saw the reappearance of the pyulcon with Jean de Vigo, the application of the trocar with Drouin, and the use of needles with Mick. In our days it has been attempted, by changing its name and appearance, to re-establish the pyulcon, but in vain; it became a bladder in the hands of Laúgier, a trocar with M. Van den Corput, and a syringe with M. Guérin. Its form changed, but the

---

* Pyulcon from πῦον, pus, and ἔλχω, I draw out.

† De la Thoracentèse par Aspiration dans la pleurésie purulente et dans l'hydropneumo thorax. Paris, 1871.

idea which gave it birth remained, with all its hereditary faults, and these different inventions, like those preceding them, fell successively into oblivion. This was seeking at a distance that which lay near at hand ; turning in the same circle without quitting it; returning to Galien when they should have thought of Torricelli or Guéricke. What have I done? I have utilized the vacuum and its aspiratory power by simplifying the air-pump for the occasion; and I have shown, by conceiving the idea of the aspirator, how it is possible to have at one's service, in an instant, a powerful vacuum capable of drawing up the thickest fluids through the finest needles. This was very simple ; it was only necessary to apply to medicine one of the most common principles of physics ; but yet, the idea must first have been conceived, and, therefore, I trust that I shall be admitted to have been the first to conceive the idea. Thenceforth the problem so long attempted, how to draw out pathological fluids, appeared solved ; the perfection of the vacuum compelled fluids of every description to rise through the extremely fine needles used. The fineness of the needles guaranteed the harmlessness of the punctures. The harmlessness of the puncture allowed us to attempt and dare that which we had never attempted before, and the applications of the new method became innumerable, whilst the principle astonished by its simplicity. A phenomenon, which inevitably accompanies every invention, occurred here also, one which must be accepted without complaint, knowing it to be the most certain test we possess in science. When a man has had the good fortune to find what he was seeking (or even what he was not seeking), his discovery is immediately disputed, and what pains are taken to prove to him that his idea is as old as the world, and devoid of value ! I had hardly made the aspiratory method public, when the question of priority arose in France and other countries; claims were urged, some good-naturedly, others with asperity, not to say more, and more than one inventor of a trocar or syringe thought himself authorized to claim for himself the discovery of aspiration. Attempts were even made to drag down the debate, and to limit to a mere question of stop-cocks an innovation which affected medicine and surgery on so many sides.

The soundest arguments do not convince those who will not see. "But," we said to these pretenders, "since you invented aspiration so many years ago, how is it that it has never been mentioned, whilst a few months have suf-ficed to spread it through every country? Where are your publications, in what books are your doctrines stated, in what papers or journals have you registered your observations? where is the question of the *previous vacuum* raised, and of aspiration applied to effusions of the pericardium, to hydarthrosis, and to cysts of the liver? Show us the results of this proceeding in strangulated hernia, and in retention of urine? How is it that you have not been able to quote a single case, *not one,* whilst now they are to be numbered by hundreds?" And thus the pretended inventors were obliged to evade the question, or to keep silence. When, however, a new idea is launched, it is not alone necessary to claim to be its originator, but also to bring forward facts and proofs. We could have wished to eliminate from the debate all personal matters, but it seems to us right to establish, once for all, the starting-point and origin of this method of aspiration, which is still so young that its genealogy might well have been overlooked.

It is a matter of small importance to us to discover if the difference be great between such a trocar and such a syringe or aspirator. We leave, for a time, these instru-mental details; that which interests us is to establish with certainty the origin of aspiration—a method entirely French—which comprises the diagnosis and treatment of pathological fluids. I therefore state the question thus : *Before* my presentation to the Academy, on the 2nd of November, 1869, was a vacuum created expressly for the purpose ever employed as a means of discovering accumulations of fluid, and was aspiration developed into a method? Had any one, at any time, or in any country, applied it to the reduction of strangulated hernia, to the retention of urine, to the treatment of hydarthrosis and cysts of the liver, and to the extraction of effusions into the pericardium? Did there exist a single recorded observation concerning it in France or in other countries? My investigations permit me to be positive and exclusive in my answer, and to these different questions I reply—No. On the other hand, what has taken place *since* the 2nd of November, 1869? The method originated in France has rapidly spread over the two Continents, and in a short time, in order to fulfil various needs, seventeen aspirators have been invented.* This idea of employing a previous vacuum and a powerful aspiratory force has been so quickly grasped, that

* The principle in an aspirator is invariable; it consists in the fineness of the needles and the creation of a previous vacuum. As to the form and dimensions of the apparatus, they of course can be modified *ad infinitum.* Among other aspirators I may mention—

Dieulafoy's Aspirateur Encoche.
Dieulafoy's Aspirateur Cremailliere.
Hamon's Aspirator.
Potain's Aspirator.
Smith's Aspirator (London).
Rasmussen's Aspirator (Copenhagen).
Weiss's Aspirator (London).
Weiss's Superposed Aspirator (London).
Castiaux's Aspirator.
Regnard's Aspirator.
Leiter's Aspirator (Vienna).
Thénot's Aspirator.
Fleuret's Steam Aspirator.
Dieulafoy's Double Aspirator.

every one is anxious to improve or invent an aspirator for himself. A vacuum has been made in bottles and bladders, sometimes by very simple means, sometimes by complicated chemical processes. In a few months I have received communications from every country.* First, Russia, the spirit of which country is progressive; then North America; and afterwards England, Austria, Denmark, Mexico, Portugal, Spain, &c., adopted this new treatment of pathological fluids, and their scientific journals have been unanimous in making it well known; since that time various learned societies have been engaged in discussing the subject.

Aspiration has provoked long discussions in the Academy of Medicine, a consequence of which has been that the treatment of effusions of the pleura has been replaced amongst the questions of the day. Since the introduction of aspiration, the retention of urine, a complication so much dreaded in diseases of the genito-urinary passages, has been reduced to an insignificant incident; the reduction of strangulated hernia is effected in the greater number of cases by means of a simple puncture with a needle; effusions of the pericardium are exhausted with as much ease as those of the pleura, and the fresh applications made every day of the invention prove that we are on ground not hitherto explored.

The start has already been made, and aspiration is everywhere on the order of the day for discussion in all the medico-chirurgical societies, in scientific meetings,

* I am happy to express my thanks to foreign physicians who, from the beginning, have had the kindness to give me their aid, and who have been so good as to give me detailed accounts of the use of aspiration in their respective countries. These physicians are MM. Kieter and Zizurin of St. Petersburg, Kleinberg of Moscow, Drs. Marion Sims and James Little of New York, Sir Henry Thompson of London, MM. Billroth and Mosetig of Lisbon, C. Chaix of Mexico, Sanchez y Rubio of Madrid, Minich of Venice, Wising of Stockholm, Zaldivar of Salvador.

and in all the hospitals. Papers published here on the subject are translated in foreign countries, and various applications of the method have already been made the subject of many inaugural theses of the Faculty of Paris.*

Since when have these facts and discussions, these numerous articles and publications, which appear on all sides, and bear witness to the new current of thought, since when have these appeared? Since the 2nd of November, 1869.

The comparison which I have made between the state of science before and after my communication to the Academy is the best argument which I can use to prove the originality of my invention of aspiration. I have given dates and facts, because I know of no more positive proofs. I have replied at once to all the pretended inventors, for it would. be too much to reply to each one in particular, and I trust I have not overstepped the limits of an ordinary discussion.

Such is the actual state of the question. What do those now think who from the outset condemned the method, without even taking the trouble of understanding it? "What is the object," they said, "of changing that which already exists; what need of sub-

* Treatment of Strangulated Hernia by Aspiration. Autun, Thèse de Paris, 1871.

Treatment of Retention of Urine by Aspiration. Watelet, Thèse de Paris, 1871.

Treatment of Effusions of the Knee-joint by Aspiration. Aubry Thèse de Paris, 1871.

Treatment of Strangulated Hernia. Lecerf, Thèse de Paris, 1872.

Different Processes of Thoracentesis. Ligerot, Thèse de Paris, 1872.

Treatment of Strangulated Hernia by Aspiration. Brun-Buisson, Thèse de Paris, 1872.

The Application of Aspiration to Medicine. Castiaux, Thèse de Paris, 1873.

stituting new methods for old; and, moreover, is it possible for pus to pass through these fine needles, or to create a vacuum strong enough to draw it out? Similar attempts have been made twenty times, and have not succeeded." They thought they must stifle in the germ an invention which wounded certain susceptibilities, and which presumed to bring itself before the public without respect for routine, and without pity for the antiquated notions of the past. But it is not necessary to insist any longer on questions already settled.*

* See on this subject a communication made by M. Libermann to the Société de Médicine des Hôpitaux, at the meeting of May 10th, 1871.

CHAPTER II.

Three months after my communication to the Academy of Medicine, I published a paper,* in which I gave more circumstantial details concerning aspiration, considered as a method of diagnosis and treatment. In the course of my medical studies I had always been struck by the insufficiency of the means of investigation in difficult and doubtful cases, and often, both in medicine and surgery, I had seen the most able men held in check, adjourn their diagnosis and defer their treatment, until more certain signs or better established probabilities appeared to render the case plainer. How, for example, were we to be certain as to the existence and seat of a deeply hidden effusion of which the symptoms were not well pronounced; how were we to know, in such a case, whether surgical interference be useful, urgent, or injurious?

To meet these wants, the exploratory trocar was invented; but this trocar, which is only capillary in name, does not, it must be owned, fulfil, in any respect, the idea which originated it. It carries in itself its own condemnation; it is at once too thick and too small. Its diameter is, in fact, large, if we compare it with the fine needles which we use for subcutaneous injections, and, in spite of its bore, it

* Concerning Aspiration, Method of Diagnosis and Treatment.

often prevents the flow of fluids, either because they are thick, or because the opening of the cannula is closed. However, for want of better, surgeons had recourse to the exploratory trocar. They introduced it in searching for supposed fluids, and unfortunately the exploration was not always attended with the best results. Take, for example, an abdominal tumour, which is supposed to be of a fluid nature, and which it is wished to diagnose; the puncture is made, the trocar is inserted, but nothing flows. Recourse is had to various suppositions; perhaps false membranes obstruct the opening of the canal; or perhaps the fluid is too thick to flow through; and at last it is asked if penetration has been truly effected down to the collection of fluid. To be brief, the trocar is pushed further forward, the tumour pressed upon in the hopes of making the expected fluid gush forth, and rarely the desire is resisted to malaxate the region under exploration. These manœuvres are not effected without some pain; the points of contact between the serous membrane and the instrument are multiplied; soon afterwards vomiting and hiccups begin, the abdomen is inflated, the sufferings become more acute, peritonitis declares itself, and death is sometimes the consequence of a mere tentative exploration.

It was to remedy the inconveniences of the exploratory trocar that I had the idea of making use of long, hollow needles, of so small a size that the most delicate organs could be traversed by them without their being injured more than by acupuncture needles, the perfect harmlessness of which is well known. These needles should not measure more than half a millimetre in diameter, but in order to make fluids as thick as pus pass through so small a channel, the fluid must be drawn out by means of a powerful aspiratory force. This force I found in the vacuum of the air-pump, which I modified to suit the circumstances, and thenceforth, I was in possession of the aspirator and the previous vacuum. What is, then, this *previous vacuum* to which I call particular attention ? for it is that which from the first has decided the success of aspiration. An aspirator, whatever it be, is nothing else than a recipient in which a vacuum is made. This recipient, or body of the pump, is furnished with stop-cocks, by means of which communication is obtained with the external air. As soon as the vacuum is formed in the body of the pump, a power of aspiration is held in reserve, to be utilized when the proper moment arrives. Thus a vacuum is first established. This vacuum, or, if preferred, the body of the pump in which it is made, is put into relation, by means of one of its stop-cocks, with the fine needle intended to be introduced into the tissues. To satisfy ourselves as to the value of this proceeding, let us take an example. Let us imagine a cyst deeply seated in the liver, and let us proceed to search for the fluid by means of the previous vacuum. The aspirator is prepared, or, in other words, the vacuum is made as a preliminary, and the needle is put into communication with the body of the pump, the stop-cocks remaining closed. This hollow needle is then introduced into the region to be explored, and when it has passed the distance of a centimetre through the tissues (that is to say, when the opening at the point is no longer in contact with the external air), the corresponding stop-cock of the aspirator is opened. What occurs ? The air contained in the needle is at this point rarefied by the previous vacuum in the body of the pump, and the needle possesses in its turn aspiratory power; it becomes an aspiratory needle, and carries the vacuum with it. Then, if pushed through the tissues, it is with the vacuum in our hands that we proceed to the discovery of the effusion. At the moment that the aspiratory needle reaches the fluid, the latter rapidly traverses the glass index, jets into the aspirator, and

the diagnosis is inscribed in the apparatus without the interference of the operator.

Owing to the proceeding thus described, and having at
our command a previous vacuum, we are certain not to
pass beyond the layer of fluid, which is of consequence if
the collection be of small extent; and we are sure not to
go too far, which is of still greater importance, if behind
the effusion there is a vital organ, such as the heart.
We may know exactly at what moment the needle
penetrates a bladder distended by urine or a hernial loop
of intestine; in one word, we have in our hands an intelligent force, which, moreover, has the advantage of
being perfectly innocent. It is by separately studying its
different applications that all the importance of the previous vacuum can be appreciated. I am content for the
present to determine its utility and mode of employment.

The previous vacuum is, above all, a means of diagnosis; it is extremely valuable in the search for a collection of fluid, and thus the exploratory trocar has been
hastily abandoned to adopt the aspiratory needles. But
when the end is attained, that is to say when our only
concern is to evacuate the fluid which has just been encountered, then very often the subsequent vacuum is made
use of. Therefore, a complete aspirator ought to be able
to produce a previous vacuum and a subsequent vacuum;
it ought even to be capable of being changed, at a given
moment, into a syphon.

By a *subsequent vacuum* I mean that which is produced in the body of a pump when the piston is raised
in such a way as to draw up the fluid as it presents itself.
It is the vacuum which is made in syringes and other
instruments of the same kind. Certain opponents of
aspiration have thought they had found in the subsequent
vacuum an argument to oppose to the previous vacuum.
" The subsequent vacuum," they say, " is far from having
the same power as the previous vacuum; thus it ought to

be preferred to it, for it exposes the patient to no consecutive accident." I own that I do not well grasp the argument. Do those who argue thus desire to establish degrees in the force of aspiration, according to the *quantity* of the vacuum at our service ? We should say, if we listen to them, that a subsequent vacuum which would not give, let us say, more than four cubic centimetres of vacuum at every stroke of the piston, ought to be ten times less powerful than a previous vacuum, which would give at one stroke forty cubic centimetres. But such reasoning would be so utterly opposed to the most elementary laws of physics, that it would not even be worth the trouble of discussing it. A vacuum is a vacuum, and supposing it perfect, it would never give an aspiratory force greater than that of one atmosphere ; thus, whether it be subsequent or previous, whether the body of the pump measures four or forty cubic centimetres, the *power* of aspiration does not vary, and the *quantity* is quite an indifferent element.

The *quality* of the vacuum, on the contrary, causes marked modifications in the aspiratory power. The more rarefied the air, the greater is the power of the vacuum. In every well-made aspirator, the mischievous space is reduced to very small dimensions, owing to the perfection with which an instrument must be constructed whose function is not only to produce, but also to preserve, a previous vacuum. The older instruments, syringes, and pyulca of every kind, which aimed only at producing a subsequent vacuum more or less good, did not require the same perfection of construction ; thus they were only capable of sucking up fluids very badly, so badly that they were modified twenty times without, what was desired being obtained. The subsequent vacuum only owed its imperfection then to a fault of construction, but it necessarily found again all its power in the aspirators, and furnishes a force equal to that of the previous vacuum.

It is thus seen that the opponents of aspiration have no

reason for preferring the subsequent to the previous
vacuum, since they have each the same aspiratory power.
But in their minds subsequent vacuum is synonymous
with imperfect vacuum, and their objection does not the
less persist in another form.   To them, a vacuum badly
made is preferable to a vacuum well made, and the reason
is that they fear the great power of the latter.   But,
as I have just shown that, in an aspirator, the subsequent
vacuum has the same power as the previous vacuum, it
follows, that our honourable opponents, in order to be
consistent with themselves, make grave charges against
aspiration, as we understand it to-day, and regret the
advent of aspirators.

Their objections do not appear to us difficult to answer;
they fear, they say, the accidents which may be the consequence of a too complete vacuum.   It is only necessary to
come to an understanding with each other.   This paradox
conceals a confusion of thought which it is urgent on us to
dispel.   That which is dangerous is not the quality or
the perfection of the vacuum, but the *dose* in which it is
used.   If I have to draw out the pus of a cyst or abscess
in the liver by aspiration, it is necessary that the
vacuum should be sufficiently perfect to allow me to draw
out the fluid, and to cause it to pass through a needle
which is only the half of a millimetre in diameter ; so far
there is no harm done, but the important point is that
aspiration be not pushed to excess, and that it be not
continued in an ill-advised way to the point of cupping
the interior of the cyst.   In such a case, indeed, the
vacuum would be prejudicial ; it would especially be so if
the thoracic cavity were operated on, without sufficient
consideration for the delicacy of the lungs, and the state
of the pleura.

Aspiration must not be blamed for making too good a
vacuum, but the operator must be condemned who makes
use of aspiration without understanding it.   It is not

sufficient to have in one's hand an aspiratory needle and a powerful force; it is, above all, necessary to know how to make use of them. To choose the diameter of the needle adapted to the case, to apply or discontinue the force at the proper time, these are essential conditions; in one word, it is necessary to know how to *manage the vacuum,* and the conclusion is, that the trouble of studying the question should be undertaken before judgment is pronounced on it. If, indeed, the previous vacuum, put into communication with a collection of fluid, must necessarily exhaust all its power, and without it being possible to arrest its effects, in that case, I understand, it would be open to reproach. Then, it is true, energetic aspiration, carried too far and continued too long in the interior of a cyst or an organ, might possibly cause accidents, such as hæmorrhage, laceration, &c., but this need not be, for the operator suspends aspiration at his will; it is sufficient to turn the stopcock of the aspirator, as the break of a machine is applied, and the quantity of the required vacuum is controlled. It can be applied, discontinued, controlled, distributed according to the organ, and according to the case; it can be employed in every way, so that every objection fails, and the previous vacuum preserves its superiority all the more because it can be regulated, and applied quite as well as the subsequent vacuum.

I have said that a good aspirator ought to be able, at a given moment, to be transformed into a syphon. The syphon is of itself an organ of aspiration, and M. Potain has made an ingenious application of it, in the treatment of purulent pleurisy. It is well not to forget the properties of the syphon. Without entering into theoretical considerations on this physical instrument, we should recollect that a syphon ought to be ten metres long to possess an aspiratory force equal to that of a pneumatic pump (water being taken as the objective), and its long arm to measure from seven to eight metres, in order that

c

its aspiratory force should equal that of a good pneumatic aspirator. By this it is seen how weak is the aspiratory power of a syphon, which only measures the space which separates the bed of the patient from the floor. Now, if this force be sufficient, when put in action, to exhaust an effusion of the pleura, it is because the lung by its expansion aids the expulsion of the fluid, and, above all, because the tube introduced into the pleura, if used for the treatment of purulent pleurisy, is often of a large size. But if, by means of this syphon and a fine needle, it be attempted to draw out the fluid of an abscess of the liver or the fæcal matter of strangulated hernia, no result is obtained.

Nothing is more simple than to change an aspirator into a syphon. The descending arm of the tube must be emptied by a stroke of the piston; the current is then established, and the stream is continuous. We shall have to discuss the value of the syphon at length when we come to speak of the treatment of effusions into the pleura. It may be stated in advance, however, that it constitutes only a very imperfect mode of aspiration.

CHAPTER III.

The tolerance of certain organs for fluid tumours is a remarkable fact; thus a hydatid cyst of the liver may develope itself for many months without its presence being betrayed, except by the most insignificant symptoms. It is the same with certain ovarian cysts and those of the spleen, and with some effusions into the pleura, which are discovered on the post-mortem table without the existence of the disease having ever been revealed by signs sufficient to attract attention. The silent progress of these fluid formations is easily explained. The slowness of their developement allows the organs to become accustomed to the gradual compression, and the symptoms of the tumour are not clearly marked until it has attained considerable proportions.

Purulent collections behave differently, according to the circumstances; in the acute stage, they are accompanied by fever, pain, and other well-marked phenomena; but when they are of a chronic nature, they only exert a morbid action in their vicinity by compression, and their growth may also remain unknown till they have acquired exaggerated dimensions.

There is then a group of fluid, serous, cystic, and purulent tumours, which increase slowly without any marked reaction, almost without signs, and which do not

c 2

betray their presence in an evident manner till they are developed to the point of impeding the functions of neighbouring organs. Then the predominant symptoms are phenomena of pain and vascular trouble. The pain is not generally acute; it consists rather in sensations of discomfort, uneasiness, and weight, unless the nervous filaments are compromised, which gives rise to actual neuralgia. The vascular trouble is characterized by œdema, and by superficial collateral circulation, which bear witness to the obstacle presented to the deep circulation. The subcutaneous veins develope themselves in an unusual manner, and little networks of vessels appear at points where they are not normally seen.

When these different symptoms—pain, œdema, collateral circulation, are pronounced enough to attract attention, we are led to seek the cause of the evil, and we search for other signs, which may allow us to complete the diagnosis; but when they are so little developed that they merely arouse suspicions, they leave considerable indecision in the mind of the observer as to their significance. Such cases are habitually deferred till the morrow, and their diagnosis indefinitely adjourned; they are the more willingly temporized with since the life of the patient does not seem directly compromised; very often the question of exploratory punctures is raised, but the exploratory trocar being so uncertain a test, and offering so few guarantees, we delay having recourse to it till the last moment. Meanwhile we preach patience to the patient, and he is submitted to a treatment in which paints, friction, and blisters play the principal part, and which lead him slowly to the day when a decision must be arrived at.

This is what most often occurred before the introduction of aspiration; the result was that, owing to the lesion being hardly ever ascertained at the outset, clinical science wanted positive facts on which to found the diagnosis of certain affections in their first period, and cysts of the liver, kidneys, and spleen, and many other fluid tumours were not suspected or recognized till the changes were far advanced. That is why it was not possible to attack these diseases early, which was all the worse, as the chances of cure diminish in proportion as the time becomes longer from the date of formation. In fact, a fluid tumour, by its increasing developement, presses upon the tissue of the organ, thickens it, atrophies it, and diminishes or annihilates its normal function. Moreover, the limiting membranes and the sac of the effusion thicken, become vascular, and, in a word, organized, and prove to be one of the most serious obstacles to the success of the treatment. Thence a twofold impotence, clinical and therapeutical, the one leading to the other. Such was often the situation of the medical man when called upon to give his advice on certain tumours at their first period, or period of formation. But now new processes do not leave any place for doubt and hesitation; it is no longer justifiable to temporize or to defer till the morrow a diagnosis which should be made to-day; explorations made by means of the aspiratory needle are the most certain and most harmless test which we possess, and the punctures made by a needle which measures but half a millimetre in diameter are quite inoffensive. I have thrust these needles into almost every part of the body, into the joints, the liver, the spleen, the bladder, the intestines, the lungs, and the meninges, and I can affirm, and a great number of observers affirm with me, that we have never seen consecutive accidents. We know with what fear a simple puncture of an articulation was regarded till lately; with what care adhesion was established before penetrating certain organs of the abdomen; with what recklessness he would be charged who would pierce the chest with a fine trocar, without first considering the wound of the lung. We had been educated in the idea, that the least wound of the lung was followed by

cysts of the liver, kidneys, and spleen, and many other fluid tumours were not suspected or recognized till the changes were far advanced. That is why it was not possible to attack these diseases early, which was all the worse, as the chances of cure diminish in proportion as the time becomes longer from the date of formation. In fact, a fluid tumour, by its increasing developement, presses upon the tissue of the organ, thickens it, atrophies it, and diminishes or annihilates its normal function. Moreover, the limiting membranes and the sac of the effusion thicken, become vascular, and, in a word, organized, and prove to be one of the most serious obstacles to the success of the treatment. Thence a twofold impotence, clinical and therapeutical, the one leading to the other. Such was often the situation of the medical man when called upon to give his advice on certain tumours at their first period, or period of formation. But now new processes do not leave any place for doubt and hesitation; it is no longer justifiable to temporize or to defer till the morrow a diagnosis which should be made to-day; explorations made by means of the aspiratory needle are the most certain and most harmless test which we possess, and the punctures made by a needle which measures but half a millimetre in diameter are quite inoffensive. I have thrust these needles into almost every part of the body, into the joints, the liver, the spleen, the bladder, the intestines, the lungs, and the meninges, and I can affirm, and a great number of observers affirm with me, that we have never seen consecutive accidents. We know with what fear a simple puncture of an articulation was regarded till lately; with what care adhesion was established before penetrating into the organs of the abdomen; with what recklessness would be charged who would pierce the chest with ... but from considering the sound of the ... been ... in the ... that th... followed it the passage of air into the cavity of the pleura, and by the terrible accidents of traumatic pneumo-thorax. I have shown how greatly exaggerated these fears were, and it will be seen in the articles on hydarthrosis, strangulated hernia, retention of urine, and pleurisy, that punctures of the articulations, intestines, bladder and lungs, are completely innocent in their effects, if care be taken to act according to the precepts laid down.

On this subject of harmlessness I foresee objections, and I hasten to answer them. I shall be told of aspiratory punctures, one of which caused arthritis after evacuation of a hydarthrosis, and the other an attack of peritonitis after the exploration of a hydatid cyst of the liver. The aspiratory needle, it will be said, is not then so entirely harmless, and though it may be superior to all other methods of investigation, it does not put the patient completely beyond the reach of accidents. To that I would reply that I know nothing absolute in medicine or in surgery; that in any case the accidents mentioned are extremely rare, and that, in fact, they are more often the fault of the operator, who has not conformed to the principles which have been established by experience. I will explain myself. We have a patient attacked by hydarthrosis of the knee-joint, for which aspiration is decided upon. The aspirator is prepared, and a No. 1 needle is thrust into the articulation. But the fluid does not flow. The operator, astonished, asks himself if the needle is not too fine, or the fluid too thick; he satisfies himself by many to-and-fro movements that the instrument has well penetrated the joint, and in the hope of aiding the flow of the fluid, he resorts to a deplorable manœuvre, and presses the joint between his hands. Then he removes No. 1 needle and replaces it by No. 3, and this time the fluid is rapidly extracted. But in the evening the patient experiences the preliminary pains of arthritis, which on the following day increases in intensity, and, from an isolated example, aspiration as a treatment for hydarthrosis is a little too hastily condemned. However, how is that which has taken place to be explained ? The starting point of the accidents is apparently very insignificant; it is none the less of great importance and worthy of engaging our attention. When the surgeon is about to make use of a needle, he is not always careful enough in assuring himself of its permeability, its opening being so fine that a few grains of dust or of rust suffice to close it.

It is not astonishing that, as a consequence, the fluid is arrested in its passage. Through this follow the manœuvres of which I have just spoken, the pressure of the articulation, the introduction of a larger trocar, the irritation of the synovial membrane, and the consequent arthritis.

Let us take another example. A patient is attacked by a tumour of the liver ; a No. 2 needle is introduced, and 1,800 grammes of the fluid of hydatid cyst are aspirated; there has been no pain, the patient is relieved, and the puncture is so fine that it is hardly possible to discover its mark on the skin. All goes on well; but the surgeon, desiring to prove the complete success of aspiration, percusses the liver to verify the diminution of the tumour, palpates the abdomen, measures its circumference, and, some hours later, peritonitis, fortunately limited, declares itself. These accidents are owing to the operator ; he was doubly wrong to empty so large a cyst at one operation, and to submit the patient to the process of measuring and percussion which caused the developement of accidents, when after the conclusion of the operation he should have left the patient in absolute repose.

We must, then, in investigations made by means of aspiration, act with method ; we must appropriate the size of the needle to the organ under exploration, assure ourselves in every case of the cleanness and permeability of the needle about to be used, avoid measuring and sound-

ing, which cannot but have bad results, and practise that
minute and almost exaggerated carefulness which ends by
becoming a habit of mind, and which, without exception,
removes all chance of failure.

When these conditions are adhered to, I have no fear in
asserting that a No. 1 aspiratory needle is entirely harmless; and we must be quite convinced of this, if we wish
to derive from aspiration all the benefit which may be
expected from it; if we hesitate or fear, we shall fall back
into the doubt and uncertainty in which the exploratory
trocar left us, and temporise indefinitely before making the
diagnosis certain. The needle must be thrust in bodily,
without hesitation, whatever may be the organs or the
region to be explored, and whatever may be the depth, with
the certainty that the exploration, if well made, is without
danger, and that the fluid will jet into the aspirator as
soon as the needle has reached it.

The confidence which I have in the harmlessness of exploratory punctures by means of needle No. 1 is based on
experience, and allows me to lay down without restriction
the following principle :——

*It is always possible, owing to aspiration, to search for
a fluid collection, without any danger, whatever may be
its seat or its nature.*

It will henceforth be easy to verify the accuracy of the
symptoms, even when the latter are ill-defined, by the existence of the lesion; observation will become more rigorous,
our clinical knowledge will gain in consequence, and many
pathological manifestations, which formerly seemed to us
insignificant at the outset, will, perhaps, acquire the value
of a pathognomonic sign, when we are able to establish the
relation of cause and effect. Our suspicions will be awakened
early, and we shall acquire greater skill in the examination
of fluid tumours; aspiration will furnish us with the means
of verifying our diagnosis, and therapeutics will have for its
mission to attack disease while it is as yet little to be feared.

Hitherto I have chiefly considered the difficulties of diagnosis in chronic and latent effusions ; but the previous vacuum may be called upon to render us not less important services in acute formations of fluid. The liver, which, by its situation, is bounded by two serous membranes, the peritoneum and the pleura, is an organ which ought to be closely watched ; for hepatic suppurations, whether they be primitive or consecutive, may develope themselves with such rapidity, that in a few weeks they may penetrate into one of these two serous membranes, where, according to the circumstances, they cause peritonitis or pneumo-thorax. In the case of abscess of the iliac fossa, and particularly in perityphitis, it is to be feared that the collection, by breaking into the peritoneum, may become the cause of fatal peritonitis ; in interlobar pleurisy, of which the progress is generally so devious and the symptoms so obscure, we have to fear vomicæ, with or without pneumo-thorax.

Thus, when percussion and palpation reveal an increase of volume in an organ or a region, whether it be the liver, the kidney, the pleura, or the iliac fossa, when this increase has been rapid and accompanied by pain or interference with the normal organic function, when to these local symptoms are joined general phenomena, such as rigors, sweating, and fever, more or less intermittent, we may be convinced that pus is forming somewhere; the fluid, infiltrated at first, begins rapidly to collect, then it seeks to find a passage for itself, to the detriment of the neighbouring organs or serous membranes, and we shall have reason to repent if, from inattention to the different phases of the disease, we have not acted opportunely. I should never finish if I were to endeavour to enumerate all the cases in which aspiration is called on to decide a diagnosis. Tumours of the iliac fossa and of the hypochondrium, perinephritic abscesses, encysted and interlobar pleurisy, swellings of the hips and of the pelvis, hydatids and abscess of the lung, abscess and aneurism of all regions, collections of fluid below the aponeuroses, hygroma of the deep bursæ, coxalgia, tumours of the liver, of the epiploon, &c. The means employed are always the same—the action of the previous vacuum; the finer the aspiratory needle, the more harmless the puncture, and the more perfectly must the vacuum be made to draw out the fluids.

Thus, the two elements of security and of certainty in diagnosis are the fineness of the needle and the power of the previous vacuum. The mode of operating does not vary. The needle is introduced into the tissues to be explored, and, thanks to its aspiratory power, of which I have explained the mechanism at length, this needle, which carries a vacuum at its point, becomes, in the hands of the operator, an intelligent force; it sucks up the liquid as soon as it meets it, and it indicates to us at the same time the presence, the seat, and the nature of the collection.

At the moment of introducing the needle into the tissues, it is always proper to ascertain its permeability by means of a silver wire and of a fine jet of water intended to remove any foreign bodies which may obstruct the canal. I repeat this practical detail once more, because it is desirable to avoid exposing one's self to failure from a cause which is so easy to remove.

CHAPTER IV.

THE formation of fluid in an organ is a very complex action, and is subject to laws which vary for every fluid and for every organ. Sometimes mechanical injury is the direct cause; it determines, according to the circumstances, hydarthrosis, hydrocele, effusions in regions rich in cellular tissue, and pleurisy, following on wounds in the lungs or fracture of the ribs. Sometimes the fluid accumulates in a serous cavity, the pleura, pericardium, or synovial articulation, in consequence of a change almost insignificant and altogether local in the serous membrane, from the influence of cold, damp, or a similar external cause. In other cases, behind the apparent local cause, is concealed a general condition, a holopathy,* diabetes, gout, tuberculosis, or rheumatism, which governs the situation and maintains the disorder in spite of all our efforts.

These differences in the causes of fluid formations explain why certain effusions disappear after a small number of aspirations, and without being reproduced, whilst others form again with incredible obstinacy; so much so, that we might classify the fluids according to the cause which engenders them, and we should see that they are formed with so much the greater ease as the cause which

* Holopathy, a disease *totius substantiœ*, a word established in use by M. Marchal de Calvi.

produced or maintains them is more concealed and difficult to grasp.

The causes of the purulence of a fluid are themselves very various. The formation of pus is owing sometimes to local irritation, sometimes to a general condition. the tendency of which is to change all the pathological serous secretions into pus. After these remarks on the production of effusion in different cases, it is easy to understand that aspiration cannot always have the same efficacy. It is sometimes necessary to associate with it other therapeutical agencies. It is powerless to attack the cause—it only destroys the effect ; but this effect may in its turn become a cause, and thus the circle of treatment is enlarged.

What is, then, the part played by aspiration in the treatment of pathological fluids ? It is difficult to reply in a. categorical manner, and for the reason that a new method undergoes improvement every day. When we considered aspiration as an element of diagnosis, we were justified in being affirmative and exclusive, because there are not two ways of treating the question, for the fineness of the needle and the power of the vacuum have limits which it is not possible to exceed ; but when the question is considered of its numerous applications to the treatment of fluids, we can but state the results hitherto obtained, reserving for ourselves the privilege of completing them as further knowledge is acquired. For the time being, then, we are involved in empiricism, but in an empiricism of a high stamp —that which exists at the outset of every science of observation, and which accompanies it far in its development.

Since the commencement of my labours on aspiration, I have ascertained that certain effusions yield at once and without relapse, and I have seen hydarthrosis, hydatid cysts of the liver, and accumulations in the cellular tissue cured at one sitting. I have not always been tempted to account these successes as the result of aspiration ; for every day we see effusions of the pleura yielding to a single evacuation by means of a simple trocar. I was not slow to perceive that the different serous membranes have various aptitudes for pathological secretion; thus, whilst the fluid of simple pleurisy has but little tendency to reproduce itself, the fluid of the synovial membrane of the knee-joint forms again, on the contrary, with the greatest ease, and the fluid of the cranial meninges is singularly obstinate. The cause of the formation of fluid is an important agent in the diversity and mode of its reproduction; the more this cause is local and direct, the less is the fluid reproduced; thus, in hydrocele and hydarthrosis, following on contusion, and in many other cases, it is not rare to find effusion, if not of long duration, overcome by a single aspiration.

But if this effusion is allowed to become chronic, without exit being given to it, the effect becomes a cause, and the situation is aggravated. The presence of exudation in a joint may have a bad influence on the nutrition of the synovial membrane and ligaments, the serous membrane thickens, the ligaments are distended, and thus arthritis becomes established.

Effused fluids undergo various transformations, of which the primitive cause is unknown to us. Why, for example, should one cyst of the liver be found to undergo five, six, ten aspirations before cure is completed, without the fluid losing any of its limpidity, whilst another operated on under the same circumstances, and with the same precautions, will pass on to suppuration after the first puncture? There are in the formation and change of pathological fluids gradations which still escape us, but the practical fact shown by experience is that a certain number of effusions, differing as to their seat and their nature, disappear after a single aspiration, undergo no change, and do not relapse. These facts are not of very frequent occurrence, and more often the fluid reappears, sometimes under the same form, sometimes under a different aspect, with the addition of leucocytes or bloodcrystals. But when one has to deal with an effusion which is easily reproduced, it is not enough to extract it, it must also be prevented from forming anew. It is to meet this difficulty that irritant injections of alcohol, tincture of iodine, &c., have been introduced. We know with what brilliancy this method was inaugurated in France by Velpeau, and with what rapidity it spread through all countries. These injections were intended to cause a vicarious inflammation, a modification of the secretion, or adhesion of the secreting walls. The results were often remarkable, and the cures in affections which had till then resisted every means, explain the well-merited popularity of this process. But in looking at it more closely, we see that side by side with incontestable results there were many cases in which the remedy was worse than the disease. With regard to hydarthrosis, for example, it is only necessary to read the four-and-twenty cases collected by Boinet, and published by Roux, Velpeau, and Bérard, to be convinced that iodine injections very often caused intense inflammatory accidents, violent pain, fever, and rapid swelling of the joint; so much so, that, to remedy these accidents, it became necessary to have recourse to an energetic antiphlogistic treatment, and which did not always succeed in overcoming these complications. Hydatid cysts of the liver have been submitted to a similar treatment, and irritant injections after previous adhesions have given, here as elsewhere, some good results; but if one takes a strict account of all the failures, it will be seen that this process had not a well-marked superiority over the others, for the eschars, incisions, and wounds, which were a consequence, too often left the door open for different forms of purulent infection.

This method of irritant injections, practised on the organs and serous membranes, with or without previous adhesions, was not without advantages when it was invented; for no practical and inoffensive means then existed of treating pathological fluids. Before the introduction of aspiration, and when the surgeon had only the simple trocar at his command, the effects of which he had good reason to fear, he did not dare multiply punctures in certain regions, and we can understand why surgeons, who saw an effusion form again after the second or third puncture, believed in the indefinite reproduction of fluid, and occupied themselves in seeking for a therapeutical process other than simple evacuation, and thus it was that irritant injections were introduced.

But with aspiration I have given means of drawing out, without danger, without the least difficulty, and every day if required, the fluids which accumulate in the serous cavities, and in the different organs. I have sometimes found myself confronted by stubborn hydarthrosis, which I have aspirated morning and evening for eight consecutive days, or by suppurating scrofulous glands, which I have followed up for many weeks. I have had to contend with abscesses and cysts of the liver, the fluid of which was reproduced as often as I withdrew it. I have continued aspiration patiently and persistently, without the use of irritant injections, and, generally, I have obtained good results. These facts caused me to reflect, and gradually I acquired the conviction that aspiration alone, without the help of any injection, often succeeds in drying up an effusion at its source, and I thought that a kind of therapeutical law might be formulated on the subject of pathological fluids, of which the following is the expression. When a fluid, whatever be its nature, accumulates in a serous cavity or an organ, and when these are accessible to our means of investigation without danger to the patient, our first care ought to be to aspirate the fluid; if it forms again, it should be again drawn out, and as many times afterwards as it is necessary, so as to exhaust the serous cavity by an entirely mechanical and absolutely harmless means, before thinking of modifying the secretion by irritant and sometimes dangerous agents.

The same method has been successively employed by M. Dolbeau in congestive abscess, by M. Bouchut in the treatment of purulent pleurisy, and it has been recently put into use by M. da Camara Cabral, of Lisbon, who has treated and cured a child attacked by congenital hydrorachis. This is, I believe, one of the most practical proceedings which aspiration places at our service : we are in possession of a purely mechanical means, which allows us to dry up a great number of fluids, without the aid of injections ; a struggle is begun between the serous membrane which secretes, and the operator who excretes, and often the membrane is tired out sooner than the operator.

Many reasons can be given to explain this mechanical drying up of fluids. First, the initial cause, producing the effusion, acts and persists with a variable intensity ; when this cause exhausts in one effort all its mischievous power, it leaves, as a sign of its course, only an effusion which it is easy to dissipate ; but when it obstinately continues, it impresses on the effusion a tendency to relapse. Moreover, with our present ignorance as to the persistence and intensity of causes, our first care should be to withdraw the exudation, without waiting till it becomes in its turn a cause of irritation. I have often seen hydarthrosis, pleurisy, hydrocele, and even cysts of different kinds, yield rapidly to a single aspiration; we ought, therefore, to give our attention to the removal of the cause, to watch the fluid, to remove it as it forms, and to follow it up till it ceases to reappear.

The organs themselves favour the mechanical drying up of fluids, and in this manner :—I take, for example, either a chronic effusion of the pleura, or a cyst or abscess of the liver ; the cavity contains, let us say, 1,000 grammes of fluid, of which 300 are drawn off, and the result is that the lung or liver, freed from part of the pressure, tends to fill up by expansion of its tissue the void left after the issue of the fluid.

If, however, 1,000 grammes are drawn off at once, the

same end is not obtained, and the interior of the cavity having been completely emptied, becomes in its turn an instrument of aspiration. But by taking care to use successive aspirations at short intervals of time, and on a small scale, the fluid has not time allowed it to re-form, and, on the other hand, the compressed and flattened organs are gradually allowed to regain their normal situations and dimensions.

I consider it, then, a grave error to empty at one operation ovarian cysts, cysts and abscesses of the liver, the pleural sac, or large purulent collections of the cellular tissue ; it is necessary to know when to stop, to proceed slowly, with patience, without producing shock, to perform five, ten, twenty, or a hundred aspirations; these are the true conditions of success. Farther on, I report the case of a woman attacked with many hydatid cysts of the liver and the pleura, and whose condition was most serious; she was subjected to many hundreds of punctures, and her health is now perfectly re-established.

We are led to ask what becomes after this process of the sacs, walls, and enveloping membranes of cysts and various effusions. Their transformation is dependent upon their age : when these membranes are recent, they disappear *in situ* by a particular process ; either they suppurate, or they undergo fatty degeneration ; but, if they are left to grow old, they become thickened, stratified, and vascularized, and it is then necessary to attack them by means which shall be detailed in each particular case. This proves to us that we generally wait too long before attacking fluid collections ; the more recent the effusion the easier it is to master ; but if it persists long, it hollows out cavities whose walls become rigid; it alters the parts and organs with which it is in contact ; it compresses and atrophies their tissue ; and, by fixing these organs in a new and abnormal position, it becomes a hindrance to their physiological functions.

D

It is necessary, then, to have this principle well understood, that the chances of cure diminish according as the
date is distant from the period of the formation of the fluid ;
whilst successive aspirations, performed early and repeated
according to the rules that I have just laid down, have
given us successes of which an account will be given when
we come to speak of the particular applications of the
method.   This method is less brilliant than other surgical
plans of treatment, but it offers more guarantees; the
operator works in a closed cavity, without danger to the
patient, and without fear of the effects, sometimes disastrous, of incisions and irritant injections.

My intention is not to condemn injections absolutely,
far from it, for they are sometimes of incontestable utility ;
but the kind of fluid used, the therapeutical indications,
and, above all, the manner of performing injections, are
destined to undergo marked changes.   Since the discovery
of the aspiratory apparatus, it is possible to introduce and
withdraw at will every kind of injection through a needle
not more than a millimetre in diameter ; the result of
which has been that, for cleansing and modifying cavities
hollowed out in the midst of an organ or tissue, it is no
longer necessary to make large openings, or to allow
sounds of a large calibre to remain *in situ*.   These
processes, which were rendered necessary by the difficulties
experienced in managing the fluids injected, left free
access to the external air, and became too often the cause
of many accidents, such as erysipelas, ulceration, fistula,
suppuration, and purulent infection.

The aspiratory apparatus, on the contrary (which, to be
perfect, ought to be at the same time an injecting apparatus), allows us to act protected from the air, since everything
takes place in the morbid cavity, and in the receiver in
which a vacuum has been made ; the fineness of the
needles, and the punctures accumulated on the same
point, allow us, when the time for operation arrives, to

establish adhesions, which take the place of tedious and painful applications of various caustics.

Thanks to the power obtained by the play of the piston in the body of the pump, the aspiratory needle is at the same time an injecting needle ; it may be adapted to two purposes without being removed, and the narrow tube which is used to draw out the pathological fluid is also used to introduce the modifying fluid. Aspiration and injection are practised by turns, with the same facility and by the same mechanism, without pain or fatigue to the patient, who can get up or lie down at pleasure, and who is not obliged to place himself in one of those sometimes uncomfortable positions, the sole object of which is to aid the issue of the fluid.

Injections after the new method have a slightly different application, according as the needle is left within the cavity or not. It can be withdrawn after each injection, for the puncture it leaves is so insignificant that no harm is done by making it every day. When the treatment, however, is of long duration, and when the washing and injections have to be repeated several times in twenty-four hours, it is preferable to allow one of the trocars constructed for this purpose, the volume of which does not exceed that of the aspiratory needle, to remain in the morbid cavity : these trocars are particularly applicable to chronic effusions. I intend them for diseases of the liver, pleura, and pericardium, and I propose to make their use general for all affections of the same kind. They have not the inconveniences of indiarubber and gutta-percha tubes ; they undergo no change by contact with liquids, and their mode of occlusion renders the access of air impossible. They are fixed without the least difficulty by means of a few drops of collodion, and their small bore facilitates their introduction so much, that by removing them many times in the course of treatment, ulcerations and fistulas may be prevented. Finally, the projection which they make on the surface of the skin is so slight, that they occasion neither inconvenience or pain to the patient, who can get up, walk about, and follow his usual avocations. A more detailed description of this will be found in the treatment of purulent pleurisy and cysts of the liver.

The trocar being introduced and fixed by means of tapes and a few drops of collodion, what is the plan to be pursued in performing the injection? Formerly the pathological fluid was evacuated at once, and replaced by an injection, which was left partly or entirely in the cavity. This proceeding does not seem applicable in every case, and I propose to substitute for it the following :—Suppose a purulent collection of 1,000 grammes ; part of the fluid is first extracted, care being taken not to completely withdraw it the first time, nor to push aspiration to the point of producing the effect of cupping in the interior of the cavity. If the trocar or the needle is obstructed at the moment of the operation, it is only necessary to drive the obstructing body back again by an inverse stroke of the piston, and to continue aspiration. Instead of evacuating, without intermission, the entire fluid collection, only a small quantity should be drawn off, about 150 grammes, and replaced immediately by 100 grammes of injection at the same sitting. This proceeding should be repeated five, six, eight, or ten times in succession, so that after this process of cleansing, by the quantity of fluid injected being each time less than· that aspirated, the cavity would contain three or four hundred grammes of fluid less, and the purulent collection would be completely replaced by the injected fluid. This is an insensible substitution. These successive aspirations and injections are very easy to execute, as the aspirator is mathematically graduated, and the quantity of fluid set in motion may be known to within a few grammes. The cleansing process over, an injection is introduced into the morbid cavity, and should be allowed to remain : the

volume of this injection, compared with that of the pathological recipient, is equal to about a fifth part.   The operation that I have just described should be performed every
day, and even two or three times in the twenty-four hours,
in urgent cases.   It is easily seen that it has little resem-
blance to other processes, which consist in emptying a
morbid cavity by one stroke of the trocar, and refilling it
with an irritant fluid, of which the quantity and result
are often imperfectly estimated.

Injections, as they were formerly used, were surrounded
with difficulties. The syringe was very often badly bored ;
it did not hold the fluid well; its extremity imperfectly
fitted the tube left in the morbid cavity ; this tube was
difficult to fix ; it provoked ulcerations ; the cutaneous
opening was so badly closed that only half the injection
penetrated, or part of it was lost in neighbouring tissues ;
and if it was desired to withdraw the injection, it could only
be accomplished with difficulty, by malaxating between the
hands the organ or diseased part—a manœuvre which
favoured the introduction of the external air.

But by means of aspiratory-injectors the fluid is, on
the contrary, easily introduced or withdrawn at the will
of the operator, without a single drop being diverted
from its true destination ; he proceeds slowly, without a
shock, and measuring the power of projection.   This power
is given by the play of the piston, which enables him to
convey to the fluid an impulse capable of carrying it into
all the anfractuosities and the most intricate parts of the
cavity.   This is an advantage over the siphon, which has
the inconvenience of establishing a current in the same
fluid layers without reaching the thickest and most
adherent layers of the effusion.

There are, then, two very distinct stages in the method
of operation just described—cleansing and injecting.
By these means the walls of the cavity are prevented
from quickly suppurating, which occurs sometimes when

a pathological fluid is evacuated at one operation and replaced by an injection. Here the modifications are effected slowly, the detritus of false membranes and the mischievous effects of the pus are neutralized every moment; we are constant witnesses of the gradual and continuous contraction of the cavity, and the surrounding tissues and organs, at first compressed by the effusion, gradually return to their normal positions. It is the duty of the operator to follow the progress of the recovery, gradually to diminish the quantity of fluid used for cleansing and injecting, in a manner commensurate with the contraction of the cavity. The choice of the fluids used is still to be pointed out, but different cases afford different indications, and this part of the treatment will be studied in detail, with the particular applications of the method.

Thus far I have only considered the treatment of pathological fluids, but there are cases in which a normal fluid causes by its exaggerated developement a very serious morbid condition. Thus, in retention of urine, the extreme distention of the bladder becomes in a short time very dangerous if issue is not given to the fluid; but aspiration always overcomes this complication, and without the least danger, and overcomes it so well, that retention of urine, considered a few years since as one of the most terrible accidents in affections of the genito-urinary passages, is in itself now nothing more than, so to speak, an insignificant phenomenon. The treatment of strangulated hernia is, again, one of the most happy applications of aspiration; the fluids and gas which accumulate in an hernial intestinal loop, are one of the principal obstacles to the reduction of strangulated hernia; but experience every day teaches us that the aspiratory needle is sufficient, in the majority of cases, to effect the reduction of hernia in cases which had resisted taxis, and which would otherwise have had to run the risks of kelotomy.

These two last-mentioned applications of the aspiratory method, the treatment of retention of urine and strangulated hernia, introduce into surgical practice modifications as remarkable as the changes brought about in medical therapeutics by the new treatment of pericarditis, pleurisy, and cysts of the liver.

In this summary I have only spoken of accomplished facts; but much yet remains to be done. Many other applications of the aspiratory method may be already foreseen. Why should the needle not be insinuated into pulmonary cavities of phthisical patients, to modify by means of aspiration and injections the walls of the cavity and the adjoining tissue? Why should we not perform direct blood-letting of the lungs and heart in desperate cases of congestion? These different questions are now in course of study, but, faithful to a self-imposed rule, we only desire to advance facts sufficiently tested by experience.

CHAPTER V.

IN the previous chapters I have pointed out the general indications of a method which is applicable to the diagnosis and treatment of all pathological fluids, and which includes one of the largest domains of medicine and surgery. In the course of this work I have avoided comparing aspiration with other methods which, at various times and in different hands, have aimed at solving the same problem ; for such a study would, by introducing foreign elements into the discussion, only serve to complicate a question which it is the object of my efforts to simplify.

Many other processes have a value which I do not deny, and I am far from pretending that aspiration may be always and everywhere preferable to them ; but the superiority of a process or method cannot be established by means of discussion in which theory too often plays the principal part ; therefore I confine myself to a simple statement of clinical facts, the only absolute proof and the only incontestable argument, and I have rejected all hypotheses and arguments of a more or less subtle character, believing that exact and rigorous observation is the only basis on which a method can be founded.

My first care has been to establish the origin of aspiration, and I have proved that it originated in France, November 2, 1869. Since then, it has spread with such rapidity through all countries, that in three years we have collected materials and cases enough to enable us to compare and judge of its value in its different applications.   Three years have sufficed to overturn old methods and reawaken discussion as to the treatment of all pathological fluids.   Before the introduction of aspiration, each fluid collection was differently treated, according to its nature, its seat, or its age ; acute and chronic pleurisy was treated by puncture, followed by empyema with large fistulous openings ; pericarditis was attacked with fear, and as late as possible, by means of the bistoury and the trocar.   Hydatid cysts of the liver required painful applications of caustic, followed by gaping wounds, and injections of every kind ; hydarthrosis was temporized with by blisters and paintings of iodine ; and in the case of retention of urine, it was doubtful which of the proceedings in use was least mischievous ; everywhere the same uncertainty of opinions reigned, and the same divergence as to the means to be employed.

By aspiration, therapeutics are simplified ; all these different modes of treatment are fused into one ; punctures made by means of the trocar, caustics and their eschars, incisions and their pathological sequences, are disappearing day by day, and giving place to the aspiratory needle.   This needle is absolutely harmless, for it is only a millimetre in diameter ; it is armed with great power ; it carries the vacuum with it ; it passes through the tissues, and searches the depths of the organs, drawing out the fluids which it meets on its passage ; it serves, according to circumstances, as a needle of injection ; in one word, it is sufficient for almost every need.

Uniformity in Diagnosis and Treatment.—This is the first result of the aspiratory method, hence, with experience aiding me and cases accumulating, I have been enabled to draw a few conclusions which I have collected and formulated in the following propositions :—

I. It is always possible, by means of aspiration, to

search, without danger, for a fluid collection, whatever may be its seat or its nature.

II. When a fluid accumulates in a serous cavity, or in an organ, and when this serous cavity or organ is accessible to our means of investigation without danger to the patient, our first care should be to aspire the fluid; if it is reproduced, to draw it off again, and to repeat the operation many times if necessary, so as to exhaust the serous cavity by mechanical means before thinking of modifying the secretion by irritant and sometimes dangerous agents.

III. When aspiration, often repeated, does not succeed in drying up the source of the fluid, or when the fluid holds in suspension solid particles, such as crystals of cholesterine or false membranes, which fill up the small opening of the needle, use must be made of successive washings and injections, so as to act slowly on the pathological tissue, and to gradually obtain the contraction of the cavity.

Thus, with a few exceptions, unity in the treatment of fluids is obtained. This is, I believe, the greatest service that the aspiratory method has rendered.

Pathology is not composed of incongruous and heterogeneous elements; different diseases group themselves around morbid units, to which therapeutical units must necessarily correspond. Thus, the large class of scleroses, so well studied and unified by the French school of the Salpêtrière, will doubtless one day find its treatment in a therapeutical proceeding, which will be the same for all the tissues and organs attacked by sclerosis, for the pathological unit necessarily calls for the therapeutical unit.

The treatment of pathological fluids, considered under this novel aspect, is no longer the exclusive property of surgery; it takes its place in the domain of medicine : aspiration is ground on which surgery and medicine may meet, and on which, I hope, they will be able to draw closer the bands that ought to unite them. The diagnosis of fluid collections is most commonly confided to the art of the physician; it is auscultation and percussion which discover to us the effusions of the pleura and pericardium, the cysts and abscesses of the liver, &c.; and I trust that this method of aspiration, in giving to medicine the means of testing diagnosis, will also enable it to institute the treatment. The sphere of operations called medical would thus be considerably enlarged; and in that I do but follow the example of my illustrious master, Trousseau, to whom medicine owes two of its highest victories, thoracentesis and tracheotomy.

We have finished the general exposition of the aspiratory method, and when we consider its rapid development and the kind reception which it has everywhere received in foreign countries, it is pleasant to us to be able to say that it was in France that it had birth and grew.

PART II.

ASPIRATION IN THE ORGANS

CHAPTER I.

DIAGNOSIS AND TREATMENT OF HYDATID CYSTS AND OF ABSCESSES OF THE LIVER BY ASPIRATION.

Summary: Article I. — The Diagnosis of Hydatid Cysts of the Liver. — Mode of Operating — Harmlessness of the Method. Article II.: The Treatment of Hydatid Cysts of the Liver.—Cases.—New Symptoms. Article III.: Critical Examination of the Method.—Purulence of the Fluid.—Significance of Accidents.—Odour of the Fluid.—Urticaria.—Regurgitation of Fatty Matters. — Deviation of the Catamenial Period. Article IV.: Abscesses of the Liver.

I HAVE applied the method which for some years I have sought to apply generally to all pathological fluids to the diagnosis and treatment of hydatid cysts of the liver. It may now be said that aspiration has taken the place of simple puncture, and that the aspiratory needle has caused the exploratory trocar to be forgotten. Numerous observations, gathered from the most diverse cases of hydarthrosis, pericarditis, retention of urine, and strangulated hernia, have proved the absolute harmlessness of the investigation of fluids made by means of No. 1 and No. 2 aspiratory needles, and have confirmed the conclusions which I enunciated in 1870, at the time of the publication of my first paper, namely, that " It is always possible, by means of aspiration, to search, without danger, for a fluid collection, whatever may be its seat or its nature." In the present part I will limit the question to hydatid cysts and to abscesses of the liver, and I will separately consider the diagnosis and treatment of each of these diseases.

ARTICLE I.

The Diagnosis of Hydatid Cysts of the Liver by Aspiration.— Mode of Operating.—Harmlessness of the Method.

UNDER certain circumstances, and principally when the disease has arrived at an advanced stage, the symptoms of hydatid cysts of the liver are so pronounced that it is scarcely possible to commit an error of diagnosis. The tumefaction of the part, the almost uniform projection of the tumour under the false ribs, or in the vicinity of the linea alba, the sensation of elastic resistance which this tumour gives, the dilatation of the lower intercostal spaces, the extent and form of the dulness, the almost constant absence of fever, icterus, and ascites, the slow march of the disease, the presence of networks of veins on the middle of the abdomen and on the thorax ; all these signs, when they are united, leave no doubt as to the diagnosis of the disease.

But we have not always before our eyes cases so complete and, so to speak, so typical ; sometimes certain signs are absent, when, for example, the cyst has been developed towards the upper part or in the deeper parts of the organ ; sometimes a rare symptom, such as ascites, predominates and masks the true lesion, leading us into error ; and again, we are often called upon to detect a cyst at an early period, and the whole of the phenomena, taken together at this time, only allow of suppositions. We remain then in doubt, we abstain from all active intervention ; we wait patiently ; the disease progresses ; the cyst becomes multilocular, or divided by septa ; its walls thicken; it invades the greater part of the organ; the general symptoms increase in intensity; and when we are obliged to interfere, we perceive that it is sometimes too late.

In these difficult and doubtful cases, as in abdominal tumours in general, and in some bastard interlobar or encysted pleurisies, we have but one means of absolute certainty, and that is the assurance of the presence of fluid. And to arrive at this result, one process was till lately the only one used, that was the introduction into the doubtful tumour of a so-called exploratory trocar. This exploratory trocar was then introduced in search for the effusion, and what occurred? Let us suppose a negative case. The puncture is made, the trocar is in its place, but nothing flows; recourse is had to various suppositions; false membranes are thought to obstruct the opening of the cannula, or the fluid to be too thick to flow through, or it is doubted whether penetration is really effected as far as the fluid collection. To be brief, the trocar is pushed farther, the tumour is pressed upon in the hopes of making the expected drops of fluid gush out, and the part under exploration is malaxated. These manœuvres are not performed without causing pain, and soon after, vomiting and hiccups commence, the abdomen becomes inflated, the pain more acute, peritonitis declares itself, and death is sometimes the consequence of this tentative exploration. It is facts of this kind, and they are not absolutely rare, it is these sometimes fatal accidents which have bound practitioners in general to cautious prudence, and which gave rise to the idea of establishing adhesions between the organ and the abdominal walls, before hazarding a search for the fluid. Thus one is placed between two alternatives, either to run the chances of serious accidents if adhesion is not previously established, or to provoke adhesion; that is to say, to undertake a long and painful operation in order to arrive at a simple exploratory puncture. Which of these two is chosen? Most frequently neither the one nor the other; inaction is preferred, and to explain this inaction, an argument is made use of that has some appearance of truth. Taking all things into account, it is said, the cyst developes slowly, very slowly; its presence does not exert a bad influence on the economy for a long time, there is no pressing call for action, and the urgency of the case allows of surgical interference being deferred. The more specious this reasoning, the more easily it is accepted; but it is dangerous; for I can show, as is indeed rational, that a hydatid cyst has the greater chance of cure the less it is developed, and if attacked at the time nearest to its first formation. In such a case, then, the confirmation of the diagnosis must be hastened, by making one's self assured of the presence and nature of the fluid; and as a means both certain and harmless, I propose to replace puncture by aspiration, and the exploratory trocar by the aspiratory needle. I shall doubtless meet with some doubts, and shall not carry conviction at once; but I hope, by means of numerous observations, to show the truth of what I advance, and to see the process which I am about to describe universally adopted.

When I proposed aspiration of gas and fluids as a means for the reduction of the intestinal loop in strangulated hernia, the process was hastily condemned, under the impression that the puncture of the intestine would involve serious dangers, without giving good results; however, a short time afterwards, a number of cases were published, showing the efficacy and innocency of aspiration as a means of reduction in strangulated hernia.

I also assert the same of the aspiration of the fluid of hydarthrosis, a proceeding which some surgeons still look upon as rash—quite wrongly, in my opinion; for I have employed aspiration in the knee-joint many hundred times without ever having to record the slightest accident, and aspiration of fluid in hydarthrosis is rapidly becoming general.

I may, however, be allowed to make some reserves on the subject of the mode of operating, which in such cases is a matter of great importance : seventeen aspirators have been made within a short time in France and foreign countries ; they, of course, effect the previous vacuum, without which they would not be aspirators ; but the calibre and size of the needles have been altered too often, which is an error. It is indispensable to know the size of the needle which should be employed under different circumstances ; this is why I always make use of needles mathematically graduated. I base all my observations on the same standard, knowing beforehand what is the exact diameter which corresponds to needles No. 1 or No. 2 ; and thus I do not expose myself to the accidents which may happen with a needle of three millimetres in diameter, when a needle of one millimetre fulfils all the necessary conditions. Therefore, for the exploration of cysts and tumours of the liver, I always make use first of needle No. 1, and subsequently, if necessary, of needle No. 2, and I have never witnessed any serious accidents.

The Mode of Operating.—In the case of a hepatic tumour, of which the diagnosis is doubtful, I should advise the following mode of exploration :—To make use of a hollow No. 1 needle, and to assure one's self previously of its permeability by means of a silver thread and a jet of water. This precaution is necessary, for the size of the needle is so small that a few grains of rust or dust are sufficient to obstruct the opening. The aspirator being ready, that is to say, the vacuum being previously made, the needle is introduced into the part to be explored by a sharp puncture; as soon as this needle has passed a centimetre into the depth of the tissues (that is to say, as soon as the opening at its extremity is no longer in connection with the external air), the stop-cock connecting it

E

with the aspirator is turned, and a vacuum is thus also produced in the needle. This needle, which carries the vacuum with it, is slowly driven forward, and with the vacuum in our hand we advance through the tissues in our search for the fluid collection. The tissues can be thus punctured to the depth of three, five, ten, or even more centimetres, and at the instant that the aspiratory needle meets the fluid, it is seen to flow into the glass body of the pump, and the diagnosis is inscribed there without the interference of the operator.

If no issue of fluid is the result of the puncture, the part under exploration must by no means be pressed ; the needle must be withdrawn, its permeability again ascertained, and the operation recommenced at another spot ; the quantity of fluid considered sufficient must be drawn off, and the flow then stopped. The puncture is so fine that it is hardly visible, the pain is scarcely worth mentioning, and no dressing is required. It is well, as an excess of precaution, for the patient to be kept at rest for some hours afterwards.

The Consequences of Exploration.—With aspiration thus performed, I have never seen any serious accident follow, but I have sometimes observed, especially with women, the following phenomena. In some rare cases, it is true, nausea is observed after the puncture, as well as radiating pains in the abdomen or the right shoulder ; these symptoms, which might be feared as the commencement of peritonitis, are of no importance ; they disappear after a few hours ; they are not accompanied by fever ; and they are rather the result of a reflex action than the consequence of phlegmasia. Moreover, the patient who has experienced these symptoms after the first puncture, does not have a return of them at subsequent explorations. Here, not less than in tumours of the spleen, ovaries, and epiploon, I can assert that I have never observed any serious accidents. There are many things which explain the almost complete harmlessness of these explorations ; first, the extreme fineness of the needle, of which the diameter is three times less than that of the ordinary exploratory trocar, the peritoneum being therefore touched only in an extremely minute point ; and, further, the simplicity of the mode of operating. The exploratory trocar is sometimes introduced with difficulty, and it then requires jerks and efforts to make it penetrate as far as the organ to be explored ; it is never known exactly at what moment the fluid is reached, and in the fear of its having passed beyond, or not having reached its destination, the trocar is often withdrawn, or pushed forward several times, and has its direction changed. Nor is this all; if the fluid does not appear at the external end of the cannula, the temptation is rarely resisted of aiding its issue by pressing on the tumour, compressing it between the hands, and asking the patient to change his position. Now these different manœuvres multiply the points of contact between the trocar, already too large, and the serous membrane, which becomes inflamed ; thus peritonitis is developed, the dangerous consequences of which we all know.

Needle No. 1 of the aspirator, which is extremely fine and pointed, is on the contrary pushed, slowly and without resistance, through the tissues, and the fluid is sure to gush out as soon as it is reached. Here, therefore, there is no longer any hesitation, no uncertainty as to the direction of the exploratory instrument, no pressure on the tumour, since a powerful vacuum draws out the fluid as soon as it is reached, and consequently there is no peritoneal irritation. Finally, at the moment of withdrawing the aspiratory needle, there is no fear of allowing a few drops to fall into the peritoneal cavity, as the fluid is held immovably by the same power of aspiration.

To recapitulate, it may be said that the exploration of tumours of the liver and hydatid cysts in particular by means of the No. 1 aspiratory needle, conducted with the precautions that I have indicated, presents no danger, and leads to a certain diagnosis. This proceeding may be used at all stages of the disease, without any necessity for inducing adhesions. It affords information as to the presence or absence of the collection of fluid, and of its seat and nature. It is, therefore, now no longer justifiable to give way to mischievous temporizing, and the diagnosis should be at once established, that the question of treatment may be considered.

ARTICLE II.

The Treatment of Hydatid Cysts of the Liver by Aspiration. Cases.—New Symptoms.

What service can aspiration render us in the treatment of hydatid cysts of the liver? In this particular case I have utilized the application of the same general idea which I formulated on the subject of all pathological fluids; that is to say, when a fluid, whatever may be its nature, accumulates in a serous cavity or an organ, and when this serous cavity or organ is accessible to our means of investigation, without danger to the patient, our first care should be to draw off the fluid; if it forms afresh, to draw it off again, and as many times afterwards as is necessary, so as to exhaust the serous membrane by a mechanical and entirely harmless means, before thinking of modifying the secretion by irritant and sometimes dangerous agents. This method has given good results in hydarthrosis, and has been employed with success in cold abscesses, in purulent pleurisy and hydrorachis, &c. We believe this to be one of the most practical results of aspiration; we are in possession of a purely mechanical means which enables us to dry up a great number of fluids. I have treated this question at length when speaking of aspiration in general.

CASE I.—HYDATID CYST OF THE LIVER—ASPIRATION—
CURE (DIEULAFOY).—A patient, aged 24, was admitted
in May, 1870, to the Beaujon Hospital, under the care
of M. Gubler, in ward St. Martha, No. 1. She was
found to have a slight tumefaction of the right hypochondrium, and a well-marked projection in the angle formed
by the rectus abdomnis muscle and the ribs. This
tumour was not nodular or indurated; to the touch it was
found to be uniform and resistent. The liver was rather
depressed, and the tumefied region was seamed by veins
which were not very apparent. The general symptoms
were not well characterized; there were no dyspeptic symptoms, no icterus, and the woman, although she believed
it was eight months since the beginning of the disease,
only complained of the size of her abdomen, and the
increasing inconvenience she experienced in breathing.

The diagnosis of the tumour was discussed, and M.
Gubler considered it was a hydatid cyst of the liver. However, to be more certain, and feeling confidence in the
innocence of the aspiratory needle, he asked me to
practise aspiration. I made use of needle No. 1, which
was introduced at the most projecting part of the tumour,
and at a depth of four centimetres the fluid was reached.
It immediately jetted into the aspirator, limpid and
transparent as distilled water. I drew off, at one sitting,
500 grammes, and I stopped when the cyst seemed exhausted. I withdrew the needle, there was no pain, and
the puncture was so insignificant that it was hardly
visible. In the fluid some echinococcus hooklets were
found, but no albumen.

After this operation the patient did not experience the
slightest uneasiness; she was able to get up the same day,
the respiration became normal, the tumour did not reappear, and a fortnight afterwards the woman asked for
her dismissal. Since then I have tried to find her again,
feeling anxious to know if the cure was complete; but I

have not obtained any further particulars. Nevertheless, this case shows us the harmlessness of aspiration, and the immediate good which resulted, enabling the patient to quit the hospital a fortnight afterwards.

It must be confessed, however, that here the most favourable conditions were combined; the cyst was but little developed, was superficially placed, and had not been long forming.

CASE II. — HYDATID CYST OF THE LIVER — TWO ASPIRATIONS—CURE—SUDDEN APPEARANCE OF URTICARIA —REMARKS ON THE URTICARIA (DIEULAFOY).—A man, æt. 30, a locksmith by trade, was admitted in the Beaujon Hospital, under the care of M. Matice, for a large tumour of the abdomen. The disease commenced two years before, with violent and continuous pain in the right hypchondrium. At this time leeches and blisters were applied to the region of the liver; the pain continued for two months and then disappeared, when the patient began to perceive an unusual developement of the abdomen. Neither ascites nor icterus were detected, and the man had never had either epistaxis or intestinal hæmorrhage. The lower intercostal spaces were not enlarged, collateral circulation was developed on the median and lateral parts of the abdomen, and the culminating point of the tumour was situated in the angle formed by the ribs and the rectus abdominis muscle. Measurement at the site of the tumour gave the following results :—

Total circumference of the abdomen   78 centimetres.
Right side   41   ,,
Left side   37   ,,

The tumour was smooth to the touch; on pressure it gave a sensation of pseudo-fluctuation, the dulness was complete, and extended forwards and upwards to the fourth intercostal space; below, it descended two fingers' breadth beyond

the false ribs. As general symptoms, the man complained of unusual weakness; that he had been obliged
to give up his business of locksmith for two months;
that his appetite was bad and respiration impeded, and
that vomiting occurred at intervals.

M. Matice, having diagnosed a hydatid cyst of the
liver, made a puncture by means of an ordinary exploratory trocar, and drew off almost 300 grammes of a
clear and limpid fluid, after which the flow ceased.
Hardly ten minutes after this operation, the patient was
seized with sickness and hiccups, and with urticaria, which
rapidly affected the whole of the right side, the leg, arm,
and thorax, without invading the left side. The patient
complained, at the same time, of intense pain in the
abdomen, and he vomited greenish-coloured matter; but
these symptoms, which raised the fear of peritonitis, were
allayed in the evening. The patient was feverish for some
days, and the tumour continued of the same apparent size
as before the puncture. The general condition was satisfactory, and aspiration of the fluid was proposed. I
performed aspiration with needle No. 2, puncturing the
tumour at the most projecting point, and drew off 950
grammes of a fluid slightly inclined to purulence, but
having no offensive odour. After this operation, the
tumour was completely dissipated, no accident occurred,
and the patient experienced neither pain, sickness, nor
urticaria, the fever disappeared, the respiration became
freer, and the appetite gradually returned. Three weeks
later, the man left the hospital, and was able to return to
his work as a locksmith. I saw him four months afterwards; the cure had not been deceptive, his health was
excellent, and the tumour could no longer be found in
the right hypochondrium.

What was peculiar in this case was the sudden appearance of urticaria, occurring a few minutes after the
puncture, and coinciding with dyspnœa, nausea, and

vomiting, like that which takes place after the ingestion
of mussels, or some kinds of shell-fish. The rash of
urticaria rapidly affected the right side of the body, and
remained limited to it for some hours ; the fever was slight,
but in the evening all these phenomena had disappeared.
Some days later, having, by a singular coincidence, performed aspiration upon a woman suffering from a cyst of the
liver who was under the care of M. Axenfeld, I witnessed
similar appearances, which I report in greater detail in
Case VII. The patient, some hours after the puncture,
was attacked by general urticaria, which persisted for
two days, sucessively invading and leaving different parts
of the body. Struck by these two incidents, I asked
myself what relation could exist between the puncture of the liver and the developement of urticaria. I
report these cases without in the least seeking to start a
theory, but I cannot prevent myself from comparing them
with facts better known. Prurigo is commonly observed
in icteric patients, and it has seemed very natural to
explain it by the action of the biliary acids upon the
termination of the nerves, which would no doubt be apt to
produce itching. Graves, on his side, struck by the relation between certain diseases, notices the union and succession of arthritis, hepatitis, and urticaria. In the course
of an articular phlegmasia, said he, a patient is seized by
hepatitis with icterus, and this is followed by urticaria ;
and as the succession of these morbid phenomena
occurred eight times under his own observation, he concluded that they were not the result of fortuitous
coincidence, but that these different affections must be
united by some causal relation. It is certain that in
the cases of which Graves speaks, the urticaria, like the
prurigo above mentioned, appears to have followed the
icterus, and pruriginous affections seem to have a close relation with icterus. But in the two patients of whom I have
just spoken, the urticaria occurred after an insignificant

puncture of the liver, and without there being a trace of icterus : in one of them the urticaria was generalized, and occupied the whole of the right side of the body before ten minutes had elapsed. It is not possible, then, in this case, to refer the developement of these accidents to icterus, and, on the other hand, the relation between the urticaria and the hepatic lesion cannot be denied. A short time since, I received, from M. May Figueira, professor at Lisbon, a letter, in which he described a case analogous to those which I have just recounted ; a patient suffering from hydatid cyst of the liver, and upon whom he had practised aspiration, was attacked three or four minutes afterwards by urticaria.

The same phenomenon has been observed by M. Lannelongue, and M. Clamoisy recently communicated to me a fact of the same kind. He practised aspiration on a patient for a voluminous cyst of the liver, and drew off more than two kilogrammes of fluid. Two days afterwards, the patient showed feverish symptoms, and urticaria with prominent eruption developed itself over the whole body, and then gave place to a generalized vesicular eruption.

Thus, in these affections of the liver, icterus is not the sole cause of the developement of urticaria or prurigo, but between certain hepatic troubles and the developement of pruriginous diseases, there is a relation which I note, but which is not yet clearly established.

CASE III.—HYDATID CYST OF THE LIVER—SEVEN ASPIRATIONS—CURE—REGURGITATION OF FATTY MAT-TERS—THE SIGNIFICANCE OF THIS SYMPTOM (DIEU-LAFOY).—A woman, æt. 30, born at Algiers, and having always lived in Algeria, was admitted, October 16th, 1871, into the Beaujon Hospital, under the care of M. Moutard-Martin. This woman, who had been ill for a year, had, as a first symptom, pain in the right shoulder and under the right breast ; laughing or talking a little loud was sufficient to bring on the pain. Some months later, she observed that her corsets were becoming tight ; she was obliged to let out her dresses ; her respiration became less free, and the least labour fatigued her excessively. From the commencement of the disease a symptom occurred which has, perhaps, not yet been noted, and on which I insist the more strongly as I have already observed it in four individuals since my attention was first called to the point. After meals, when this woman had eaten of fatty food, such as butter or broth, she was seized with a true regurgitation, and without any nausea or retching her mouth filled with the fatty particles of her food, and they were rejected with her saliva. I noticed this symptom still more markedly in the patient of Case VI. This regurgitation of fatty matters (without vomiting) was with her so marked at the commencement of the disease, that she spat them out immediately after her meals, and all her handkerchiefs were impregnated with them. She compared the appearance of her saliva to what is commonly called " eyes of fat" on broth, and her sputa on paper gave the appearance of a spot of oil. For many weeks this symptom existed alone, to the exclusion of any other digestive trouble ; it afterwards disappeared with the progress of the disease. I again saw the same phenomenon in a man, with all the symptoms of hydatid cyst of the liver, who came for consultation to the Hôtel Dieu. When I questioned him minutely as to his digestion, he gave me, on the subject of the fatty matters, details entirely analogous to those of which I have just spoken.

A few days ago M. Clamoisy told me of a similar case. A patient suffering from a hydatid cyst, whom he was called to attend, gave him details on the subject of fatty matters in his alimentation, like those I have just mentioned. At present, I do not attempt to explain this phenomenon, nor to lay stress on its value. I am content to bring it forward.

The day of her entrance into Beaujon the patient in this case presented the following phenomena :—The hepatic region was slightly tumefied ; the dulness was rather extensive ; in front, the tumour was plainly felt below the false ribs. The collateral circulation was not marked on the median line, and slightly developed in the right axilla.

Measurement at the level of the tumour gave the following results :—

Total circumference . . . . . 75 centimetres.
Right side . . . . 39 ,,
Left side . . . . 36 ,,

The dyspnœa was intense, there was marked dyspepsia, and hardly any appetite. Whenever the patient attempted to walk she vomited bile, and the pain in the right shoulder reappeared. M. Moutard-Martin diagnosed a hydatid cyst of the liver, and asked me to perform aspiration, which took place the following day, October 17th.

Having chosen the most protruding point of the tumour, I assured myself of the permeability of needle No. 1, which was introduced with a sharp stroke. I drove it slowly forward, and at a depth of three centimetres reached the fluid. It had the limpidity which is observed in hydatid cysts that have undergone no change. I drew off 700 grammes, and stopped before the fluid was completely exhausted.

The relief was immediate ; no accident occurred ; and the patient got up the same day, without having any vomiting. In the evening, however, she, being nervous about herself, was restless and slightly feverish. My colleague, M. Foix, the house surgeon on duty, gave her a soothing draught, and administered for the few following days weak doses of sulphate of quinine. After the first operation M. Moutard-Martin had the extreme kindness to place the patient under the care of M. Axenfeld.

The tumour, which had greatly decreased after aspiration, in a few days again attained a considerable size. The patient had some shivering fits, much restlessness and sleeplessness. The catamenia occurred scantily on Nov. 1st, and on the 3rd of the same month I performed aspiration for the second time. The puncture was made with needle No. 1, and very near the preceding puncture; 450 grammes of a slightly purulent fluid was drawn off, having an odour of sulphuretted hydrogen, and containing no trace of echinococci. The amelioration was decided during the day, but in the evening there was an attack of fever, which lasted two hours. On Nov. 5th the size of the abdomen at the level of the tumour was 73 centimetres; that is, two centimetres less than at the beginning. The patient got up every day, went into the garden, slept well, and enjoyed her food. Nov. 10th, the size of the tumour had increased, but without our noticing an aggravation of the general symptoms. Fresh aspiration of 400 grammes of fluid, decidedly purulent, and with a strong odour of sulphuretted hydrogen. The puncture was made with needle No. 2, and very near the other punctures, within a space the size of a franc. These punctures converging towards the same point, have the advantage of producing by their number adhesion which might at any moment be very useful, if it became necessary to insert a large trocar into the liver. This mode of producing adhesion, utilized in such a case so as to be prepared for every eventuality, is analogous to acupuncture practised by Trousseau.

After this aspiration the patient experienced neither shivering nor fever, but for some days following felt very acute pain in the lower region of the liver.

Nov. 15*th.*—Aspiration of 350 grammes of pus by needle No. 2. Disappearance of pain; no shivering or fever.

Nov. 17*th.*—Pain in the lower intercostal spaces, and in the right axilla. Aspiration of 200 grammes by needle No. 2. The pus consistent and thick, without any particular colour, but still preserving its characteristic odour. The condition of the patient was excellent; the tumour had almost entirely disappeared, collateral circulation was no longer observable, and the appetite was very good.

Nov. 20*th.*—Aspiration with the same needle. I could find but 120 grammes of pus.

Nov. 25*th.*—Notwithstanding the total absence of pain and the complete disappearance of the swelling, a puncture was made a centimetre below the usual spot. I penetrated rather deeply without meeting any fluid, and aspirated only a little blood, after which I withdrew the needle.

Nov. 30*th.*—A fresh attempt at aspiration, which drew only a small quantity of blood.

Dec. 4*th.*—The patient menstruated well; her condition improved every day; she left the hospital on the 15th.

To sum up, we see here a hydatid cyst of the liver treated and cured in two months, by means of seven aspirations performed with needles Nos. 1 and 2, without accident, and following a gradual course towards convalescence. It is probable this cyst was unilocular, but there is nothing to prove that in the principal sac there were not secondary cysts in process of developement. From the first aspiration the cyst became purulent, the different parts of the cyst were destroyed little by little by the inflammatory process which took place within the organ protected from the air. As soon as the fluid was formed again, I drew it out; and it is a singular circumstance that, though the pus was thick, and in a cavity where false membranes were certainly undergoing a process of decomposition, the needles were seldom blocked up. Thus, by purely mechanical means, without previous adhesions, without irritant injections, it was found possible to exhaust this cyst, after it had been transformed into an abscess.

CASE IV. — HYDATID CYST OF THE LIVER—THREE ASPIRATIONS—CURE.—This case, published by Dr. L. Monod, is extracted from the *Gazette Hebdomadaire*, of July 19th, 1872.

The patient, L——, a concierge in L'Avenue de la Grande Armée, æt. 49, married, and father of a family, had enjoyed, till the end of the year 1866, robust health, and had had no serious illnesses before that time. On Oct. 21st, 1866, whilst employed at the Lyons Railway Station, he was violently struck by a luggage van in motion. The blow was directed against the back and lower part of the chest, on the right side, and at the level of the liver. L——, after this accident, kept his bed, and afterwards his room, for three months. Vomiting and spitting of blood, with frequent cough, gave reason to fear, at first, an injury to the lung; but nothing further justified this fear. When, at the end of three months, L—— was able to return to work, he still coughed a little, and often felt rather severe pains in the side. He had not, moreover, recovered his former strength. At the commencement of the year 1867, he remarked that his " stomach " began to increase in size, and that his digestion was often feeble and troublesome. From that time he grew thin and weak, but slowly, so that he did not feel himself constrained till the end of 1868 to change his usual work for a sedentary occupation.

I had occasion to see L—— for the first time, and temporarily, in January, 1870. For six months he had been the subject of very acute icterus, and at the same time the dyspepsia was becoming more frequent and troublesome. His face had the characteristic colour of icterus, he had a look of suffering, and his features were drawn, which contrasted with his apparent stoutness, due to great distension of the whole of the superior abdominal region. Examination of the abdomen enabled me to ascertain the following particulars :—

The liver filled the whole of the right hypochondrium, and descended below the false ribs for many centimetres, and on its anterior surface there was a round, regular tumour continuous with the liver about as large as the fist, dull, without sensible fluctuation, rather hard to the touch, but presenting a certain degree of elasticity towards its centre. My impression was that I had to deal with an encysted fluid collection, caused by the accident which occurred in 1866. Two or three days afterwards Dr. Potain, under whose care I was anxious to place the patient, examined him and diagnosed a cyst. He proposed to L—— that it should be punctured, which the latter acceded to at first; but doubtless, on reflection, the prospect frightened him, for not only did he not come into the hospital, but he even left for the country without seeing me again, and I did not hear anything of him for eighteen months. On the 23rd of June, 1871, my advice was again asked by L——, and I was then enabled to study his case more thoroughly than I had done before. I give my notes of the second examination.

I was at first struck by the change which had taken place in my patient. He looked yellower, more suffering and fatigued than ever. He could not undertake any work requiring expenditure of strength.

His general condition was that of a serious, slowly but continually increasing cachexia ; the emaciation was much increased, and the icterus persistent, and was even more marked. He had no longer his former pale yellow colour, but the more decided colour of gamboge, and the icterus was spread equally over the whole body. The indigestion had been, and was still frequent. There were alternations of constipation and diarrhœa, but the constipation predominated. The fæces were gray ; the urine, scanty and often loaded, was of the characteristic brown colour. Vomitings were frequent ; they were generally of a watery character, seldom after food, and occurred almost always on rising in the morning. The appetite was capricious ; soon appeased, and returning quickly ; thirst was great and continual ; the tongue was slightly furred, but red at the edges. With regard to the circulatory system, there had been two attacks of a serious character. In November, 1870, and in February, 1871, L—— was taken with epistaxis, for which medical aid was required. Recourse was had to perchloride of iron, ice, and finally to plugging, anteriorly and posteriorly. The first time the epistaxis continued for almost twelve hours ; the second time for seven hours, and its intensity seemed to have placed the patient's life in danger. Since then he had not had even slight hæmorrhage. Other troubles of the circulation had been of a purely local character ; thus, there had been a swelling of the legs, but I found no positive trace of it. The pulse was a little soft and slow, but regular ; the heart was healthy ; there was only a slight blowing murmur at the base of the large vessels.

There was nothing to note with regard to the chest, except the difficulty of breathing, due to the distention of the sub-diaphragmatic part of the thorax. He had never suffered from any nervous disturbance, properly so called. He suffered from fever, from sleeplessness, and had very frequent and intense headache. L—— did not complain of much tenderness of the liver; he said, however, that he sometimes felt fugitive pains there. What he complained of most was a fixed, painful spot, situated in the right shoulder.

The skin was generally dry, but exercise, or the heat of the bed, caused profuse perspiration. He had often, from the same causes, excessive itching. We must add, finally, to the number of these sensory troubles, that not uncommon perversion of taste, which gives to food an earthy taste, and, what is more remarkable, a true hemeralopia. By daylight the patient clearly distinguished objects, which only appeared yellow to him ; but as the day declined his vision began to fail, and when the night came, he said that he felt "almost blind."

His treatment, for a year and a half, had been purely palliative. It had consisted externally of five or six applications of flying blisters, applications of a lenitive inunction, and some Baréges baths. Internally, the patient had taken Vichy water, purgative pills, and various cooling drinks, but all without producing any marked result.

Local Condition.—The abdomen, above the umbilicus, was, as I have said, considerably distended. This segment of the abdomen was at least 1·10 metre in circumference ; the liver was enormous ; it extended beyond the false ribs for 11 or 12 centimetres, and its height was 20 centimetres. By percussion, the superior limit was almost 2 centimetres below the nipple ; whilst, below, its inferior edge was clearly felt above and to the right of the umbilicus. To the left, the liver occupied the whole epigastric region, and the dulness continued 4 or 5 centimetres beyond the vertical median line. The left hypochondrium was filled by the stomach, which was habitually tympanitic ; the sound was clear in every part of the abdomen below the umbilicus ; there was no trace of ascites.

The projection formed by the tumour of the liver was much more marked than it was at my first examination. Its convexity was no longer round, but oblong in the horizontal direction. This convexity was, however, tolerably regular, without furrows or depression, and did not appear to be formed by several prominences placed side by side. Its culminating point was nearly at the extremity of a vertical line of 14 or 15 centimetres in length, drawn downwards from the right nipple. The tumour, moreover, was pro-

F

longed less towards the right from this point than towards the left, where it reached the median line. Its limits were difficult to fix, and its size impossible to estimate, as it lost itself in the substance of the liver. It was continuous with the liver, and the skin, which was perfectly healthy, glided freely over its surface. Indolent to pressure, this tumour possessed a tolerably well-marked elasticity over a small space. Percussion gave everywhere a dull sound, without thrill; but if, placing the hand flat to the right of the most projecting point, I percussed on the left and at some distance from this point, a rather obscure sensation of fluctuation was felt, which I had not hitherto observed. Auscultation combined with percussion gave only a negative result.

Such was the condition in which I found the patient in June, 1871. My excellent friend and colleague, Dr. Leroy, was good enough to examine him with me; he confirmed me in the opinion that it was a large cystic tumour, and advised me to attempt puncture. This seemed to us, in fact, indicated as the starting-point of active treatment, as well as a means of assuring ourselves of the diagnosis. We agreed to perform it with Dieulafoy's instrument, which offered us every possible chance of success, and by the aid of which we relied on obtaining, by many operations, the complete evacuation of the cyst, if the first attempt succeeded.

We consequently made—July 1st, 1871—the first puncture at the culminating point of the hepatic tumour; that is to say, $4\frac{1}{2}$ centimetres below the lower border of the liver. This puncture yielded, in a quarter of an hour, 2 litres of a perfectly clear and colourless fluid, which is the fluid of hydatid collections.

The puncture was made with a No. 3 exploratory trocar (old system, the trocar independent of the canula). Aspiration was easily effected, without any loss of time. The cyst was far from being emptied at this first sitting;

but we had thought it necessary to stop the flow, because the patient felt a sensation of weakness and emptiness in the epigastric region, and we feared syncope.

After the operation, repose in bed. Broth twice the same day, light food the next day. On the third day, L—— got up and ate with an appetite; except the sensation of void which has been mentioned, there was no disturbance to be noted. At the end of three or four days the urine became clearer, the stools were coloured by bile: the eighth day I observed a marked diminution of icterus; the appetite improved. The abdomen, moreover, decreased in size, its circumference at the level of the tumour measuring 1 metre. The tumour itself, the volume of which was visibly reduced, still, however, contained fluid; and, as it was no longer so much distended, fluctuation was perceived in it very plainly.

July 11*th.*—Encouraged by the first result, we made a second puncture 3 centimetres beyond the first one, and on the same horizontal line. We made use of the needle canula No. 2 of M. Dieulafoy's instrument. Issue was given to a rather denser fluid, mixed with bile, and containing white membranous débris in suspension. The flow became suddenly slower, and stopped spontaneously after the evacuation of 300 grammes of fluid. We concluded from this that we had penetrated this time into a cavity distinct from that which we had partly emptied at the previous puncture. L—— felt neither pain nor weakness immediately after this operation. We ordered repose, and compressed the hepatic region by means of a bandage round the body.

In the evening, pains in the stomach, accompanied by vertigo and nausea, obliged us to loosen the bandage.

July 12*th.*—In the morning the patient was doing well, but as a matter of prudence I ordered him to keep his bed.

July 13*th.*—He passed the day in his arm-chair, and ate a little food. The stomach distended by flatulence, and he complained of frequent eructations. (Magnesia and charcoal administered.)

July 13*th*–14*th*.—Five or six fluid stools relieved him much.

July 14*th*.—The general condition excellent.

July 14*th* to 24*th*.—L—— became an out-patient, and returned to his work, though he still remained rather weak, and the appetite was indifferent. The digestion was, nevertheless, much better ; the stools, as many as two or three a day, were soft and coloured with bile ; the icterus had almost entirely disappeared ; the sclerotic was still, however, of a yellowish colour.

The improvement in the local condition was marked ; the circumference of the body at the level of the liver was 96 centimetres ; the height of the liver from 16 to 17 centimetres ; the distance from the border of the false ribs to its inferior edge, 8 centimetres ; from its inferior edge, by a horizontal line passing through the umbilicus, 35 millimetres. Percussion from above assigned to the liver the same limits as at the commencement of the treatment, 2 centimetres below the nipple.

On the left, the organ no longer filled the epigastric region. Percussion gave a dull sound as far as the median line ; beyond that, the resonance of the stomach, which was not pressed into the left hypochondrium, was perceptible ; in short, the tumour seemed to have contracted ; it was no longer elongated, but had become more globular, with a marked projection in its centre.

July 24*th*.—The third puncture was performed 3 centimetres distance within the second, and with the same No. 2 canula. We obtained almost 1½ litres of a fluid coloured by bile, but less dense than that of the last evacuation. This operation, like the preceding one, was borne well. The following night, however, L—— had some slight shivering fits, followed by profuse perspiration. The 25th passed well, but on the 26th I found the patient suffering. He had complained since the morning of shooting pains compared to pinching and dragging in the lower edge of the liver, below and a little beyond the punctured points. Pressure provoked the pains; they increased or recommenced on the patient turning on his left side; he felt then, he said, as if the liver became displaced, and the dragging pains grew more intense; there was no general sensitiveness of the abdomen, no desire to vomit. He had had three stools since the evening, and the appetite was good. Pulse, 84. He had had sweats again during the night, but without the preceding shivering fit. I attributed this pain to the formation of peritoneal adhesions in the neighbourhood of the punctures, and prescribed painting with laudanum, and poultices.

July 27*th.*—The pains persisted; and I found even the sensitiveness on pressure extended. The general state continued satisfactory. (Painting with tincture of iodine, *loco dolenti.*)

July 29*th.*—The pains had greatly diminished, but the patient was obliged to lie on his back for fear of exciting them. The nocturnal sweats still profuse; little sleep. (Prescription: pills of extrait thébaïque, and of agaric.)

July 31*st.*—The pains no longer continued, except when lying on the left side. The general condition excellent. The circumference of the body, at the level of the liver, not more than 94 centimetres. There was nothing to note from the 1st to the 6th of August; from the 7th to the 11th, the patient was much tried by a sharp attack of diarrhœa (mucous), with some griping. He had from ten to twelve evacuations a day; treatment, saline purgatives and opium. On the 12th, the diarrhœa stopped, and the patient went on well.

Towards the 20th of August, an eruption of *herpes zona* appeared, including the whole of the right half of

the body at the level of the liver.   Two or three little
groups of herpes appeared at the points of puncture.
Superficial and rather acute pains, compared to the prick
of a lancet, accompanied this eruption, which disappeared
completely at the end of August.

From this time no complication hindered the general
and local progress of our patient.   In the last days of
August the circumference of the body at the level of the
hepatic region had decreased to 92 centimetres, the
height of the liver to about 13 centimetres.   The organ
did not extend more than 5 centimetres beyond the ribs,
and to the left the dulness, instead of passing beyond the
median line from the xiphoid appendix to the umbilicus,
did not even reach it, and the whole epigastrium was
resonant on percussion.

September 7th.—I note the following details :—The
abdomen of L—— has diminished in size, since the first
of July, in a manner which has surprised all who know
him.   Circumference, 91 centimetres ; height of the
liver, 12 centimetres ; distance from the lower border to
the false ribs, 4 centimetres ; from the lower border to
the horizontal line passing through the umbilicus, from
7 to 8 centimetres.   The aspect of the organ is greatly
changed, the projection lately formed by the cystic
tumour has disappeared, and palpation does not find any
elastic or resistent point.   The surface of the hepatic
gland, always slightly convex, is hard and of uniform
resistance.   At the same time the condition of L—— is
most satisfactory, and he considers himself cured.   He
begins to grow fat ; his cheeks are visibly filling out ; the
icterus has left no trace ; his colour is returning, and
his appetite excellent.   L—— does not yet feel himself
capable of great fatigue, but he is on his feet all day.
He says that he still sometimes has a dragging sensation
when lying on his left side, but that it can hardly now
be called pain.

After about a month and a half, towards the month of November, I saw L—— for the last time, and a fresh examination showed me that he was still in the same condition. He had grown fatter, and I attributed to this cause a slight increase of the circumference of the body, which measured 93 centimetres instead of 91, for the liver had rather diminished than increased in size; its height, measured by percussion, hardly exceeded 11 centimetres. Thus, the amelioration still continued four months after the commencement of active treatment.

Five months after the publication of this case, the state of the patient was still improving, and the cure was considered established.

CASE V.—SEROUS CYST OF THE LIVER—ONE ASPIRATION—CURE.—I extract this case, published by M. Bouchut, from the *Gazette des Hôpitaux* of Feb. 13, 1872.

Reine B——, æt. 11, was admitted Dec. 3rd, 1871, to No. 49, St. Catherine ward.

This child, generally in good health, had suffered in the region of the liver for six months. She felt a continuous deeply seated pain there without any shooting, increased by pressure with the hand; the abdomen was tumefied, and under the right false ribs there was a rather large and deep tumour. The child had had no jaundice, she was growing weaker by degrees, eating little and becoming thinner, without having either vomiting or diarrhœa. Many flying blisters had been applied to the right hypochondrium, but the pain persisted, and she was therefore obliged to go to the hospital. The child was small, thin, pale, without being yellow; her tongue white and pasty; she had no appetite, no desire to vomit, and no diarrhœa.

The skin was healthy, without heat, and there was fever only at irregular intervals.

There was no disturbance of the respiratory, sensory, or

motor functions. The disease seemed to have originated in the right hypochondrium.

The abdomen was swollen, and the swelling chiefly occupied the hepatic region. There was there a deep, continuous, and dull pain, increased by pressure.

The false ribs formed an evident projection and were raised by the liver, which extended three fingers' breadth beyond them. That organ gave rise to dulness, extending for 15 centimetres at the side, and 12 at the anterior part under the rectus muscle. The large lobe was evidently increased in size, and its edge could be felt; in the small lobe there was a considerable projection, which formed a movable tumour, deeply seated, and raising the skin and the cartilages of the false ribs. Deep down it was a tumour, externally it was only a projection of the hypochondrium. The skin was neither hot nor red. Pressure was painful but bearable, and there was a perceptible dulness, though the swelling was elastic throughout its whole extent. Below this there was the tympanic resonance of the intestines as far as the pubis, and there was no water in the abdomen.

This tumour was very large, elastic, fluctuating, without hydatid thrill, but it vibrated under the finger like a bladder much distended with water.

Auscultation alone or combined with percussion revealed no abnormal sound.

Considering these symptoms, which revealed the existence of a fluid cyst occupying the small lobe of the liver, we thought that it was a hydatid cyst with echinococci, or a serous cyst.

The fluctuation, elasticity, resistance, and vibration of the tumour made this probable. A puncture was consequently made with the hollow needle of Dieulafoy's aspirator, without adhesions between the tumour and the walls of the abdomen being previously established.

The needle had scarcely been introduced when a jet of fluid sprang out to the distance of 20 centimetres;

it was as colourless and transparent as spring-water. I drew off almost 85 grammes. It was of a chlorinated, saline taste, and did not precipitate albumen by heat. After having allowed it to settle, we looked to see if there was no deposit to be examined, and we studied the deep layers with a microscope without finding any débris or hooks of echinococci. It was a fluid formed of chlorinated water. After the operation the child had for twenty-four hours acute pain in the right hypochondrium, increased by the least pressure, also a desire to vomit, and fever with great prostration. All this disappeared under the influence of laudanised poultices, and the next day she seemed cured. She was soon able to get up and leave the hospital. She had hardly gone home when she was attacked by fever, lost her appetite, began to cough, and complain of a slight pain in the right side under the breast.

She was brought back to the hospital, and it became evident that she had on the right side a pleuritic effusion reaching to the lower angle of the scapula. The child had a dry cough, want of appetite, and a little fever, dulness at the base of the right lung, absence of vesicular murmur below a whispering sound, and œgophony towards the angle of the scapula.

This effusion did not increase, and under the influence of a blister and tincture of bryonia it was gradually absorbed. For the second time the child was cured.

She afterwards took scarlatina, which ended well; and she left the hospital.

M. Bouchut concludes this case with some reflections on the consecutive accidents of the puncture, and on the pleurisy with which this child was attacked. He seems to regret not having established previous adhesions. I have already sufficiently explained, in the article on *Diagnosis,* the slight gravity of the accidents which sometimes follow puncture in the exploration of cysts of the liver, by means of the aspiratory needle; we ought not, I think, to exaggerate their importance.

CASE VI.—HYDATID CYST OF THE LIVER—ONE ASPIRATION—CURE (CHAIROU).—I was consulted in June, 1871, by a woman, æt. 43, whose pallor and cachectic aspect might have led one at first to suppose the existence of some malignant affection. For six years the digestion had been bad, the appetite had diminished, constipation was the normal condition, and the patient, owing to increasing weakness, had been obliged to keep her room for six months.

I examined her, and found a marked hypertrophy of the liver, with pain in the hepatic region. This pain, which had existed for a long time, became, after a few days, so acute that I was obliged, in order to ease it, to give frequent injections of morphia. Though the increase in the size of the liver seemed to be general, it appeared to me that a tolerably well-defined tumour existed, towards its lower border.

I performed aspiration on the 21st of July, by means of needle No. 2 of Dieulafoy's aspirator, and drew off 150 grammes of a limpid and transparent fluid. This fluid, examined under the microscope, contained hooks of the echinococcus, and it was neither more nor less than that of a hydatid cyst. I had hardly performed the operation than the woman was seized with syncope, which was, however, only fugitive.

Dating from this time, the pain disappeared, the digestion improved, and convalescence was perfectly established.

Six months afterwards the cure was complete, and it has not since been disturbed.

SUMMARY OF THE SIX PRECEDING CASES.

In these six cases, it may be seen that the treatment of

cysts by aspiration was simple and innocent to a degree rarely met with in other proceedings. It was not necessary to previously establish adhesions, nor to use irritant injections; it was sufficient to exhaust the fluid by a mechanical and entirely harmless method. Sometimes this fluid continued to the end in a limpid and transparent state during the whole time of treatment; sometimes it became purulent, and the cyst was changed into an abscess of the liver, which did not prevent the exhaustion of the fluid being effected without difficulty. But we must expect to meet cases of a less simple character; the liver may be invaded, in a great part, by multiple cysts of ancient date, which pass successively or simultaneously into suppuration, and which only disappear by the intermediary transformation of their products into crystals of margarine and chloresterine.

When a case of this kind is met with, what is the course of treatment to be followed? This point I will try to establish in the following case.

CASE VII.—HYDATID CYSTS OF THE LIVER AND THE PLEURA—THREE HUNDRED ASPIRATIONS—EFFECTS OF THE CATAMENIAL PERIOD—WASHING OUT THE CYST—TROCAR LEFT IN SITU—CURE (DIEULAFOY).—A woman, æt. 43, was admitted, July 8th, 1871, into the Beaujon Hospital, ward St. Paul, No. 14, and was under the care of M. Axenfeld. This woman came to be treated for an enormous abdominal tumour. She believed the disease commenced five years previously. At that time she had some digestive trouble, characterized by loss of appetite, inflation of the abdomen, and a peculiar regurgitation of fatty food, a phenomenon to which I have drawn attention in Case III. After each meal the fatty parts of the food returned into her mouth by a movement of regurgitation, whilst the rest of the food was kept down;

butter and fatty soups particularly provoked it. This intolerance of the stomach towards fatty aliments only lasted some months. Since my attention was first drawn to this symptom, I have observed .it in three patients attacked with hydatid cysts of the liver ; it particularly appears at the commencement of the disease, and ceases with its progress ; I do not seek to explain it, I content myself with pointing it out.

As symptoms occurring at the commencement of the disease, we also noted pain in the right hypochondrium, looseness of the bowels, and a noticeable emaciation. Then, the strength decreasing, the patient was many times obliged to interrupt her household duties, and it was not till eighteen months later that a tumour appeared in the epigastric fossa. From that time her complexion became slightly icteric, the menses were suppressed, the tumour made slow and imperceptible progress, until it attained its present size.

Actual Condition.—The hepatic tumour was extremely voluminous ; it descended as far as the right iliac fossa, reached the umbilicus, passed beyond the linea alba, and its most projecting point was at the epigastric fossa. This whole region was one of absolute dulness. Measurement gave these results :—

Total circumference	.	.	.	79	centimetres.
Right side	.	.	.	41	,,
Left side .	.	.	.	38	,,

The reason there was not a greater dimension on the right side was that the tumour passed beyond the median line, and encroached on the left side. Collateral circulation was developed; no icterus, no ascites; the menses very irregular. To the touch, the tumour was resistant and elastic. No hydatid thrill was perceptible, but fluctuation was manifest. The general symptoms were strongly marked ; digestion bad, dyspnœa extreme, and the patient had great difficulty in going upstairs. M. Axenfeld did not hesitate to diagnose hydatid cyst of the liver, which only confirmed the opinion which he formed two years previously, when he had occasion to see the same patient at the St. Antoine Hospital. Aspiration of the fluid was decided upon.

July 11*th.*—The puncture was made with needle No. 1, and I reached the fluid at the depth of two centimetres; it had the appearance and habitual limpidity of that of hydatid cysts : I stopped the flow at 480 grammes, so as not to leave too great a vacuum in the interior of the sac. The circumference of the abdomen, after this evacuation, diminished 1½ centimetres; but the process of measuring, which I was wrong in practising, was doubtless partly the cause of the ensuing accidents. About an hour after the puncture, the patient had pain in the abdomen and right shoulder, with nausea and diarrhœa; in the evening, about five o'clock, these painful accidents improved, and an irritation appeared in different parts of the body.

The next day urticaria with fever developed itself, and successively attacked the thighs, abdomen, chest, and arms : the diarrhœa continued. This urticaria, showing itself without icterus and after the puncture of the liver, was a phenomenon which struck me the more as a few days before I had observed another example of it, occurring ten minutes after puncture, in a patient under the care of M. Matice, and who is the subject of Case II. With this woman the urticaria persisted three days, disappearing and attacking all parts of the body, with febrile exacerbation in the evening, tumefaction of the left side of the face, as in the case of dental fluxion; extreme and very painful dysphagia, so that the patient was not able to swallow a single mouthful of liquid for twelve hours. The soft palate and the posterior-superior part of the pharynx were dry and intensely red. After the third day these accidents disappeared.

August 7th.—New aspiration 1 centimetre from the preceding : 700 grammes of a fluid slightly turbid, and having the smell of sulphuretted hydrogen, drawn off. This second aspiration was followed by no accidents ; neither vomiting, fever, nor urticaria. The appetite began to return, but the pain persisted in the right shoulder.

August 14th.—Drew off 600 grammes of fluid, which had returned to its limpid appearance, and lost all odour. Two hours after this puncture, a rather violent fever declared itself, and persisted till the next morning.

The patient feeling relieved, asked to be allowed to spend some days at her home. She went, but returned twelve days afterwards, suffering and coughing much, and with the tumour, which had almost returned to its original size.

September 3rd.—Aspiration, with needle No. 2, of 450 grammes of a slightly purulent fluid, with a very decided odour of sulphuretted hydrogen. Stopped the flow ; relief ; no fever.

September 5th.—Aspiration of 800 grammes of a purulent fluid ; very visible improvement the following days. The total circumference not more than 72 centimetres ; which was 7 centimetres less than at the first puncture. But the dulness, in the posterior part of the chest and the right axilla, remained still at the same level, without modification.

September 11th.—A new puncture at the same spot. I drew off 350 grammes of pus. The patient got up and ate with a tolerably good appetite.

September 16th.—The tumour developing again, but slowly and without fever. 300 grammes of a thick greenish pus, with a very decided odour, drawn off. The circumference of the body not more than 68 centimetres, which was 11 centimetres less than at the beginning.

September 21st.—200 grammes of pus.

September 23rd.—40 grammes of pus. Here concluded the first part of this case, in which the steady improvement of the patient, and the gradual drying up of the purulent source made us hope for an approaching cure. But soon accidents occurred afresh. On the left side of the linea alba, below the xiphoid appendix, a little red tumour was perceived, pointed like a phlegmon in course of formation. The patient had fever and acute abdominal pain, was seized with accesses of cough, and respiration became extremely difficult. By auscultation, sibilant and snoring *râles* were heard in both sides of the chest; the dulness, before observed on the right side, increased sensibly; there was diminution of the thoracic vibrations without œgophony. There was no doubt that a fluid collection existed at this spot, but of what nature?

October 3rd.—A puncture was made with needle No. 2 in the sixth right intercostal space, a little behind the axilla, and I drew off 800 grammes of a fluid as limpid as that which was drawn off from the first hepatic cyst. Had we to do with a cyst of the pleura, or of the upper surface of the liver? A question difficult to answer. After the operation the dyspnœa diminished, but the fever persisted, and the next day the patient complained of pain in the side at the level of the left breast: auscultation discovered an extremely distinct friction sound at the base of the chest at the left side, whilst nothing analogous was heard in the right side.

A blister was applied to this spot. Morphia draught. The patient was fed with milk and broth. The new abdominal tumour, however, making progress, 150 grammes of pus, situated deeply in the liver, were aspirated.

October 8th.—The friction in the left side had partly disappeared, but the dyspnœa was violent, and by auscultating the right lung an amphoric murmur was heard, the respiration was metallic, the maximum of which was the middle part of the sub-spinus fossa. The patient, moreover, spat purulent mucous, coloured with blood and mixed with the débris of false membranes. The cough was incessant. The patient was then attacked by pneumothorax in the right side, which had been preceded by dry pleurisy in the left. But what was the starting-point of this pneumothorax ? Did the lung communicate with the liver and the pleural cavity, or only with the pleura ? It was certain that, the initial cyst of the liver having been dried up, this fresh purulent hepatic collection did not seem to have any communication with the bronchial tubes; it was, therefore, probable that the liver was not concerned in the pneumothorax.

November 1st.——Apart from the extreme prostration of the patient, and her incessant debilitating cough, her general state was no worse, and under the influence of numerous aspirations, repeated four or five times a week, the purulent collection of the liver was diminishing. But a fortnight later the size of the organ again increased ; punctures made to some depth in different points showed that there were many collections in course of formation, and distinct one from the other. In fact, according as the punctures were made towards the small lobe of the liver or towards the lower border, fluids of different appearances and colour were aspirated, either purulent or hematic.

I then decided to perform many aspirations every day, exactly as with certain patients punctures are made with Pravaz's syringe. Many hundred aspirations were therefore made with needles Nos. 2 and 3, and often the needle did not meet with fluid till at a depth of 8 or 10 centimetres, which indicated that the liver was suppurating over a great extent.

To recapitulate, the second phase of this disease was characterized by a pneumothorax which endangered the life of the patient for many days, and by the developement of new abscesses in different parts of the liver

December 1st.—The pneumothorax remained very limited without formation of fluid, and air entered the whole of the upper part of the lung ; the multiple abscesses of the liver tended to unite into one focus, which was deeply situated, and was frequently aspirated. The patient no longer spat false cystic membranes.

January 1st.—When I left the Beaujon Hospital to enter the wards of M. Tardieu, at the Hôtel Dieu, M. Axenfeld kindly asked me to take this patient, and to continue my observations to the end of this interesting case. But it happened that the punctures made with needles No. 3 and No. 4 no longer allowed pus to pass, the canula becoming obliterated every moment. This obliteration was owing to little white concretions, which at the first glance might have been taken for phosphate of lime, but which, when analyzed by M. Yvon, resident apothecary, were found to be composed of agglomerations of margarine and cholesterine. In the presence of this unforeseen accident, it was found necessary to give exit to the pus which formed every day by a larger aperture. We had no occasion to establish adhesions between the liver and the abdominal walls, for the number of punctures, which had been accumulated at one point, had already produced this result.

A gutta-percha sound, 12 centimetres long and 5 millimetres in diameter, was introduced and allowed to remain in the hepatic cavity.

Every morning the aspirator was applied to the aperture of this sound, and thus the pus could be removed as it formed, and the cavity cleansed by injecting and aspirating at stated times a liquid composed of water and a few grammes of alcohol. Owing to this manœuvre, rendered extremely convenient by the rack aspirator, which is an injector at the same time, a great quantity of white concretions could be drawn out, and the cavity gradually diminished.

G

February 2nd.—The improvement seemed to be positive, when on the morning of February 2nd, after the aspiration of the fluid, which on that day was coloured with blood, the patient was seized with a long shivering fit, followed by heat, sweating, and complete prostration. In the evening there was another shivering fit ; and the next day, in performing aspiration, I remarked that the fluid drawn off was sanguineous, not homogeneous, and of a fœtid odour ; the face of the patient was much altered, the pulse was miserable, and the first impression of the dressers was, that these were the initiatory symptoms of purulent infection.

Nevertheless, in spite of the apparent gravity of the case, my prognosis was not very unfavourable, for I hoped that these accidents would subside in the evening or the next day. A gramme of sulphate of quinine was administered. Another shivering fit occurred during the day ; after which the patient was attacked with pulmonary congestion, accompanied by slight hemoptysis, which lasted two days. The attacks of fever did not reappear, and after this relapse the course of improvement was slow and progressive.

What had occurred? I thought from the first there had been no question of purulent infection, and I referred these symptoms, apparently so serious, to the approach of an abortive catamenial period. I had all the more reason for forming this opinion, as a few days before I had seen an analogous case in a young woman under our care and that of Dr. Linas, for purulent traumatic pleurisy, and whom we treated by means of successive aspirations and injections. In the case of this young girl, at two different times, a month apart, the disease, which was proceeding towards cure, was suddenly arrested in its march by an access of fever simulating purulent infection, and coinciding with hæmorrhage of the pleural cavity. The patient menstruated by the pleura.

The same thing doubtless occurred in our patient, and the ordinary accidents which accompany hemoptysis and hæmorrhage of the cyst might be repeated, according to all appearance, the following month. This is what, in fact, took place.

February 28*th.*—Although the cavity of the cyst hardly contained 60 grammes of fluid, shiverings came on again, and a new hæmorrhage by the cyst and the bronchi. But we knew then the cause of these troubles, and were not much alarmed, as we hoped to be able to lessen them the following month, by establishing a healthy derivation by means of leeches, and by administering aloes for several consecutive days.

In the month of April the patient left the hospital to enter on her convalescence at home. I saw her during this time, and though her improvement was very slow, she was able to get up and even to occupy herself with her household business. Every trace of pneumothorax had disappeared, the liver had almost returned to its normal size ; menstruation was not yet re-established, but every month slight hemoptysis occurred.

To recapitulate. This case may be divided into three phases. In the first, an enormous cyst was dried up by successive aspirations ; in the second, new accidents occurred—pleurisy, pneumothorax, formation of multiple abscesses ; in the third period, the union of these abscesses into one purulent collection, concretions of margarine and cholesterine, introduction of a gutta-percha sound into the cavity, cleansing of the cyst, and accidents occasioned by the deviation of the catamenial periods.

This was the conclusion of this case, when I published it in the *Gazette des Hôpitaux.* For some time the gutta-percha tube, which still remained in the liver, served for administering injection, the quantity of which was diminished every day, and I considered the woman as certain of cure, when she was seized, in May, with new

G 2

accidents, and a second pneumothorax in the right side; there was intense pain, extreme oppression of breathing, and stethoscopic signs. The symptoms were complete. An enormous quantity of false membranes came from her, thick, stratified, and of such dimensions that many reached the size of 3 or 4 centimetres square. This was the sac of the cyst, which had made a new path for itself through the bronchi. This terrible complication was happily the last. In June I withdrew the tube, which had become useless. The appetite returned, but menstruation was not re-established till September.

The patient is now completely cured, the hepatic region has returned to its normal size, and air passes through the whole extent of the lungs.

ARTICLE III.

Critical Review of the Method.—Purulence of the Fluid.—Signifi-
cance of Accidents.—Odour of the Fluid.—The Urticaria.—
Regurgitation of Fatty Matters.—Deviation of the Catamenial
Period.

. If we consider these different cases in a general manner, we see that in the first six the treatment and the termination were uniform; the fluid was dried up by successive aspirations, but this fluid behaved differently according to the circumstances. Thus, in the Cases I., V., and VI., purulence was not produced, as a single puncture sufficed to ensure cure. In Case IV., the end was attained by three aspirations, and without the fluid having lost any of its limpidity to the last.

In Case II., on the contrary, the fluid was slightly turbid from the second aspiration, but it had not time to be completely changed into pus, as cure was effected after this second puncture.

Case III. shows us the fluid of the hydatid cyst becoming more and more purulent, and diminishing at the same time in quantity, so that after the sixth aspiration, that is to say, in six weeks, the source was completely exhausted. Each time that purulence occurred, the fluid had the odour of sulphuretted hydrogen. This odour, without being exclusively peculiar to hepatic pus, was here acquired to such a degree, that its cause and significance as an element of diagnosis in a difficult case should be inquired into. The formation of pus in the cyst sometimes causes a febrile condition, more or less acute, with loss of appetite, pain in the hypochondrium or in the right shoulder, and a sensation of weight in the liver or region of the same side.

It is worthy of remark, that the issue of the fluid through a needle as fine as No. 2 is never, so to speak, interrupted, in spite of the presence of hydatid sacs, which are theoretically supposed to obstruct the flow. It would be difficult to explain why the cyst sometimes suppurates, and why at others purulence is not shown in the course of treatment; it is probable that in the first case the sac of the cyst undergoes fatty degeneration, and afterwards disappears.

The change of the sac of the cyst is doubtless connected with its age: when the envelope is young it easily disappears, whether it suppurates or falls into a state of fatty degeneration; but in growing old it thickens, as in Case VII., becomes stratified and vascularized, and the chances of cure are less as the age of the cyst is more advanced.

All the patients of whom we have been speaking were operated on without it having been necessary to establish previous adhesions between the liver and the abdominal walls, and the puncture never caused serious accidents. Pain, nausea, vomiting when they occurred, had no bad results, and I should rather consider that they were more often the result of the excitability of the peritoneum than a consequence of phlegmasia of the serous membrane.

Moreover, I am not very certain that these accidents were not sometimes caused by the operator without his knowledge. We ought to carefully avoid every manœuvre other than aspiration pure and simple, and when the operation is over, the tumour must on no account be percussed under the pretext of proving the diminution of its size; the patient also must not be turned about for the purpose of submitting him to fresh measurements. These proceedings, are quite useless, only inconvenient, and can be deferred till the next day; the puncture once made, the patient should recline on his back, and repose for some hours.

I speak here particularly of the precaution to be taken after the first operation, for experience shows us that in subsequent punctures tolerance is established.

From a clinical point of view, the cases which I have reported are instructive, for they call our attention to the new considerations which I have developed.

The regurgitation of the fatty parts of the food is a symptom which seems to belong to the first period, or the period of formation of hydatid cysts of the liver.

The developement of urticaria, occurring after the hepatic puncture, is a curious phenomenon, the origin of which is still unknown, but which deserves to be specially studied, because of the relations which exist between affections of the liver and the developement of cutaneous eruptions, with or without icterus.

The deviation of the catamenial period is an accident important to know of; it puts us on our guard against an erroneous impression which would lead us to suspect the developement of purulent infection, and it leads us, at the same time, to show more reserve in our prognosis.

As to the odour of sulphuretted hydrogen which is observable from the time that the purulence is established in the cyst, this phenomenon is not peculiar to hepatic pus, but I have nowhere met it developed to such a degree of intensity ; it ought to be a valuable sign in a case of difficult diagnosis.

The formation of concretions of margarine and cholesterine was only observed in one of the seven cases which I have reported.

ARTICLE IV.

The Mode of Operating.—The Cleansing of the Cyst.—The Method of Successive Injections.—The Hepatic Trocar.

When performing aspiration on a hydatid cyst of the liver, the most projecting point of the tumour is chosen, and the puncture made by means of No. 1 needle, according to the directions given in the previous article on *Diagnosis*. If the cyst is not large, that is to say, if it does not contain more than 400 grammes of fluid, it may be completely emptied at once.

In the opposite case, it is better to stop after having drawn off 400 grammes, and to begin again some days later. It is wise to proceed gradually, for the organ more easily fills up the void left by the issue of a small quantity of fluid, and the entire sac is not exposed to the sudden invasion of suppuration. In withdrawing small quantities by successive aspirations, at short intervals, the fluid has not time allowed it to reform, and the liver, which has been crushed and flattened, is enabled to slowly regain its original position and dimensions.

The punctures ought to be made as near as possible on the same spot, that is to say, in a space about as large as a franc piece ; the reason for which is, that owing to the number of punctures, an inflammatory process occurs in the tissues of the serous membranes, which, repeated many times in the same place, ends in causing adhesions which allow, at a given time, of the use of a large trocar.

From the time of the second or third puncture, needle
No. 1 can, without fear, be replaced by needle No. 2,
which facilitates the flow of the pus.

The number of punctures is extremely variable; the
fluid collection may be dried up by the first aspiration,
whilst in other cases it is necessary to puncture a great
number of times; but this is an insignificant consideration, if it is remembered that these aspirations are neither
more painful nor more difficult to perform than the
punctures which can be repeated many times a day with
Pravaz's syringe. It is then only a matter of patience
and perseverance for the medical man; he acts under
cover, without danger, without fear of the terrible
effects of incisions and large openings. He works by a
means entirely mechanical, and without running the
risks, sometimes so disastrous, of the eschars produced by
caustics, and of the irritant injections of alcohol and
tincture of iodine.

The method is less brilliant, but it is more sure.
Aspiration is not the exclusive appanage of surgery, it
belongs still more to medicine, it is the ground on which surgery and medicine will meet, and on which, I hope, they will
tighten the bonds that should unite them. The diagnosis
of fluid collections is usually confided to the art of the
physician; it is auscultation and percussion which lead us
to the discovery of effusions of the pleura and pericardium,
of cysts and abscesses of the liver, &c.; and I could wish
that the aspiratory method, by giving to medicine the
means of accurately testing its diagnosis, should also
enable it to institute the treatment.

When successive aspirations do not succeed in drying
up the source of the fluid, or when false membranes and
concretions of cholesterine obstruct the channel of the
needle, another means must be had recourse to to give issue
to the pus. I advise neither caustic applications nor large
openings; I prefer permitting a tube to remain *in situ* in the

liver, by means of which the cavity can be frequently washed out ; this was the process I followed with the patient in Case VII. For this purpose a gutta-percha sound, from 10 to 15 centimetres long, and about 5 millimetres in diameter, is chosen ; or, better still, one of the hepatic trocars that I have had made for this object.

The sizes of these trocars are various ; No. 1 can be first used, and afterwards replaced by Nos. 2 or 3. The hepatic trocar may be introduced at the spot where the aspirations have been made, for the punctures accumulated at the same place have already established adhesions between the liver and the folds of the serous membrane. As soon as the puncture is made, the canula is fixed firmly by means of tapes passed through the openings of the shield, and made to adhere by many layers of collodion. These preparations being ended, the evacuation and the cleansing of the tumour begin.

It will be understood that to perform this operation it is indispensable to have an aspirator that can be used for injection as well as aspiration.

The cleansing of the cyst and injection are two things which require certain precautions. By the old methods, the cavity was emptied at one sitting of the pathological fluid, which was replaced by an injection, left partly or wholly in the cavity. I propose another process, which I will describe. Suppose a purulent collection of 1,000 grammes. I would commence by extracting a part of the fluid, taking care not to exhaust it entirely, nor to push aspiration to the point of producing the effect of cupping in the interior of the cavity. If the trocar is blocked up at the moment of the operation, it is sufficient to push back the obstructing body by a reverse stroke of the piston, and to continue aspiration. Instead of emptying at one stroke the entire collection, but a small quantity should be drawn off, about 150 grammes, which should be replaced immediately by 100 grammes of injection, and at the same sitting this process may be repeated five, six, eight, or ten times, so that, after the cleansing, the quantity of the fluid injected at each stroke of the piston being less than the fluid aspirated, the cavity would contain 300 or 400 grammes of fluid less,

DIEULAFOY'S HEPATIC TROCAR.

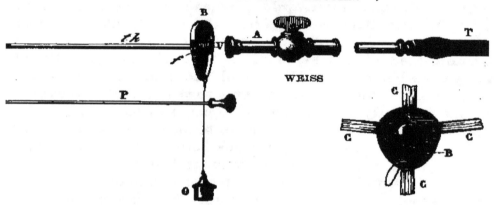

WEISS

Th. Hepatic trocar.
A. Intermediate fitting between the trocar and the aspirator.
T. Tube of the aspirator.
B. Shield of the trocar.
V. The screw to which the intermediate fitting and the obturator are adapted.
P. The needle of the trocar.
O. Obturator.
CC. The tapes retaining the hepatic trocar (front view) in its place by means of collodion.

and the purulent collection would be completely replaced by the injection. This is an insensible substitution. These successive aspirations and injections are very easy to perform, since the aspirator is mathematically graduated, and thus the operator knows to within a few grammes what is the quantity of fluid put into motion.

In performing this process of cleansing, various fluids may be used according to the case, either simple water, or water mixed with thymic acid, carbolic acid, or permanganate of potash. The cleansing over, fluid may be injected and left in the morbid cavity ; the volume of the former should be about one-fifth the size of the latter. For this use, I advise the following solution :—

Distilled water, 400 grammes; sulphate of zinc, 1 gramme.

This operation may be performed every day. It may be seen that it has little analogy with the other processes, which were beset with difficulties. First, the hepatic abscess was difficult to empty, and the pus remained in the intricacies of the cavity, and use was often made for injection of badly made syringes, which retained the liquid imperfectly, and the extremity of which fitted badly to the tube inserted in the morbid cavity. This tube was difficult to fix, it was injured by contact with the fluids, it provoked ulceration, and it filled up the orifice in the skin so indifferently that only half of the fluid was injected; and if desired to be withdrawn, it was done with difficulty, and by manœuvres which allowed of the free access of the external air.

By means of the aspiratory-injector the fluid is, on the contrary, completely introduced or drawn off at the will of the operator, without a single drop escaping its true destination ; he proceeds slowly, without shock, and measuring the force of the projection. This force is afforded by the play of the piston, which enables him to give to the fluid an impulse such as sends it into the most intricate recesses of the cavity. The changes are brought about slowly, the detritus of false membranes and the effects of the pus are neutralized continually, and every day he watches the cavity gradually and progressively contracting, and the tissue of the liver, at first compressed, gradually returning to its original position.

It is the duty of the operator to note the progress towards recovery, and to progressively diminish the quantity of the fluid in a manner proportioned to the contraction of the cavity.

Conclusions.—The following conclusions may be drawn from the cases here related :—

1. It is always possible with needle No. 1, armed with a previous vacuum, to investigate without danger hydatid cysts of the liver ; and if the first puncture gives no results, a second and a third may be made in the substance of the organ.

2. Aspiration often repeated with needles Nos. 2 and 8, enables one to dry up the fluid of the cyst by a mechanical means.

8. The fluid may remain clear and limpid till completely dried up, but more often it acquires various degrees of purulence. The treatment is the same in both cases.

4. If complications arise, as in Case VII., or if aspiration is not sufficient, the best course is to leave a hepatic trocar *in situ,* by means of which the washing out of the cavity, and the injection of an appropriate fluid, can be practised every day, or twice in the twenty-four hours.

5. It is unnecessary to propose adhesions by caustics, for this result is obtained by the punctures accumulated at one point.

6. The size of the hepatic trocar should be modified according to circumstances.

ARTICLE V.

Abscess of the Liver.

If I have placed in the same division the diagnosis and treatment of cysts and abscesses of the liver, it is because the mode of operating in both cases is exactly the same ; moreover, as most of the cysts change into abscesses under the influence of treatment, it follows that they may be confounded with one another in therapeutics.

Primary suppurations of the liver are rare in European

countries; we more often observe secondary suppurations occurring after embolic metastasis, or which are the consequence of pre-existing cysts. But, whatever may be their origin or cause, the purulent formations and transformations of the liver may take an acute course calling for all our attention. The liver, which, by its situation, is limited by two serous membranes, the peritoneum and the pleura, is an organ which ought to be closely watched, for hepatic suppuration developes itself sometimes with such rapidity that in a few weeks it ends in penetration of one of these serous membranes, and peritonitis or pleurisy with pneumothorax, according to the circumstances, is the consequence.

Also, when palpation and percussion disclose an increase of volume in the liver, when this increase has been rapid and accompanied with pain in the lower border of the organ and in the right shoulder, when these local symptoms are connected with general phenomena, such as sweats and fever, more or less intermittent, we may be convinced that pus is forming; the fluid, at first infiltrated, collects rapidly, then it seeks to make a passage for itself to the injury of the neighbouring organs or serous membranes; if we do not attend to the different phases of the disease, we shall have to repent not having acted in time.

CASE I.—ABSCESS OF THE LIVER—TWO ASPIRATIONS—CURE (DIEULAFOY).—A male patient, æt. 28, was admitted, in November, 1871, into the Beaujon Hospital, under the care of M. Moutard-Martin. He had a slightly icteric tint, though the examination of urine did not disclose the least trace of the colouring matter of the bile; he sometimes had shivering fits followed by heat, and an access of fever ill characterized, and which for about a month had returned at irregular periods. The appetite was bad, and sleep disturbed.

In the region of the liver, towards its inferior edge, and approaching the rectus abdominis muscle, a rather voluminous tumour was found, hard and very slightly elastic. Collateral circulation was not very much developed. He had never had hepatic colic or vomiting. He was not explicit as to the commencement of his disease. Its progress had, however, been rapid, as he said, two months before, no tumour had been apparent.

At the request of M. Moutard-Martin, I performed the first aspiration, with the assistance of Dr. R. Blache, the house surgeon. The puncture was made with needle No. 2, and gave issue to a purulent, tenacious fluid of a greenish-yellow colour, and without odour. The flow was stopped after 550 grammes had escaped.

This operation was followed by no accidents of any kind, the tumour diminished about two-thirds; the patient, much relieved on the following days, got up for a few hours, and sleep and appetite partially returned.

Seven days afterwards I performed a second aspiration, which yielded 300 grammes of pus, after which the abscess was exhausted. The improvement continued. Fresh aspirations were needless, the tumour disappeared completely, and the patient became a servant at the hospital, where I saw him for many months, and thus I am enabled to affirm that his cure was complete.

CASE II.—ABSCESS OF THE LIVER—DIFFICULTY OF THE DIAGNOSIS—MULTIPLE ASPIRATIONS—(DR. LAFFAN, PHYSICIAN TO THE UNION HOSPITAL, CASHEL).*—In this case, the author's aim is to show the superiority and harmlessness of the aspiratory method. He used it with a patient whose symptoms led him to suppose an abscess of the liver. The diagnosis being very difficult, Dr. Laffan resolved to make use of the aspirator. Needle No. 1 was

* Observations illustrative of the Use of Dieulafoy's Aspirator. Dublin Journal of Medical Science, March, 1872.

introduced several times, and at some days' interval, at different points, and in such a way as to circumscribe the supposed lesion. No pus was found, but none of these explorations caused the slightest accident. The author, who has in many other cases made use of aspiration, confirms in every particular the proposition which I have put forth on the harmlessness of the method, and I cannot do better than quote his own words :—" The positive result which this case goes to establish is the perfect safety with which the most important organ may be traversed, not in one, but in several directions, by these delicate instruments."*

* At the moment of concluding this article I received a letter from Dr. Chaillou of Tourney, informing me of a fresh success of hydatid cyst of the liver cured by a single aspiration.

CHAPTER II.

The Treatment of Retention of Urine by Aspiration.

Summary.—Article I.: History.—The Harmlessness of the Aspiratory Puncture in Retention of Urine.—Comparative Value of this Proceeding.—Article II.: Indications and the Mode of performing Aspiration in the Treatment of Retention of Urine. —Article III.: Cases.

ARTICLE I.

The Harmlessness of the Aspiratory Puncture in Retention of Urine.

WHEN I began my investigations on aspiration I was, above all, struck by the harmlessness of the aspiratory punctures, and seeing that the aspiratory needles could be introduced with impunity into the most delicate parts, I thought immediately of puncturing the bladder and evacuating the urine in the case of retention.

I tried it first experimentally. Operations performed on dogs proved to me that the bladder of the animal could be punctured, the fluid it contained drawn off, and this repeated many times a day, without the slightest accident resulting. In the animals destroyed, a few moments after the operation, it was not possible to discover traces of the puncture on the external surface of the organ ; internally, small, reddish, ecchymotic spots having the appearance and size of flea-bites were barely visible.

I attributed the innocence of these punctures to the contractility of the bladder and the extreme fineness of the needle, which was not more than a third of a millimetre in diameter, and I became convinced that the evacuation of urine by aspiration would prove to be one of the most useful applications of the method. Thus, in my presentation to the Academy of Medicine (at the meeting of November 2nd, 1869), mention was made of this new proceeding, and three months later, in a paper intended to give a more detailed account of aspiration, I formulated the following ideas :—" The retention of urine has given rise to operations rather difficult to perform, and but little anodyne in result ; these are forced catheterization, the boutonnière, and rectal and suprapubic puncture. Far be it from me to deny the services rendered by these different means ; but I may be allowed to bring forward the results given by aspiration : Needle No. 1 is introduced through the abdomen above the pubis, and the urine aspirated ; the puncture is so fine and the walls of the bladder are so contractile, that the contact of the urine with the peritoneum is not possible. When aspiration is ended, it is well to withdraw the needle quickly, or previously to aspirate the few drops of urine which it may still contain.

" Time may be taken to overcome the obstacle to the flow of the urine, for the same proceeding can, without the least inconvenience, be repeated many days in succession. "

The entire harmlessness of the vesical puncture, and the possibility of indefinitely repeating the operation, can be confirmed by numerous pathological facts.

On the 26th of February, 1870, M. L. Labbé first applied aspiration to retention of urine. It was tried upon an old man with a large prostate, and with whom many attempts at catheterization had been unsuccessful.

M. Labbé thrust needle No. 2 into the bladder, and drew off the urine ; accidents were immediately averted,

H

and the patient recovered. Since that time a number of cases has been collected ; many are cited in the thesis of M. Watelet,* others have reached us from England,† from Russia,‡ and the United States,§ and it is relying on these clinical facts that I proceed to answer the objections that have been made, to consider the subject as a whole, to lay down the principles of the new method, and to discuss the questions connected with it.

1. Is aspiration of the urine an operation easy to perform, and harmless in result ?

2. In what case, and at what time, should aspiration be performed ?

3. What is the mode of operating ?

These are the propositions which we have to develope.

To establish the harmlessness of aspiration in retention of urine seems to me the principal point of the question under consideration, since all other methods hitherto in vogue have been accompanied with real dangers ; and it may be asserted, that if puncture of the bladder is not more often performed when necessary, it is not because the operation is difficult (for nothing is more simple than suprapubic puncture), but because the operator dreads, and with reason, the accidents which are too often the consequence. It is in attempting to guard against these accidents that perineal, recto-vesical, subpubic and hypogastric punctures have been recommended in turn ; but it is only necessary to read the works published on this subject, to be convinced that not one of these methods

---

* Ponction de la Vessie par Aspiration. Thèse de Doctorat. Paris, 1871.

† Illustrations of the Surgical Uses of the Aspirator, by Jessop. British Medical Journal, Dec. 7th, 1872.

‡ Report of Prof. de Kieter on the Uses of Dieulafoy's Aspirator in Russia, December, 1872.

§ Puncture of the Bladder by Dieulafoy's Aspirator, by J. Little. New York, 1872.

had any decided superiority over the other, for they were all capable of provoking the most serious complications.

Thus, in the presence of a patient suffering from retention of urine, it was not easy to come to a decision. What to do—perform perineal puncture? But M. Voillemier's opinion on this proceeding is :—" The surgeon, most certain in his knowledge, is never certain of the course his instrument follows in traversing a region so complicated as the perineum ; if he inclines the handle of the trocar a little too much one way or another, he may wound the prostate, or the rectum, and sometimes not penetrate the bladder."*

What can be said of the recto-vesical puncture ? It presents the same inconveniences, the same dangers, without offering greater guarantees. The hypogastric puncture is most generally employed, but the patient is none the less exposed to the chances of urinous infiltration, either because the cannula leaves the bladder, or because the urine trickles along the walls of the instrument left *in situ;* the inflammation of the wall of the· abdomen, and the cellular tissue of the pelvis, attains sometimes an alarming proportion ; the bladder itself may be inflamed to gangrene, as a result of the use of unsuitable instruments (Pouliot†), and if the patient escapes these primary accidents, he is still exposed to urinary fistulæ, and to adhesions which are established between the bladder and the walls of the abdomen.

Retention is, therefore, in consequence of the difficulties met with in overcoming it, a very serious complication ; it causes in a great degree the developement of urinary infiltrations, and purulent collections of the

* Traité des Maladies des Voies Urinaires.

† Ponction Vésicale Hypogastrique. Thèse de Doctorat. Paris, 1868.

pelvis; it exposes the patient to the accidents of catheterization, to false passages and laceration of the canal, and when the question of treatment arises, the greatest indecision reigns as to the means to be employed. For these different reasons, it is easy to understand how desirable it would be to change retention of urine into an insignificant accident, no longer dangerous, and it is to this end that I propose a process easy to execute, and entirely harmless in result. This process is aspiration.

To support my opinion, and to make it accepted, I have had recourse to facts, without resting on theory. I appeal only secondarily to vesical contractility, and the results obtained by physiological experiment, and I base my proofs on the examination of pathological facts, and on clinical observation, the only incontestable arguments.

If I succeed in showing the complete harmlessness of the vesical puncture, it will be evident that retention of urine, a complication so frequent and grave in diseases of the genito-urinary organs, is no longer anything more than an insignificant phenomenon; and if I am able to prove that we have in our hands a simple and harmless means of guarding against the accidents of retention, we shall no longer have to occupy ourselves with the means, sometimes so dangerous, of averting this complication, but may spend the time in attacking the cause.

I have collected twenty cases of retention of urine treated by aspiration; in some patients eight, twelve, and twenty-four punctures of the bladder have been made in a few days, and by adding up the various cases, a total of ninety-eight aspirations is given.

These different operations are collected in the following table; I dispense with all commentary, as they are an incontestable proof of the complete harmlessness of aspiratory punctures in retention of urine.

TABLE OF OPERATIONS PERFORMED BY MEANS OF ASPIRATION IN RETENTION OF URINE.

Operations.	Authors.	Nature of the Disease.	No. of Punctures.	Result.
I.	L. Labbé	Hypertrophy of the prostate in a man, æt. 65; retention of urine; catheterization impossible	1 aspiration	Without Accident.
II.	Guyon	Multiple strictures in a man, æt. 72; retention	23 aspirations performed in a few days	,,
III.	Blache	Stricture of the prostatic part of the urethra; retention	2 aspirations	,,
IV.	Dieulafoy	Hypertrophy of the prostate; retention	1 aspiration	,,
V.	L. Labbé	Traumatism; retention	8 aspirations	,,
VI.	Guyon	Hypertrophy of the prostate; retention	4 aspirations	,,
VII.	Chuzeau	Stricture; retention	6 aspirations	,,
VIII.	Houzel	Cancer of the prostate; retention	11 aspirations	,,
IX.	Cusco	Stricture; retention	3 aspirations	,,
X.	Labbé	Retention	1 aspiration	,,
XI.	Dieulafoy	Hypertrophy of the prostate; retention	3 aspirations	,,
XII.	Le Bêle	Hypertrophy of the prostate in an old man.	1 aspiration	,,
XIII.	Lannelongue	Many strictures; hypertrophy of the prostate	11 aspirations	,,
XIV.	Ziembicky	Retention of urine; catheterization impossible	1 aspiration	,,
XV.	Kieter	Retention of urine	1 aspiration	,,
XVI.	Little	Hypertrophy of the prostate	14 aspirations	,,
XVII.	Jessop	Hydatids of the prostate; retention of urine	1 aspiration	,,
XVIII.	Jessop	Stricture of the urethra	1 aspiration	,,
XIX.	Dublin Journal	Retention from traumatism	4 aspirations	,,
XX.	,,	Hypertrophy of the prostate	1 aspiration	,,

On these twenty patients aspiration was performed ninety-eight times. In order to judge correctly of the value of the process employed, it is of no use to make a statistical table of the persons cured and of those who died since the treatment for retention, which is in point of fact only the treatment of a complication, and has nothing in common with lesions, such as stricture, wounds, or ruptures of the canal, which determine the gravity of the case.

What we have to do is to take each patient separately, in order to study the good or bad results of aspiration. What interests us is to know in what measure aspiration was harmless and useful, and after a detailed examination we shall be able to arrive at a conclusion as to the exact value of the process.

Its harmlessness does not seem to us difficult to establish; it strongly recommends itself if, after ninety-eight punctures of the bladder, there is not a single accident to record. In reading the detailed cases of these patients, it will be seen that in not one of them was found a trace of peritonitis, abscess, hæmorrhage, or infiltration of urine; some of them were operated on two or three times in the twenty-four hours, and for many successive days, without ever experiencing the least morbid symptom.

In Case II. (Guyon) twenty-three aspirations were performed in eight days, and the most simple catheterization could not have been more harmless. In Case VII. (Cluzeau) the urine was aspirated on three successive days, which enabled a sound to be passed on the fourth day. In Case VIII. (Houzel) ten aspirations were made on a spot not larger than a half-franc piece. In Case XIII. (Lannelongue) eleven aspirations were performed. Little, in Case XVI., practised fourteen, and everywhere the observers have been unanimous in declaring the complete benignity of these operations.

How, indeed, should accidents occur? The puncture of the peritoneum and the bladder is so minute that there is no danger to fear from it; the true source of danger would be the contact of the urine with the peritoneum, for peritonitis might be the consequence; but the passage even of a few drops of urine into the peritoneal cavity is really impossible if we reflect on the fineness of the needle and the contractility of the bladder. I have already said that, in animals killed immediately after the operation, it was often difficult for me to discover traces of the vesical puncture, and in the patients who were examined after death, " the mucous membrane of the bladder, at the spot of the capillary punctures, only showed very small dark points without abscess or sanguineous infiltration into the vesical walls." (Muron.)

The absolute innocence of the vesical puncture and of aspiration seems to me, therefore, a settled question, and my conviction is based on physiological experiments, on anatomical examinations, and above all on pathological facts. Can any one have the least fear of an operation which, performed ninety-eight times, has not provoked a single accident, even when repeated several times a day on the same person ? Need one hesitate for an instant to make use of a process so harmless and so painless ? The pain is, in fact, next to nothing, it is the sensation of the prick of a needle, and how much less disagreeable is this sensation to a patient than the passage of a sound or bougie through the urethra.

Thus, owing to aspiration, we need no longer to worry ourselves as to the means of fixing the sound and retaining it in the punctured bladder; nor have we to concern ourselves with the passage of the urine into the peritoneum, with abscess of the pelvis, nor with fistulæ following the operation. There is no longer hesitation in the choice of a process, no longer difficulty in its execution, and no longer the delay so often dangerous to the patient.

ARTICLE II.

Indications and Method of Aspiration in the Treatment of Retention of Urine.

THE harmlessness of the vesical puncture by aspiration being an established fact, we proceed to reply to the second question—" Under what circumstances should aspiration be used ? " When vesical puncture was a really dangerous operation, recourse was only had to it, as was natural, as a last resort, after having tried the series of palliative means, and in many cases this is what took place : a man not having passed water since the previous day presented himself with one or many strictures of the urethra ; the passage of a catheter was first tried once or twice without success ; then drinks were forbidden, in the hope of gaining time; the patient had a bath, but in spite of every treatment the volume of the bladder increased, accompanied by the most acute suffering. Catheterization, with sounds and bougies of different forms and diameters, was again tried, and it was not sufficiently seen that the mucous membrane, contused and irritated by these manœuvres, swelled, and helped to render the stricture still more impassable. Thus we moved in a vicious circle, out of which it was not easy to find our way. Pain and vesical distention still increased, not to speak of the false passages, the rupture of the mucous membrane, the accesses of urethral fever, and urinary infiltration—accidents which were often the consequence of a lengthened delay, or of a too violent process of catheterization.

This picture is not at all overdrawn ; those who have had to deal with analogous cases know how difficult it is to arrive at a decision ; one always hopes to be able to reduce the stricture ; one temporizes, asks one's self if one ought to persist in employing the means to avoid operation, or have recourse to a puncture, the consequences of which are dreaded, or to urethrotomy, which presents serious difficulties. And yet this question should be decided promptly, for a delay of some hours may cost the patient his life. What is to be done? To perform urethrotomy?—a difficult operation, which not everybody is able to perform, for it requires a thorough knowledge of surgery, not always met with in the country and in small towns, where surgery is far from being as extensively practised as medicine. Perform the suprapubic puncture? But the possible consecutive accidents must be thought of —infiltration of urine, peritonitis, urinary fistula; in short, the situation is a difficult one; we hesitate, and the result of these reflections too often is to induce us to seek in expectation a remedy which is not to be found in it.

Let us suppose that an analogous case presents itself, now that we have aspiration at our service. This new proceeding requires neither especial skill nor surgical knowledge; it presents not the slightest difficulty, and puts us out of the way of any danger. Thus, if a patient is suffering from retention of urine, from whatever cause, aspiration should be performed whenever the first and second attempt at catheterization, aided by the other usual means, has failed to overcome the obstacle. There is no use in temporizing; it is useless to expose the patient to new sufferings and to the risks of false passages and febrile attacks, when we have in our hands a therapeutic means of such efficacy. Let us begin first by removing the complication, and we shall then have plenty of time to treat the cause of the evil. The evacuation of the urine has other advantages besides those of meeting the difficulties of the moment. It is of great use in long and laborious labours which produce retention by compression of the urethra.

In the case of a man suffering from hypertrophy of the prostate, vesical puncture is often at once palliative and curative of the retention. M. Sappey has, indeed, demon-

strated that there exists a notable difference in the direction of the prostatic portion of the urethra according as
the bladder is empty or distended ; whence the possibility
of sounding a patient when the bladder is empty, although
catheterization was impossible when the organ was full.
The more the bladder fills, the higher it rises, leaning
at the same time towards the abdominal wall ; and in this
double movement of ascension the urethra is drawn along,
and the anterior concavity of the canal is so exaggerated
that the sound, in spite of its curve, is often unable to
penetrate into the bladder.

Cases I. (Labbé), IV. (Dieulafoy), XII. (Le Bêle), are
the confirmation of these anatomical indications.   These
were three cases of old men with voluminous prostates, and
in whom micturition became impossible without any other
appreciable cause.   Catheterization, which could not be
performed while the bladder was full, was easy enough
after the evacuation of the urine.   The same fact is
observed sometimes in strictures ; a stricture which was
impassable during retention of urine permits the passage
of a bougie when the bladder has been emptied.   This may
be observed in Cases X. (Labbé), and XIV. (Ziembicky).

Aspiration in retention of urine fulfils, then, a double
object ; not only does it avert immediately and without any restriction the accidents due to extreme distention of the organ, but it further places the canal in conditions favourable to catheterization : thus the question of
opportunity seems to us easy to decide ; and the complete harmlessness of the aspiratory puncture, as well as
the immediate benefit derived from it, are two conditions
which allow of sharply deciding the question,—That, if, in
a case of retention, catheterization, practised systematically,
has twice failed, whatever was the cause of the retention,
we must have recourse to aspiration without persisting
in the use of sounds and bougies.   When we had
only the choice of proceedings equally bad, because

they were all dangerous, there were reasons for waiting till the last moment, and for exhausting the whole series of possible means, before deciding to puncture ; but now that the aspiratory needle removes all dangers and all scruples, it would be an error to torment the urethra, to multiply tentative efforts, and to leave the patient a prey to the pangs of retention and the risks of the unforeseen.

The mode of performing aspiration in retention of urine is extremely simple. The operation having been decided on, the spot for the puncture is chosen, which is the same chosen for suprapubic puncture ; that is, one or two centimetres above the pubis on the median line. Before making the puncture, it is necessary to assure one's self of the permeability of the needle about to be used, for it is so long and its calibre so small that a few grains of rust or dust are sufficient to block up the opening. Care must therefore be taken to examine the needle with a silver thread and a jet of water, at the risk of failure. By introducing an obstructed needle, believed to be permeable, the operator is in danger of piercing the bladder from one side to the other, for he keeps pushing the needle forward, expecting to meet the urine, which does not appear.

The long needle No. 1 is to be preferred. Its diameter, which is only one-third of a millimetre, allows perfectly of the passage of urine, and its length, which is twelve centimetres, enables it to reach the bladder through the layers of the abdomen and the adipose tissue, which is sometimes so thick in this part.

I advise the use of needle No. 1 as an excess of prudence, for needle No. 2 has often been employed without the slightest inconvenience.

The aspirator being ready, that is to say, the previous vacuum being made, the needle is introduced sharply at the spot pointed out. Before the needle has penetrated a

centimetre into the tissue, that is, as soon as its opening
is no longer in contact with the external air, the stop-cock
connected with the needle is opened, and
the vacuum is thus formed in the needle
itself. This needle, carrying the vacuum
with it, is slowly, very slowly, pushed in
the direction of the bladder, until the
urine flowing over the glass index shows
that the bladder is pierced. Owing
to this proceeding, and having the previous vacuum at our command, we
know the precise moment the fluid is
reached. At the same time, care must
be taken to push the needle two centimetres further, and for this reason : the
bladder, in emptying, contracts, and if the
point of the needle is only caught in its
walls, it would probably be driven out by
the contraction of the organ. It is, therefore, necessary to note these two parts of
the operation : the first part consists in
slowly pushing the needle forward till
it has penetrated the vesical cavity; and
the second, in introducing the needle to
the depth of two centimetres. This precaution being taken, the operation is continued ; a litre of urine is evacuated in
ten minutes ; time must be taken, and
the abdomen of the patient must not be
pressed upon under the pretext of aiding
or hastening the issue of the fluid. Such a proceeding
cannot but be harmful, it is also useless, for the urine is
doubly induced to flow by the aspiratory power and by
the contraction of the bladder ; and it is also dangerous,
for it might displace the needle and permit the contact of
a few drops of urine with the peritoneum.

When the bladder is emptied, that is to say when the liquid no longer flows, all that is necessary is to quickly withdraw the needle. There is no fear of the urine passing into the peritoneum, for it is held immovable by the aspiratory force. The operation over, there are no precautions to be taken, no dressing to be made ; the puncture is fine, not to say invisible, and the patient can get up and walk as easily as after the most simple catheterization. The operation, moreover, can, as we prove by the cases collected in this book, be performed daily, and for a long time if necessary, without the patient feeling the least discomfort.

What difference is there between this aspiratory puncture and the old methods ? Here the patient passes without transition from a most serious condition to one of complete well-being, and a dreaded complication disappears in a few minutes by a means so painless that the responsibility of the operator is completely covered. Formerly, the result of the puncture was a matter of doubt ; it was necessary to take into consideration the mobility of the sound allowed to remain *in situ ;* the escape of the urine, peritonitis, and other accidents ; now, apprehensions and fear have given place to an absolute security, both to the patient and the medical man.

Conclusions.—Thus I have described an operation which is harmless, painless, easy to perform, and certain in its result. This new proceeding, which I propose to substitute in place of those which preceded it, seems to me one of the most directly useful applications of the aspiratory method. For the old operations, full of danger and uncertainty, I substitute a means which exacts neither special anatomical knowledge nor special surgical skill ; it is within reach of all, and a patient in a pressing case could, strictly speaking, perform it on himself as easily as he can inject morphia into himself by Pravaz's syringe.

The ease with which we shall, in the future, ward off the dangers of retention will cause infiltration of the urine, false passages, and other accidents which cause so large a proportion of the mortality in diseases of the genito-urinary passages to become circumstances of rare occurrence ; for aspiration of urine can henceforth be practised without fear of peritonitis, and without having to provide means of maintaining in its place the sound left after puncture *in situ.* Retention of urine is thus no longer an accident ; it is only an incident, without serious consequences. A factitious passage is created for the urine, the needle becomes a canal which provisionally replaces the urethra, and the patient is able to pass water by the aspirator as often as necessary, and as long as the cause which provoked the retention continues.

ARTICLE III.

Cases of Aspiratory Punctures in Retention of Urine.

CASE I. (Labbé), HYPERTROPHY OF THE PROSTATE— ONE ASPIRATION.—On February 26, 1870, M. Labbé was called to a man, æt. 65, suffering from complete retention of urine. This old man had a very voluminous prostate, and various attempts at catheterization had for two days been made without result ; these attempts had not, however, been entirely harmless, for the patient had lost a rather considerable quantity of blood by the urethral mucous membrane, and much pain had been caused.

M. Labbé immediately put aside all idea of a fresh catheterization, and, considering the enormous distention of the bladder and the alarming state of the patient, he resolved to puncture the organ. For this purpose he used Dieulafoy's aspirator. The hollow needle No. 2 was introduced a little above the pubis. (This needle, mathematically bored, was not more than a millimetre in diameter.) Almost 500 grammes of fluid were drawn off. The relief was instantaneous. Two hours later it was possible to pass a rather large bougie into the canal. All the accidents disappeared ; it was not necessary to interfere again, and the patient recovered without having the slightest accident or the least pain in consequence of the operation.

Case II. (At the Necker Hospital, under the care of M. Guyon)—Multiple Strictures—Considerable Hypertrophy of the Prostate—Laceration of the Urethra—Twenty-three Aspirations (Thesis of M. Watelet).—M. X., æt. 72, entered the hospital, August 10, 1871, with retention of urine. For twelve years he had not passed water without the aid of a sound, and he had often caused himself to bleed in using it. The bulbous sound No. 15 was stopped in the middle of the penile region ; No. 14 passed through the stricture with great difficulty ; No. 12 reached the bladder easily. There was a circular induration at the level of the stricture.

August 16th.—M. Guyon, to enable the patient to better perform catheterization, decided to perform divulsion. The operation was very painful, and blood flowed freely, but he did not succeed in passing a permanent sound. The bulbous bougie No. 15 and smaller ones, when passed into the urethra, projected under the skin 5 or 6 centimetres behind the meatus. All the instruments introduced passed into this false passage, and projected under the skin, at the root of the scrotum. The urethra continued to bleed freely. Prescription : bath, poultices, and 60 centigrammes of sulphate of quinine.

August 17th.—By digital examination by the rectum considerable distention of the bladder was felt (trocar ½ of a millimetre in diameter). Puncture, in the morning, with Potain's apparatus, and 1,100 grammes of pale urine drawn off. An hour after the puncture the patient was taken with a shivering fit, followed by profuse sweats. In the evening, the left kidney was painful to pressure. A fresh puncture, and a shivering fit in the night.

August 18th.—Puncture in the morning and evening; each time 900 grammes of urine drawn off. In the night, shivering fit, with sweat.

August 19th.—Puncture, in spite of the extreme resonance of the hypogastric region. Bilious vomitings and colic. At 3 P.M. another puncture, 1,000 grammes of clouded urine; a noticeable quantity of pus at the end of the operation.

August 20th.—Puncture at 9 A.M., 900 grammes; and at 6 P.M. 1,100 grammes.

August 21st.—At 6 A.M. 1,100 grammes; urine clear, containing less pus than the previous day. The patient taken with diarrhœa.—Tea and rum; 60 centigrammes of sulphate of quinine. Puncture at midday; 600 grammes. Not a drop of pus. Dysentery characterized by bloody stools. Puncture at midnight; 1,000 grammes.

August 22nd.—From this date the dysentery increased: 40 stools a day. Tisane of rice, julep of s. nit. bismuth. Two punctures in 24 hours; 2,000 grammes of urine.

August 23rd.—Three punctures; urine a little thick.

August 24th.—Two punctures.

August 25th.—A puncture of 500 grammes, and two punctures of the abdomen, because of the suprapubic resonance.

August 26th.—The patient grew weak; the same severity of the dysentery; only one puncture of 500 grammes in the morning.

August 27th.—One puncture of 780 grammes.

August 28th.—Inflammation of the mouth. Puncture in the morning; clyster with nitrate of silver.

August 29th.—Puncture in the morning; 500 grammes.

August 30th.—The dysentery persisted; the patient was

almost voiceless, cold at the extremities, pulse weak and thready. Two injections of nitrate of silver. For the first time, during the night, the patient passed water by the urethra in the efforts of defecation. In the morning, on pressing on the meatus, some drops of limpid urine came out. The different pricks of the punctures left no more trace than a red dot like a flea-bite. The skin was very mobile over the subjacent tissues.

August 31st.—The patient passed half a litre of limpid urine. He died on the 2nd of September. The stools were sanguineous and numerous to the end.

The autopsy was made by M. Muron, the house surgeon.

The Kidneys.—In the left kidney was a series of superficial abscesses about the size of a nut. The right kidney presented, under the capsule of Glisson, on the surface of the cortical layer, small miliary abscesses. The ureters were slightly dilated.

The Bladder.—It was slightly congested on the internal surface. The vesical mucous membrane, at the spot of the capillary punctures, showed four very small blackish marks; but there was no abscess, and no sanguineous infiltration into the vesical walls. The anterior part of the bladder had contracted no adhesion with the corresponding abdominal wall. The prevesical cellular tissue showed here and there in its substance some indurated points, which were found again in the sub-peritoneal cellular tissue of the abdominal wall. This coloration was evidently the result of slight infiltration of blood, which had taken place at different times. There was, however, no sanguineous collection, and no abscess.

Urethra.—In its canal there were three lacerations, one at the level of the navicular fossa. It was covered with a reddish tissue of new formation, with different portions of the mucous membrane adhering in such a way that a sound could freely traverse this part. The two other lacerations were longitudinal, of 2 and 5 centimetres

I

in length.   One was found at the commencement of the
perineal region, on the left side of the urethra ; the other
was on the right side, and in the scrotal region.

Prostate.—It was extraordinarily voluminous, particularly its two lateral lobes, which formed, at the side of
the membranous region of the urethra, a great mass almost
3 centimetres high ; the same mass on the side of the
bladder.   The middle lobe was moderately developed, and
made a slight projection on the side of the bladder.   On
the summit, and on the sides of the verumontanum, there
were three false passages, one of which led into the bladder.
There was no abscess, either in the prostate or in the
false passages.

Intestines.—The large intestine presented, throughout
its whole extent, an extreme vascularization of the mucous
membrane.   Principally in the rectum and in the
descending colon, little reddish ecchymotic projections
were seen, which were only the partial thickening of the
mucous membrane ; here and there, also, were a series of
yellowish spots, representing a fibrino-epithelial layer,
besides a great quantity of transparent miliary points,
which seemed to be hypertrophied closed follicles.   The
intestinal mucous membrane was remarkably thickened,
and glided with difficulty over the subjacent tissue ; in a
word, considerable lesions from dysentery in the second
stage were found ; this was as evident as possible.

This case is extremely interesting.   The patient underwent twenty-five punctures in twelve days, without any
accident being produced.   It shows, by inspection of the
parts, the harmlessness of the capillary puncture, and it
is almost certain that, but for the dysentery, the patient
would have been cured.

The specimen which I prepared was deposited in the
Necker Hospital, in the collection of M. Guyon, No. 43.

CASE III. (BLACHE).—STRICTURE OF THE PROSTATIC

PORTION OF THE URETHRA—RETENTION—TWO ASPIRA-
TIONS.—M. C., æt. 83, in excellent health, had for some
years been suffering from stricture of the urethra, at the
level of the prostatic portion. On the 6th of June, at
two o'clock in the morning, he wished to urinate, but found
it absolutely impossible. Catheterization was performed
at six o'clock, by means of a soft sound of the finest
calibre; a complete barrier was met with in the prostatic
region. More voluminous sounds were used with the same
result. No dribbling. On the 10th, fever set in, and his·
general state became serious. Dr. R. Blache pierced the
bladder, at some centimetres above the pubis, with the
hollow No. 2 needle of Dieulafoy's aspirator (this needle
is 1 millimetre in diameter), and about 500 grammes of
urine were drawn off by this apparatus. The night and
the following day were satisfactory, but, three days later,
symptoms of uræmic poisoning appeared. A new aspiration was performed on the 14th, followed by marked
relief. Afterwards, fever and delirium attacked the patient,
and he succumbed.

This case is intended to show the harmlessness of
aspiratory punctures of the bladder, and the relief which
follows the operation.

CASE IV. (DIEULAFOY).—HYPERTROPHY OF THE PROS-
TATE—ONE ASPIRATION.—A man, æt. 65, was taken,
after a rather heavy meal, with a difficulty of passing
water, which progressively increased to complete retention. He was in the habit of passing the sound
himself, but after trying in vain to perform catheterization, he called me in. I found the same difficulty, and
after many unsuccessful attempts, and seeing the accident increasing in intensity, I resolved to puncture the
bladder by aspiration. No. 1 needle was sharply introduced above the pubis, and I drew off 800 grammes of
urine. The relief was instantaneous, and immediately

afterwards I was able to pass a sound almost without difficulty.

CASE V. (LABBÉ).— TRAUMATIC RETENTION — EIGHT ASPIRATIONS. (Extracted from the *Gazette des Hôpitaux,* September 19th, 1871 ; reported by M. Hubert, house surgeon.)

January 4th.—A mason, called A——, entered the St. Antoine Hospital. An hour before, the man, who was mounted on a scaffolding, was precipitated from a height of about two yards. He had fallen astride on to a beam, and had very severely contused the perineum and the anterior abdominal region.

The next morning, on visiting him, a rather considerable effusion of blood was observed behind the root of the scrotum. The patient complained of severe pain in the belly, which was very sensitive to the touch. The skin was hot, the pulse 120 ; poultices were applied to the abdomen. Since the accident the patient had been unable to urinate, in spite of repeated efforts, and the distended bladder had risen to three fingers' breadth below the umbilicus. Almost immediately after the accident, about a teaspoonful of blood had escaped by the urethra. Catheterization having been attempted without success by the house surgeon, M. Labbé tried to introduce bougies of different sizes into the canal. These attempts being fruitless, he made an incision in the perineum, in order to give issue to the sanguineous collection, hoping that, after having removed the pressure on the urethra exerted by this effusion, catheterization would be easier ; besides, he thought this perineal incision might allow of the introduction of a sound directly into the vesical extremity of the urethra. But in spite of lengthened attempts, it was found impossible to penetrate to the bladder. A prolonged bath was ordered, and half a gramme of sulphate of quinine administered.

Intervention was nevertheless necessary to empty the bladder, and for this end M. Labbé made a puncture with Dieulafoy's long No. 1 needle; the vacuum was previously made in the instrument, and the needle was slowly introduced into the tissues above the pubis. At the instant that the needle, which carried the vacuum with it, penetrated the bladder, the urine was seen to flow into the body of the pump. The needle was progressively pushed forward as the bladder emptied itself, till it had reached the depth of 8 centimetres, and thus about 400 grammes of urine was drawn off. The puncture only caused insignificant pain at the moment of piercing the skin.

January 6th.—The fever was acute, and, as on the previous evening, the abdominal pains intense. M. Labbé attempted catheterization again, and, not succeeding, performed a fresh aspiration of urine, and made the puncture almost at the same point as the day before. Being anxious to profit by the urethral expansion which sometimes takes place after puncture, he immediately tried catheterization, but the obstacle was not removed. Two more aspirations in the day.

January 7th.—Peritonitis, occasioned by the fall of the patient, continued to make progress; the pain was still acute, and the abdomen inflated; the pulse 140, small, and thready; the tongue dry; the facies changed. Three fresh punctures in the day.

January 8th.—The patient became worse; another aspiration was performed during the day. In the evening he died.

Autopsy.—Generalized peritonitis, little fluid, considerable injection of the serous membrane, agglutination of the intestines. The anterior surface of the bladder showed on its external surface small red ecchymotic spots, similar to flea-bites on the skin. It was at these spots that the punctures were made; on the internal surface of the bladder it was not possible to find the slightest trace of the passage of the needle. The urine in the bladder was perfectly normal and limpid, with neither blood, clots, nor pus.

This case, together with the necropsy, confirms the entire harmlessness of the aspiratory punctures.

CASE VI. (GUYON, NECKER HOSPITAL).—SPONTANEOUS FRACTURE OF THE FEMUR—PSEUDARTHROSIS—PROSTATIC HYPERTROPHY—RETENTION OF URINE — DIFFICULT CATHETERIZATION—FOUR ASPIRATIONS—(Thesis of M. Watelet).—François Nilles, mason, æt. 66, entered the Hospital in February, 1871. He had pseudarthrosis of the thigh, and chronic bronchitis; he had never had blennorrhagia, but for fifteen years he had passed water with difficulty.

On the 24th of October, 1871, he was suddenly taken with acute retention. Repeated attempts at catheterization were made with bougies Nos. 3 and 4. They were stopped in the deep part of the urethra, and our impression was that at this point a narrow stricture existed. The bladder was as high as the umbilicus on the evening of the 25th. The first aspiration was made with M. Potain's apparatus, and 1,000 grammes of clear urine drawn off.

October 27th.—In the morning visit bougie No. 4 was passed, and retained until the morning visit of the 28th. The patient did not urinate in spite of this contrivance.

October 28th.—In the evening a new puncture was made, and 1,000 grammes of urine drawn off. The patient found himself much relieved after this puncture, which he did not find painful. He had a shivering fit two hours after midday, which lasted half an hour.

October 29th.—He had not passed water since the previous evening: bougie No. 4 was passed again. In the evening a fresh aspiration, and 1,500 grammes of urine drawn off. He was taken to the St. Vincent ward to be methodically examined with bulbous bougies.

October 30th.—M. Guyon diagnosed prostatic hypertrophy. No. 12 sound was afterwards passed and retained.

October 31st.—The sound was removed and he was catheterized twice a day.

CASE VII.—RETENTION OF URINE—SIX PUNCTURES OF THE BLADDER BY DR. CLUZEAU, OF GISORS.

I was called, July 28th, 1870, to a man, æt. 68, a farmer at Neaufles. For three days he had not been able to pass water, except a few drops from overflowing. He told me that for a long time micturition had been difficult, and by touch I diagnosed an enormous prostate. He had had, moreover, for ten or fifteen years, two very large and irreducible inguinal herniæ.

On the 28th, danger being imminent, the size of the bladder having attained large proportions, I attempted catherization many times, but without any success. I then had recourse to Dieulafoy's needle No. 1, which I thrust in above the pubis, and completely emptied the bladder, to the great relief of the patient.

The next day, the 29th, I tried again, but in vain, to introduce a sound into the bladder. I then performed aspiration, and employed this time needle No. 2, in order to obtain a rather more rapid flow than the evening before. On the 30th and 31st I repeated, in the evening, the same operation, and at length, on August 1st, I succeeded in passing an olive-shaped bougie with perfect ease. I had thus, in four days, performed six aspiratory punctures of the bladder without the shadow of an accident. The operation is one of the most simple. I taught the patient to sound himself, and after this time I did not see him again.

CASE VIII. (HOUZEL).—CANCER OF THE PROSTATE—

ELEVEN ASPIRATIONS.—On July 6th I was called, in consultation with my friend, M. Huchette, to Montcavrel. For eight months the patient had suffered much in the hypogastrium and experienced great difficulty in passing water. His skin was pale and earthy, his appetite was almost gone, and at the level of the fourth dorsal vertebra a tumour was felt: it was not ulcerated but cancerous, and of about the size of a turkey's egg; there were similar tumours on the top of the head, the temple, the cartilage of the sixth right rib, and the abdominal walls.

By digital examination of the rectum a voluminous, hard, uneven tumour was diagnosed at the level of the prostate, which rose to the back of the neck of the bladder. The fæcal excretions were flattened and riband shape. The patient dated the commencement of his disease four months back. For some days the pains in the bladder had become intolerable, micturition was difficult, and since the previous evening the urine had been charged with blood and clots. I diagnosed an ulcerated cancer of the prostate, and of the neck of the bladder. I prescribed pills of the extract of hemlock and friction of the abdomen to overcome the tympanitis.

July 11*th.*—The pain was less, but the incessant desire to pass water resulted only in passing a little urine and blood.

July 13*th.*—Complete retention of urine. I tried catheterization in vain; the pain was terrible. I made a puncture at the linea alba, 3 centimetres above the pubis, with Dieulafoy's No. 1 needle, and drew off a litre and a half of urine.

July 14*th.*—Œdema of the legs. The puncture of the previous evening was no longer visible on the skin. Fresh aspiration. I drew off a litre of fluid.

July 15*th.*—A new puncture.

July 16*th.*—The œdema invaded the trunk and the face.

July 18*th.*—New attempts at catheterization, without

result; the fever was violent, the tympanitis considerable. A fresh puncture.

July 19*th.*—Aspiration.   One litre of urine.

July 21*st.*—A fresh puncture.

July 22*nd.*—The general state considerably aggravated. I made another puncture.

July 24*th.*—Aspiration of half a litre of urine.

July 25*th.*—General œdema of the body.   Aspiration.

July 26*th.*—Delirious ; pulse 104.   Aspiration.

July 27*th.*—Delirium continued ;· aspiration.   Death was imminent, and the patient succumbed the next day.

To sum up, I was able to make eleven punctures at 8 centimetres above the pubis, without provoking the least inflammation of the peritoneum or of the bladder.   These eleven punctures were made within a space not larger than a half-franc piece.

CASE IX. STRICTURE OF THE URETHRA—RETENTION— TWO ASPIRATIONS—UNDER THE CARE OF M. CUSCO (Case reported by M. Labarraque, House Surgeon).—A patient, æt. 31, entered July 27th, 1872, the Hôtel Dieu, and was placed under the care of M. Cusco.   This man had contracted blennorrhagia in 1869, and (had since experienced some difficulty in passing water.   In December, 1870, he ·underwent internal urethrotomy, was cured in thirteen days, and felt nothing particular till July, 1872, the time he entered the Hôtel Dieu.   He stated that, during the last three months, he had passed water with increasing difficulty; moreover, his prepuce was the seat of soft chancres, which prevented one from finding the meatus. There was also, in the median part of the passage, a fluctuating tumour and urinary abscess, which further interfered with the issue of the urine.   Catherization was impossible.

July 28*th.*—The patient had a bath, but he was still unable to pass water.

July 29*th.*—The retention gained ground, and catheter-

ization was attempted many times in vain. At six o'clock
in the evening, the surgeon on duty was called in haste.
He found the patient in such agony that he decided to
perform the hypogastric puncture with Dieulafoy's aspirator. The finest needle was introduced a centimetre
above the pubis, and a little to the right of the median
line. A litre and a half of urine was drawn off, and
relief was instantaneous.

No accident occurred in consequence of the puncture,
and the mark was hardly visible on the skin. The following evening, at the request of the patient, the surgeon
on duty repeated aspiration with the same success and the
same harmlessness.

July 31*st.*—The amelioration was marked. M. Cusco
opened the abscess, and resolved to perform external
urethrotomy without a conductor. From that time the
patient, who had a sound left *in situ,* became better and
better, and was discharged in the middle of September.

CASE X. (DIEULAFOY).—HYPERTROPHY OF THE PROS-
TATE—STRICTURE OF THE URETHRA—RETENTION—THREE
ASPIRATIONS.—M. X—— had suffered for a long time from
stricture, which had never attained exaggerated proportions,
but which decidedly diminished the calibre of the urethra.
Three days after some excesses, M. X—— was attacked by
a slight urethral swelling, and a certain difficulty of passing water. The retention of urine was complete on his
admission, the bladder greatly distended, and the pain
most acute.

By examination I discovered a voluminous prostate; I
attempted catheterization with a metallic sound, and with
bougies of different diameters, but it was absolutely impossible to penetrate into the bladder.

I then made a puncture above the pubis, by means of
a long No. 2 needle and drew off 900 grammes of urine.

After this operation there was the same difficulty of performing catheterization.

The next day another aspiration, but I tried in vain to introduce a bougie into the bladder. The day after a third aspiration, after which I reached the bladder by means of a fine bougie. From this time gradual dilatation was continued, and the accident of retention did not again occur.

CASE XI.—(LE BÊLE, OF MANS).—RETENTION OF URINE—ONE ASPIRATION.—I was called to an old man attacked with retention of urine, and with whom various attempts at catheterization had failed. I was not successful in my attempt, and considering the extreme distention of the bladder, I decided to perform aspiration of the urine.

I made use of needle No. 1, and obtained about a litre of fluid, but the flow was slow, on account of the small size of the conduit. This aspiratory puncture did not cause the slightest accident, and the next day it was easy to introduce an india-rubber sound by the urethra.

CASE XII.—RETENTION OF URINE—ONE ASPIRATION (BY M. ZIEMBICKY, THE HOUSE SURGEON).—A patient, æt. 40, a watchmaker by trade, was admitted the early part of June, 1872, into the St. Louis Hospital, and was placed under the care of M. Tillaux. He was attacked with retention of urine, and did not even pass any water by urethral dribbling. Many attempts at catheterization had already failed; the general condition was serious, the pain was acute, the bladder had risen as far as the umbilicus, and the patient, covered with sweat and in a state of extreme nervous excitability, asked for an immediate operation.

M. Ziembicky, the surgeon on duty, after having vainly tried to introduce a metallic sound and filiform bougies, decided, after half an hour of fruitless efforts, to puncture

the bladder by aspiration. The puncture was made by
means of needle No. 2, and the bladder was completely
emptied.

This operation was not followed by any accident,
pain ceased immediately, a good night was passed, and
the next day it was possible to perform catheterization
with bougie No. 8. From that time progressive dilatation
of the canal was commenced.

This case proves the harmlessness of aspiration, and
the therapeutic results which may be expected from it, in
averting the accidents of retention.

CASE XIII.—RETENTION OF URINE—ELEVEN ASPIRA-
TIONS—VESICAL PUNCTURE—INTERNAL URETHROTOMY—
RECOVERY (BY DR. LANNELONGUE).—*April 7th.*—I was
called to Neuilly by Dr. Putel to a patient, æt. 50, who
had not passed water for three days. Attempts at catheterization had been made without success by many medical
men, and had been followed by very abundant urethral
hæmorrhage. Putel had ascertained the existence of a
false passage, and, in my turn, I easily concluded that this
false passage occupied the inferior side of the prostate,
and that at this spot my catheter passed into a rather
large artificial cavity.

The desperate condition of the patient made me think
of having immediate recourse to suprapubic puncture, which
I performed with the No. 2 needle of Dieulafoy's aspirator.
The relief was immediate, and no accident followed aspiration. I then sought to discover the causes of the retention of urine. M. L—— denied all previous urethral
disease, and especially blennorrhagia. However, a medical
man, who had formerly sounded him, had declared the
existence of a stricture. After aspiration, I made many
fruitless attempts to penetrate into the bladder. These
attempts, which I renewed for eight days, sometimes for
one or two hours, never enabled me to reach the bladder by

the finest of bougies. For a week recourse was had every day to the aspiratory puncture, and it was sometimes necessary to perform it many times in the twenty-four hours.

After eleven punctures, which caused no kind of accident, I observed a little tenderness of the abdominal wall at the level of the spot where these punctures had been made, with œdema of the part. M. Gosselin was consulted, and we resolved to make the puncture with a large trocar, for which an india-rubber sound was substituted, which was retained seventeen days. It was not till then that I was able to introduce a fine bougie into the bladder.

The general condition of the patient had been excellent during the whole of the first period; it began to change after the sound was allowed to remain constantly *in situ.* Thinking, therefore, that having removed the obstacle, that dilatation—an excellent method under ordinary conditions—would compel us to leave the sound inserted for too long a time, I performed internal urethrotomy.

The suprapubic sound was removed, an urethral sound was kept in for eight days, and the recovery became complete.

CASE XIV.—HYPERTROPHY OF THE PROSTATE—RETENTION—FOURTEEN ASPIRATIONS (BY DR. JAMES L. LITTLE, OF NEW YORK, SURGEON TO ST. LUKE'S HOSPITAL).—Mr. Ramond, æt. 68, began to experience, five years previously, some difficulty in micturition, and the first retention of urine was overcome two years previously by the introduction of a sound.

September 6th, 1872.—I was called to Mr. R——, and I found him suffering from complete retention, with acute pain. Rectal palpation indicated hypertrophy of the prostate. I tried catheterization with various sounds, but in spite of all my efforts, it was not possible to reach the bladder. The patient was, however, suffering tortures, so I proposed to Dr. Dana to perform puncture of the bladder by means of Dieulafoy's aspirator, and Dr. Robert F. Weir, who very kindly lent me the apparatus, assisted me in the operation. The puncture was made above the pubis with needle No. 2, and I drew off 800 grammes of fluid; the same evening, towards ten o'clock, I drew off 500 grammes by another puncture.

September 7th.—The patient was much relieved; I performed two aspirations during the day; the first 500 grammes, the second 480 grammes.

September 8th.—A fresh puncture was made just above the pubis, and the needle meeting no urine, I made a puncture a little higher and drew off 400 grammes of fluid. After the greatest difficulty I passed sound No. 12, but the pain was so great that I agreed with Dr. Dana to make use of the aspirator again, and I performed the eighth puncture, which gave issue to 490 grammes.

September 9th.—Fresh puncture, 420 grammes; later, the tenth puncture, 500 grammes, and at eleven o'clock the eleventh puncture, 300 grammes.

September 10th.—Twelfth puncture, 320 grammes; and in the same day the thirteenth and fourteenth punctures. An india-rubber bougie of small size could then be introduced into the bladder, and I continued this treatment without being obliged to have recourse to fresh punctures.

Dr. James L. Little appends some remarks to this case: he asserts the complete harmlessness of the method, and he congratulates himself on having had at his service a proceeding which allowed him to make fourteen punctures, and to avoid the old and always dangerous operations.

CASE XV.—RETENTION OF URINE—ONE ASPIRATION (BY DR. T. JESSOP, OF LEEDS).—In an article* in which

* The *British Medical Journal*, December 7th, 1871. Illustrations of the Surgical Uses of the Aspirator.

the author has accumulated facts of various kinds to illus-
trate the usefulness of aspiration and its superiòrity to
other methods, we find a case of retention of urine which
we here abstract. A patient entered the Leeds General
Infirmary in December, 1870, and was under the care
of Dr. Jessop. After many useless efforts at catheterization, aspiration was performed with needle No. 1, and
88 ounces of urine drawn off. The accidents of retention
were averted, and treatment for stricture of the urethra
was undertaken.

CASE XVI.—RETENTION OF URINE—ONE ASPIRATION
(BY M. DE KIETER, OF ST. PETERSBURG).—In this case, of
which I have only the abstract, an old man suffered from
retention, due chiefly to hypertrophy of the prostate. Catheterization was not possible, and aspiration was performed.
The relief was immediate, and a sound could be introduced
into the bladder.

CASES XVII. AND XVIII. (Extracted from the *Dublin
Journal*).—The *Dublin Journal of Medical Science*
reports many cases of puncture of the bladder which
prove that M. Dieulafoy's aspirator can be made use of
with advantage and security in the treatment of retention
of urine.

A man having fallen from the height of about six
feet astride on to a plank, so bruised the perineum and
the anterior part of the abdomen, that on the day following the accident, a considerable extravasation of blood
occurred at the back of the scrotum. The abdomen was
painful and very sensitive to the touch, the skin hot, the
pulse 120. In spite of reiterated efforts, it was impossible for the patient to pass water after the accident, and the
distended bladder rose to within three fingers' breadth of
the umbilicus. Almost immediately after the accident
about a spoonful of blood was passed by the urethra.

Catheterization was attempted in vain, then a hot bath for a length of time, and finally incision of the perineum without any results. The necessity to empty the distended bladder was urgent ; the organ was punctured above the pubis with needle No. 1 of the aspirator. Four ounces of urine were drawn off ; care having been taken to push the needle farther as the bladder emptied itself. The puncture gave the patient no more suffering than that caused by piercing the skin. The operation was repeated many times at various intervals, and always with success. The patient succumbed to peritonitis, resulting from his fall. At the autopsy, on the external surface of the bladder small red ecchymoses were observed like gnat-bites on the skin, and corresponding to the points where the needle entered. The internal surface of the organ bore no trace of the punctures. The urine found in the bladder was normal, and contained neither blood, clots, nor pus.

An old man, æt. 65, whose prostate was hypertrophied, suffered from complete retention of urine. The efforts which he had made to pass water had succeeded only in causing pain, and leading to a loss of blood. After having fruitlessly tried catheterization for two days, needle No. 2 was introduced above the pubis, and sixteen ounces of urine drawn off. The relief was immediate. Two hours afterwards, a large sound was easily introduced, and all suffering disappeared. The patient was left to himself, and no accident resulted from the operation. (*Bordeaux Médicale,* Oct. 20th.)

CHAPTER III.

IF medicated and modifying fluids are not more frequently employed in chronic cystitis, catarrh, and other affections of the bladder, it is because the means at our disposal of managing these fluids are imperfect. It is rare that the syringes that are used in such circumstances are well constructed; they draw badly; the quantity of the fluid injected or withdrawn is not regulated; an assistant is needed to keep the injecting sound in the urethra; in short, the mode of operating is slow, inconvenient, and unpractical. The mucous membrane of the bladder would gain as much as the mucous membrane of other parts by a local treatment, provided always that care be taken to spare the urethra; that is to say, to avoid all contact between the mucous membrane of the urethra and the topical applications intended for the bladder.

For the insufficient means hitherto employed, I propose to substitute the simple and easy system of aspiration and injection which our new apparatus affords. For this end an aspiratory injector is selected, and the mode of operating is found to be extremely simple. A sound is introduced into the bladder, and put into communication with one of the tubes of the body of the pump, by means of a conical nipple, whilst the other tube is plunged into the medicated fluid. This nipple is intended to fit the aspirator with sounds of every size.

K

The action of the piston allows of the fluid being injected forcibly or gently. If we have to deal with cystitis

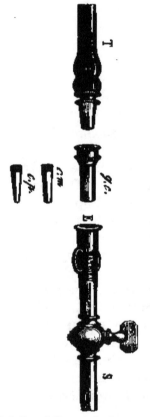

with purulent secretion, a force is given to the injection sufficient to penetrate into the anfractuosities of the bladder, and to wash out every part of it ; if, on the other hand, it is only wished to bring the mucous membrane into contact with a modifying liquid, it is injected slowly. The quantity of the fluid injected is known to within a few grammes, as the aspirator is mathematically graduated. The injected fluid can be left in contact with the mucous membrane as long as it is thought necessary, or it can be drawn off to the last drop without the mucous membrane of the urethra suffering the slightest injury. The facility with which this operation is performed, and the simplicity of the mode of operating, allow of the cleansing of the vesical cavity ; the injection may be effected every day, or twice in the twenty-four hours,

T, tube of the aspirator.
S, sound. gc, cp, intermediate
fittings.

if necessary. I believe that chronic inflammation of the mucous membrane would be rapidly ameliorated by the oft-repeated contact of a modifying fluid, such as a solution of sulphate of zinc, or of nitrate of silver, of graduated strength.

If a patient is attacked with vesical catarrh and stricture of the urethra, two affections which frequently coincide, the bladder is emptied incompletely and with difficulty, for the stricture interferes with the passage of the thick and muco-purulent portions of the urine. It is in such cases that the usefulness of my method will be recognized. It is only necessary to pass a sound, however minute its size, into the canal, and the bladder can be easily cleansed, and the situation of the patient quickly improved.

CHAPTER IV.

ARTICLE I.

THE cavity of the stomach can be reached by the natural
passage of the œsophagus, or by artificial passages, by
puncturing the organ through the abdominal walls at the
level of the epigastric fossa. It is to be remarked that
catheterization of the œsophagus has only been used till
now for treating the diseases of that tube, whilst it has
been singularly neglected in diseases of the stomach.
The cavity of this viscus is, however, as accessible to surgical means as the cavity of the bladder; catheterization of
the œsophagus is not more difficult to practise than that
of the urethra; and the mucous membrane of the stomach
is, like all mucous membranes when in a pathological
condition, susceptible of modification under the influence
of local treatment. But the reason that this mode of
therapeutics has not been employed before is because
the means at our service were insufficient. An operation
of this kind is delicate, the œsophagus must be treated
carefully, as its mucous membrane differs entirely from
that of the stomach, and does not bear the medicaments
destined for the latter without injury; it is also necessary
to exactly measure the injection intended for the stomach,
and it must be managed in such a way that its action can
be prolonged at will, or that it can be withdrawn to the
last drop when required. Owing to the apparatus which

we now possess, this is all quite easy to execute; the aspiratory injectors fulfil these ends, and the mode of operating is so simple and harmless, that henceforth it will be possible to intervene more usefully and directly in diseases of the stomach than has been done hitherto.

There are many applications of this method. For instance, if we have to deal with a chronic disease, such as ulcer, it seems to us that daily cleansing and injection of the cavity with appropriate fluids are clearly indicated. Instead of administering centigrammes of nitrate of silver in pills, would it not be preferable to apply it *loco dolenti* just like a collyrium, to allow it to remain for the time desired, neutralizing the ulterior effects by a saline injection? There would be analogous indications for gastrorrhagia. But one of the most practical and directly useful applications of this method is in the treatment of poisoning. The following interesting case, for which I am indebted to the kindness of Dr. Paul, confirms what I have stated, and shows the benefit to be derived from this new process.

POISONING OF AN INFANT, SIX HOURS AFTER BIRTH, BY A DESSERT-SPOONFUL OF LAUDANUM—THE EMPLOY-MENT OF M. DIEULAFOY'S ASPIRATORY APPARATUS— RECOVERY (BY DR. PAUL, OF DAUVILLE).—Last January I was staying at Bona, in Algeria, with a relative whose wife was about to be confined; her sister, Madame L——, who occupied the same rooms, was in the same condition. These two ladies were taken at the same time with the first pains, but Madame L——'s labour was short, and in an hour and a half she was delivered of a healthy girl. The infant was given to a friend to be washed and tended to, and I returned to Madame P——, whose labour was much slower. A very experienced midwife, Miss Mareschal, who was assisting, considered it desirable to give the little girl, five or six hours after birth, a small

dose of syrup of chicory. The lady who was taking care of
the infant undertook to administer it. In the darkness she
unfortunately mistook the phial, and gave, instead of the
syrup of chicory, a full dessert-spoonful of laudanum. The
father, entering the room at the same instant, perceived by
the odour the mistake that had been made. Terrified, he
rushed to tell me, and as the rooms were only separated
by one other, I was with the little patient immediately.
There was then no time to be lost. I found some syrup
and powder of ipecacuanha, which I administered directly,
but whether the dose was insufficient, or that poisonous
effects had already begun, ten minutes after ingestion there
was still no vomiting. I tried in vain to provoke it by
introducing my finger into the throat, by titillating the
uvula with a feather; nothing succeeded. I then concluded that the child was lost unless I could instantly
find some means of drawing off the poison from the
stomach. I could think of only one mechanical means to
give this result. I introduced an india-rubber sound by
the œsophagus, and to this first I adapted a second,
and by creating a vacuum with my mouth, I had the
satisfaction of finding that the tube was immersed
in the liquid contents of the stomach. I drew off thus
about a dessert-spoonful of the poison, and I injected by
the same means half a glass of lukewarm water, so as to
wash out what remained, and to render aspiration easier.
But matters proceeded slowly for such a pressing case.
The accident had occurred hardly more than forty minutes,
and the child was already in a state of coma, respiration
had fallen to ten inspirations a minute, and later on to
eight. The pupils were extremely contracted, the limbs
completely flaccid, and the head rolled on the shoulders as
if it was quite detached from the trunk.

In the presence of such rapid progress of the poisoning,
I endeavoured to draw out the fluids of the stomach as
quickly as possible by means of my mouth; whilst doing

this, in the midst of the trouble which the heartrending cries of the poor mother caused us, the despair of the lady who had made the fatal mistake, and the distress of the sister-in-law to whom they had been imprudent enough to tell the accident, I felt, nevertheless, that I had something at hand which would enable me to do better. But it is always thus when anxious to find something. I had thought of all the pumps, of all the instruments that I had in my box; nothing more practical or active occurred to me. At last, like a ray of light, I remembered Dieulafoy's aspirator; to fetch it and adjust the sound was the work of a minute. As we had a large coffee-pot of black coffee on the spot I used this excellent beverage to wash out the stomach. In the course of ten minutes I had performed injection and aspiration a dozen times, taking care to use fresh liquid every time. I ended by leaving a cupful of very strong black coffee, with which I had mixed a few drops of rum, in the stomach. We then passed to accessory means; mustard poultices were applied to every part of the body, a purgative injection followed by a coffee clyster, artificial respiration was kept up by alternate compression and dilatation of the ribs, then by electricity, &c. At the end of six hours the respiration became nearly normal, the muscles recovered their tonicity, the head ceased to roll on the shoulders, and the infant felt the pinches and slaps which from time to time we pitilessly administered, in spite of the distress of the young mother. Thirty-six hours after the accident the state became quite normal, with the exception of the contraction of the pupils, which persisted for three days, and the infant, whom we had hitherto had to sustain by teaspoonfuls of milk given from time to time, took the breast and got on pretty well. A few days afterwards a papulo-vesicular eruption came out over the body, but disappeared in a week, causing a slight epidermal desquamation. The infant is now a very pretty little girl, and an extreme nervousness is the only trace left of the accident. This was very marked the first week of the child's existence; the slightest noise or touch caused her to start and tremble in a manner really remarkable in so young an infant.

I hope that in a similar case the aspirator would be thought of immediately; for my part, I am convinced that it was by its use, and the promptitude with which it enabled me to act, that success was obtained in this case, on the gravity of which I have no need to insist.

ARTICLE II.

Mode of Operating.

This case shows all the benefit which may accrue from this proceeding. It is certainly not applicable to every case, but it may render us great services. It may be objected, perhaps, that it is often easier to procure an emetic than an aspirator; I reply that one does not interfere with the other, and that in poisoning one cannot take too many precautions to avert accidents. In such a case, the first thing is not to allow time for absorption to take place. Now, the action of an emetic is sometimes slow and often incomplete; aspiration, on the contrary, enables us to wash out the stomach, and in a few seconds to get rid of the poisonous substance to the last drop.

The mode of operating is very simple. Catheterization of the stomach is first performed, then an œsophageal sound is adapted to one of the tubes of the aspirator, and injection and aspiration of an appropriate fluid, according to the nature of the poison, are repeated many times. One circumstance, however, ought to be foreseen. Suppose that a medical man finds himself in the presence of a poisoned person, and that he has neither an emetic nor a sound wherewith to perform catheterization of the œsophagus at hand; he need not hesitate, but must pierce the stomach through the abdominal walls by means of the No. 1 aspiratory needle. To perform this operation, he must commence by ascertaining the limits of the cavity of the stomach by percussion at the level of the epigastric region, and having decided on the point at which the puncture is to be made, the patient should be made to drink two or three glasses of water, or some other beverage, so as to slightly distend the cavity of the stomach, and to facilitate the operation. The aspirator being prepared, that is to say, the vacuum being previously made, needle No. 1 is introduced at the spot indicated, to search for the liquid the patient has swallowed. Owing to the previous vacuum, it is known precisely when the stomach is penetrated, and there is no danger of piercing the organ through. Care must be taken to aspirate only a part of the liquid swallowed, in order to avoid the needle being pushed out by the walls of the cavity closing under the influence of the vacuum, and the washing of the cavity must be performed gradually, with a fluid varying according to the poison swallowed.

CHAPTER V.

MATERIALS are deficient for estimating the use and value of aspiration in the treatment of ovarian cysts. I only know of two cases, of which I give a summary without attempting to draw any conclusion from them.

CASE I.—UNILOCULAR OVARIAN CYST—ASPIRATION—RECOVERY (BY M. DUPLOUY).—I was consulted by a young girl, æt. 20, for an enormous ovarian cyst, which had attained such proportions that the patient was in a state of emaciation and dyspnœa approaching death.

Examination of the abdomen, palpation, and the sensation of fluctuation, which was equally perceived at all points, induced me to believe I had to deal with a unilocular cyst. I decided to evacuate the fluid of this cyst by aspiration, though the patient was in an almost desperate condition from excessive weakness and violent dyspnœa, vomiting being incessant.

The operation was performed June 23rd, 1871. At that time, the abdomen measured 1 metre 20 centimetres in circumference. I drew off 4 litres of fluid, though the size of the abdomen had led me to suppose that the cyst contained 8 or 10 litres. The fluid was very limpid, not albuminous, and contained an abundance of chloride of sodium.

After this operation, the health of the patient gradually improved, the circumference of the abdomen fell to 88 centimetres. Use was made of iodine paint and elastic compression, and three months later the patient left for Paris, in a very satisfactory state, without the fluid having been reproduced.

CASE II.—MULTILOCULAR OVARIAN CYST—FIFTEEN ASPIRATIONS—DEATH—(DIEULAFOY).—A young woman, æt. 23, came to consult me for a voluminous abdominal tumour. The examination of the region, the limited fluctuation perceived in places, the deep induration felt by palpation, led me to diagnose a multilocular ovarian cyst.

The tumour, the origin of which was dated two years back, had in the last three months attained such proportions that different functions were deranged by it. The patient could hardly walk, her digestion was bad, she breathed with difficulty, and felt at times acute pain in the abdomen.

I performed three aspiratory punctures at different points in the abdomen, and I felt that the needle penetrated into a hard and resisting tissue; I drew off three different kinds of fluid; one was rather limpid, and proceeded from a pouch situated in the left side of the abdomen, whilst two punctures on the right side gave issue to an extremely thick fluid, strongly coloured by a sanguineous exudation.

I advised the patient to have recourse to ovariotomy, but she rejected every idea of this kind, and asked for punctures, which afforded her a certain relief.

Fifteen aspirations were performed at different intervals for three months; but the abdominal tumour made rapid progress, and rose towards the epigastric fossa. The patient was seized with vomiting, and the rejected matters, being entirely analogous to those contained in the cyst, led me to suppose that perforation of the stomach had taken place. The patient succumbed three days later, with symptoms of peritonitis.

Remarks.—From these two cases, it is impossible to say what is to be the part played by aspiration in the treatment of ovarian cysts, but it may be argued *à priori* that this process would not have the same efficacy in multilocular as in unilocular cysts. The former, it seems to us, must be attacked by only one means, that is, by ovariotomy ; the latter might, on the contrary, be treated with advantage by successive and repeated aspirations, or by aspiration aided by injection after the method which I have described in the treatment of hydatid cysts of the liver.

CHAPTER VI.

The Treatment of Hydrocephalus by Aspiration.

ARTICLE I.

Hydrocephalus in the Infant.

I HAVE had occasion to perform aspiration on children attacked with hydrocephalus three times, and I have each time been unsuccessful: Dr. Jessop, of Leeds,* reports two cases equally unsuccessful. This seems to prove that in this disease aspiration, up to the present time, is not superior to other processes. I think, however, that we must not found a definite judgment on these five cases, for in the history of these little patients it will be seen that a very marked amelioration several times followed the first part of the treatment.

CASE I.—HYDROCEPHALUS—TWENTY-THREE ASPIRATIONS —DEATH (DIEULAFOY).—February 17, 1870, Dr. Blache proposed to me to perform aspiration on a child aged six months, who was attacked with hydrocephalus. Its head began to increase in size a few days after birth, and in a few months it had attained enormous proportions. The general condition was bad, the child was emaciated, often vomited, and was taken with convulsions at intervals. Death seemed imminent, and Dr. Blache and I resolved to perform aspiration.

* Illustrations of the Surgical Uses of the Aspirator, in the *British Medical Journal*, December, 1872.

The first puncture was made at the level of the anterior fontanel, outside the median line, so as to avoid the sinus. I made use of needle No. 1, and drew off only half the fluid (about 80 grammes), so as not to deprive the organs suddenly of the pressure to which they had become accustomed. No accident followed this operation, and a second aspiration, performed four days later, gave issue to 100 grammes of fluid. This fluid was as limpid and transparent as that of a hydatid cyst; it contained a slight quantity of albumen.

In consequence of these two operations the child sensibly improved, the convergent strabismus which formerly existed partly disappeared, the convulsions diminished in intensity and frequency, and the vomiting decreased. We took care to exactly measure the size of the head, which sensibly diminished; the bones, at first far apart, tended to approach one another, and we exercised a moderate compression on the cranium by means of thin bands of india-rubber.

Under the influence of this treatment, the child became somewhat fatter, but the fluid reproduced itself with such desperate obstinacy, that it became necessary to make two or three aspirations a week. The fluid always had the same appearance; it was sometimes a little coloured, and had a few drops of blood mixed with it. Twenty-three punctures were made nearly at the same spot, at the level of the anterior fontanel, to the right and left of the median line.

But the little patient was seized with broncho-pneumonia and succumbed. The autopsy was not made.

CASE II.—HYDROCEPHALUS (under the Care of M. Matice, at the Beaujon Hospital)—EIGHT ASPIRATIONS —DEATH (DIEULAFOY).—A child, aged eighteen months, came with its mother under the care of M. Matice. The mother stated that the child had good health till it was three months old. From this time the head began to increase in size, and on admission hydrocephalus was observed, which, according to the conformation of the head, seemed especially to have invaded the left ventricle of the brain. The child uttered hydrencephalic cries, and had convulsions many times a day.

I performed aspiration and drew off 50 grammes of fluid. The improvement was marked, and the convulsions disappeared immediately. The second aspiration was performed five days later, and I drew off 70 grammes of a limpid and transparent fluid, containing a very small proportion of albumen. But the improvement of the first few days did not continue long; the fluid was reproduced so rapidly that it became necessary to practise aspiration four times a week. The child was seized with fever and succumbed rapidly.

Case III.—Hydrocephalus—Ten Aspirations—Death (Dieulafoy).—Madame X—— came to beg me to see her child, who was suffering from hydrocephalus. I found a child who recalled the one spoken of by Pierre Franck, whose head measured 1 metre 30 centimetres in circumference. This one was not far from it, since the head of the child that I saw measured 1 metre 10 centimetres. The parents took the greatest care of the little patient. This phenomenal head, which filled the largest part of the cradle, was carefully guarded by many pillows, and it was only necessary to lightly touch the surface to set in movement a fluid, the waves of which could be seen through the integuments. I was convinced that it was useless to attempt the cure of such an affection, but, on the parents insisting, I consented to perform aspiration. The first puncture was made with needle No. 1, and I drew off 250 grammes of fluid; that was about one-fifth of the whole quantity. The child bore the operation perfectly, and was taking the breast whilst I aspirated the fluid. It was arranged that I should perform one aspiration a week, unless special circumstances counterindicated it. Eight days after I had begun aspiration, I was surprised to find, from measurement, that the size of the head tended to diminish. For two months the same course of treatment was followed ; each time I drew off 100 or 150 grammes of fluid, and the circumference of the head, which formerly measured 1 metre 15 centimetres, was then no more than 75 centimetres. At this time, without any appreciable cause, the fluid was reproduced with marked intensity, the child was taken with fever and convulsions, and succumbed in a few days.

CASE IV.—HYDROCEPHALUS—TWO ASPIRATIONS—DEATH (JESSOP).—On a child, aged five months, suffering from hydrocephalus, I performed one aspiration, on May 18th, 1871, by means of the finest needle, which I introduced into the anterior fontanel, and drew off six ounces of fluid ; and on the 22nd of the same month, twelve ounces. The child died on the 22nd, in convulsions.

CASE V.—HYDROCEPHALUS (JESSOP).—From a child aged three months, suffering from hydrocephalus, I drew off by aspiration, on the 22nd of July, 1871, five ounces of fluid ; on the 25th of the same month, three ounces ; on August 1st, one ounce and a half; and on different occasions I aspirated the same quantity of fluid.

Death occurred from convulsions, on September 13th. The autopsy was made in these two last cases to find out the effects of the introduction of the needle. No trace was found of it either in the meninges or in the cerebral substance.

These were the five cases in which aspiration was used ; the failure which was the result proves to us how little we can count on the curability of hydrocephalus. The opinion of M. Giraldès, which was true concerning simple capillary punctures, holds good also on treatment by aspiration. West, in 1842, says M. Giraldès, collected the cases of fifty patients on whom capillary punctures had been performed. Of these fifty, sixteen were successful. However, on examining these statistics closer, we find these sixteen successes reduced to four, and even one of these looks suspicious. Besides, another patient cited as cured, by West, succumbed after a short time.*

ARTICLE II.

Hydrocephalus in the Fœtus.—The Use of Aspiration.

If aspiration has given us hitherto no favourable result, in the treatment of hydrocephalus in the child, it can render us great services when we have to deal with hydrocephalus in the fœtus at the time of parturition. I quote the article on this subject by Dr. Hamon, which was published in the *Tribune Médicale*, Oct. 15th, 1871 :—

"When the fœtus is attacked with hydrocephalus, it would be well for the accoucheur to be able to recognize at once the true cause which opposes the descent of the head, so that his course should be defined. It is sufficient to give issue to a certain quantity of the fluid to diminish greatly the size of the organ, and thus to facilitate its descent. But it must be admitted that this diagnosis presents greater difficulties than the treatises set forth.

"Dr. Chassinat, of Hyères, has collected twenty-eight cases of hydrocephalus, of which twenty-one coincided with head presentations, and seven with breech presentations.

"In these twenty-eight cases, the accoucheur asserts that only in seventeen the disease was not recognized, but I

* Clinical Lessons on the Surgical Diseases of Children.

L

am convinced that this figure is much below the truth. As
far as concerns myself, in the only case which has come
under my observation, I never thought, notwithstanding
the difficulties of extraction, of the nature of the obstacle
which paralyzed all my efforts.   Many medical men whom
I have consulted on this subject, have made the same
avowal.   These errors of diagnosis are explained by the
rarity of these particular cases,—a rarity such as to render
the inattention of the accoucheur excusable.

"According to books, what are, then, the signs by means
of which hydrocephalus can be suspected or recognized ?
The finger meets a large and slightly convex flattened surface, according to some authors, which covers all the points
of the superior strait, without being caught in it.   This
surface is of various consistency in different parts of its
extent.   It is hard and resisting throughout during the
pains, but soft and fluctuating, on the contrary, in some
points during the intervals of contraction.   The soft and
membrane-like consistence of the bones may also be
ascertained, the largeness of the commissures, and the
fontanels.   Such signs are sufficient to at once explain
the position to adepts, but by the greater number of
practitioners we are fain to acknowledge that they are
less easily appreciated.   Their diagnosis is only really
made after the extraction of the child.

" When such an affection is suspected, there is a mode
of investigation which we owe to the progress of modern
science, one which may be applied without the least
danger and with the greatest advantage, I mean the
application of the long aspirator.   At the present time two
aspirators* are known, Dr. Dieulafoy's and mine.   In
using one or the other, it would suffice to plunge a trocar
needle as obliquely as possible, in order to avoid any
cerebral lesion, through the first accessible suture.   The

* This essay was written in 1871, and at that time many aspirators had already been proposed.   (Author's note.)

employment of these almost capillary needles would be without danger to the child, even if the point penetrated some distance into the superior part of the cerebral lobes.

" The suspected affection having been revealed by the operation of the instrument, this may now render a triple service. 1stly, It would enable the diagnosis to be cleared up ; 2ndly, it would facilitate delivery ; 3rdly, it would render the fœtus viable as *post-partum* experience proves, so far as concerns hydrocephalus of the second category.

" Now that some years' more practice has somewhat increased my experience, I should pursue another course than that which I followed in the subjoined case, and which my distinguished colleague, Dr. Phéllippeaux of St. Savinien also followed in the two cases which I borrow from him.

" If I found myself in the presence of a case of dystocia, shown by the inability of the forceps to grasp the head, a characteristic sign, I should soon suspect hydrocephalus. I should endeavour to ascertain some of the signs which characterize it—softness, want of resistance of the bones, abnormal size of the sutures and the fontanels. These objective signs once ascertained, I should not hesitate to take my long aspirator to practise an exploratory puncture. If such a method had been employed by my skilful colleague and myself, it is beyond doubt that we should have been spared in any case very painful efforts, and that we should at the same time have avoided all possible dangers resulting from forcible manœuvres for the extraction of a head of disproportionate size."

CHAPTER VII.

WE possess only two reports of cases of spina-bifida treated by aspiration ; the one is due to Dr. Camara da Cabral, of Lisbon, the other was forwarded to me from Dr. Rasmussen, of Copenhagen.

In both cases cure was obtained ; in the first patient, by simple aspiration, and in the second by aspiration with iodized injections.

CASE I.—CONGENITAL SPINA-BIFIDA—HYDROMENINGO-CELE—CURE BY EVACUATION OF THE FLUID BY M. DIEULAFOY'S ASPIRATOR.—Communication made to the Society of the Medical Sciences of Lisbon at a meeting on February 17th, 1872, by Dr. Camara da Cabral.

On November 21st, 1872, a female child was brought to me at St. Joseph's Hospital, æt. 25 days, born in Bareiro, and living in the same city.

My opinion was asked as to the nature and treatment of a tumour which originated in the lumbo-sacral region. The mother informed me that, after a normal pregnancy, she gave birth to a child bearing on the lower part of the lumbar region, in the median line, a tumour the size of a nut, which had grown to its present size. The tumour was large, oblong, its long diameter corresponding to that of the vertical column, its circumference 40 centimetres, its largest diameter 17 centimetres, and its smallest only 10. The tumour blended insensibly with the neighbouring surfaces; a slight constriction, however, resembling a pedicle, was observed near the base. The skin was shining, and presented a multitude of vascular arborisations without any depression. The great distention of the skin rendered the tumour more than ordinarily transparent; fluctuation was very distinct, and compression gave pain, which made the child cry so that it was not easy to ascertain whether the tumour. was reducible, and whether there was any reflux of the fluid into the hollow of the bony shell. When the finger was placed on the anterior fontanel a wave of liquid was felt; but the cause of this motion was not easily recognized. Was it due to the compression of the tumour or to the crying of the child?

By pressure on the tumour, the existence of another tumour, deeply attached, was easily perceived. It was somewhat resisting, and had in its upper part a portion which was easily depressible. The finger, in penetrating, was surrounded by a ring of fibrous consistence. The tension of the contained liquid rendered the examination imperfect and prevented the investigation of the state of the vertebral arches. The diagnosis given was spina-bifida.

This diagnosis was confirmed by the discovery of the existence of a deformity which generally accompanies spina-bifida. The child had varus of the right foot. It was necessary, for the purpose of treatment, to discover what anatomical variety this tumour belonged to.

The child had never had convulsions, pressure did not provoke them, and there was no paralysis. These characteristics, and the good general condition, led us to conclude that the tumour was a hydromeningocele.

The examination of the cranium showed a perfect state of developement, and we decided that the radical cure might be attempted without fear of seeing the terrible complication of hydrocephalus arise. As to the therapeutical means to be employed, that was a question to be decided; the most urgent thing was the extraction of the fluid, for it was feared the skin would break. This was the opinion of Professors Barbosa, Abel Jordas, and Silva Amado ; but the relatives of the child, in face of the prognosis, deferred the operation, and did not return to me till November 29th to ask for surgical interference. Aided by MM. Alvez, Branco, Arnaut, and Agostinho das Silva, I thrust Dieulafoy's trocar into the interior and posterior part of the tumour. All the fluid, that is 400 grammes, was drawn off.

During the operation I remarked that the canula met with no lateral resistance, but in the anterior part it was arrested by the tumour, which had been observed by palpation. This second tumour was caused by the spinal aponeurosis which had been displaced.

After having given all the fluid exit,* and having ascertained the want of median union of the arches of the fourth and fifth lumbar vertebræ, we applied strips of adhesive plaster to keep the internal walls of the tumour in contact.

The child went home without any accident having occurred. Six days afterwards, on the 5th of December, she was brought to me again ; the fluid had formed afresh, and the skin had become thicker from contraction.

The first operation had caused vomiting, which disappeared without active treatment. These good results determined us to continue the treatment of aspiration. With the assistance of MM. Alvez, Branco, Ferraz de Macedo, and Clemente dos Santos, I drew out by means of

---

* The fluid was clear and transparent, and gave an albuminous precipitate with nitric acid. This fact made me hesitate for a moment as to my diagnosis, remembering that, according to the most recent analyses, the cephalo-rachidian fluid contains no albumen. But I had seen, a short time before, an albuminous precipitate thrown down in the fluid taken from a hydrocephalitic patient who was under the care of M. Branco at the hospital.

aspiration all the fluid (250 grammes) that the tumour contained : it presented the same characteristics as the first.

As the plaster had produced excoriations, we abandoned its use and filled up with cotton-wool the anfractuosities which the skin presented after the emptying of the tumour. December 14th a third aspiration was performed. The fluid had been reproduced in greater quantity, and the tumour was of its original size. Aspiration gave exit to 425 grammes of a slightly turbid fluid. Six days afterwards, on the 20th, I thought it advisable to prevent the tissues being again distended, to draw out the fluid reproduced, which was only 250 grammes, and analogous in appearance to that aspirated the last time. The same dressing. For the first five days following this operation the fluid did not reform, but it soon began to increase till December 30th, when, with the assistance of M. Babreto Perdigao, I drew off 175 grammes of fluid. The general condition was good ; the same dressing. The child returned to Bareiro. Thirteen days afterwards, on the 12th of January of the following year, aspiration of the fluid, which was reduced to 125 grammes, was performed for the sixth time. In this operation, in which I was assisted by M. Bento de Sousa, I thrust the trocar further through the spinal aponeurosis, and penetrated in consequence into the diverticulum of the watery hernia guarded by this membrane.

It is easily understood that this last time, aspiration resulted in establishing a more perfect contact between all the points of the serous surfaces. The same dressing was applied.

Thirty-five days after the sixth and last operation, the fluid had not been reproduced, and the child's health was pretty good ; all the functions were performed regularly. Instead of the voluminous tumour which occupied the lumbo-sacral region, the skin was found at the level of the fifth and sixth lumbar apophyses, of an almost normal colour, and raised by a tumour about the size of a nut. This deeply-seated tumour contained no fluid, and was not as hard as a purely fibrous tumour.

Such was the communication which I had the honour to make to the Society of Medical Sciences. I had the child examined by the Associates, and I had the satisfaction of not being contradicted as to the reality of the cure. My readers will allow me to make two reflections on the subject of this case. Taking my stand upon the rigorous examination of the symptoms, I do not think I deceived myself as to the diagnosis of the disease ; and I think the cure which I obtained was not the result of chance. The therapeutic method employed was rational, and I feel disposed to repeat it under similar conditions. The time is already past when children who came into the world with a spina-bifida were considered not viable. The observation of certain cases of spontaneous cure has caused this erroneous belief to disappear, and since then other methods and processes of cure have appeared. We are persuaded that there is no general method for a disease which presents such distinct anatomical varieties, from the simple tumour with a well-marked pedicle, easily isolated, to a veritable deformity against which therapeutics are powerless.

In the case which I have been considering, it seems to me that, after the result of the first puncture, it was right to continue the punctures, modified as they were by the improvements which our surgical arsenal now places at our disposal. Not having discovered on the tumour any portion of the spinal axis, the best proceeding was to destroy the serous cavity of the tumour by the adhesion of its walls.

After the first aspiration there was an inflammatory process, which was rendered apparent by the general condition of the child ; after the second, a certain turbidity of the fluid ; and after the last aspiration, the adhesion of the surfaces took place.

I do not propose to revive an old process which has been condemned by the majority of pathologists, on account of it always producing bad results, and causing suppurations which rapidly spread to the meninges ; but the punctures made with Dieulafoy's instrument do not cause these troubles, and they have, moreover, the advantage of determining an inflammatory process by the congestion which must necessarily follow a powerful aspiration of fluid ; this proceeding also favours adhesions by the forced contact of the internal surfaces of the tumour.

Thus is explained the superiority of this process over iodine injections, which, first performed by a Chicago surgeon, won the applause of many of the most distinguished surgeons of Europe.

Iodine injections are as inconvenient as other methods ; they often cause rachidian meningitis, in spite of all the precautions taken to close the orifice that connects the cavity of the tumour with the rachidian cavity. To sum up, it seems to me that when hydromeningocele can be diagnosed in such a condition as science admits to be susceptible of treatment, the best thing to do is to undertake the complete aspiration of the fluid as often as the case will allow.

Almost three months have elapsed since the last operation, so we can rest assured that the cure is definitive. The child is strong and well, the solid tumour continues to atrophy, and is reduced to a very small size.

CASE II.—SPINA-BIFIDA—EIGHT ASPIRATIONS—IODINE INJECTIONS—CURE.—I owe the report of this case to the kindness of Dr. Rasmussen, of Copenhagen.

O. C——, æt. one month, came under my care on March 4th, 1871, with her mother. The infant was puny,

and on the lumbo-dorsal region there was a spherical tumour, not so large as an orange ; the diameter at the base
was 8 centimetres.   Across the walls of the tumour white
striæ were perceived, and on the top a superficial ulceration,
about the size of a two-franc piece, was found.   To the
touch, the tumour was fluctuating, and did not seem
compressible ; pressure did not produce any marked
change.   No incontinence of urine or of fæcal matter,
but the movements of the lower limbs were almost
annulled.

March 5th.—The first aspiration.   The trocar was
introduced at the base of the tumour, at a spot where the
skin was normal, and 50 grammes of a quite limpid fluid
were drawn off.   The tumour decreased, and it was then
possible to perceive the separation of vertebral laminæ ;
compression was applied by means of cotton-wool and a
circular bandage.

March 7th.—The tumour had resumed its former
size.   On the 9th I performed aspiration, and drew
off 30 grammes of a fluid looking like the first ; at
the same time I injected a solution of iodine, one part
in a thousand ; the injection was withdrawn after three
minutes.

March 11th.—The tumour had decidedly diminished.
I performed aspiration, and drew off 10 grammes of a
limpid fluid ; it was replaced by an iodine injection, which
was aspirated after a few minutes.

March 13th.—The child was doing well ; the tumour
was not much increased in size.

The aspirations were repeated on the 16th, 22nd,
26th, and each time only a few grammes were found.
On the 18th feeble movements of the feet were observed
for the first time.

On the 4th of April the child left the hospital, and in
the place of the tumour only a thickening of the integu-

ments was observed, which scarcely allowed of the state of the vertebræ being ascertained.

The mother has brought me the child since, and the last time on September 15th, 1872 : she was then as well developed as children of her age ; she did not yet walk, but the movements of the feet and legs were normal.

CHAPTER VIII.

THE TREATMENT OF STRANGULATED HERNIA BY ASPIRATION

Summary:—Article I. History, Origin, and Application of the Method.—Article II.: Harmlessness of Aspiration in Strangulated Hernia.—Article III.: The Use and Value of Aspiratory Punctures in the Treatment of Strangulated Hernia.—Article IV.: The Opportuneness of Aspiration.—New Applications of Taxis.—Article V.: The Mode of Operating.—Articles VI., VII., VIII.: Cases.

ARTICLE I.

History.—Origin and Application of the Method.

THE nature of our labours on aspiration has led us to enlarge the circle of the operations called medical, and to encroach on surgical ground, in order to place the treatment of all pathological fluids on the same footing.

Certain operations which were some years ago the exclusive appanage of the surgeon, have become by their extreme simplicity the property of all medical men : puncture of the bladder in retention of urine, the extraction of effusions of the joints, are now as easy to perform as aspiration of the fluid of pericarditis or pleurisy ; and even strangulated hernia can be reduced by this new process by the hands of a medical man the least versed in the arts of surgery. At the same time, aspiration applied to the treatment of strangulated hernia is a more complicated operation than simple puncture of the chest. It is thus well to study it in every detail, to establish its

indications and contra-indications, to discuss its opportuneness, its advantages and inconveniences; in fact, to
simplify and popularize the use of a method which renders
us real services.

The application of aspiration to strangulated hernia is
of recent date. I believe I was the first to indicate this
process as a means of reducing strangulated hernia. This
is pointed out in the inaugural theses of MM. Autun,[*]
Lecerf,[†] Brun-Buisson;[‡] and recently M. Dubreuil, at one
of the meetings of the Surgical Society,[§] did me the
honour of attributing to me the initiative of this operation.
When I brought the aspirator and aspiration before the
Academy of Medicine (at the meeting of November 2nd,
1869), I took care to point out that this method, with
its many applications, "was destined to expel the gases,
which accumulate in such quantities in intestinal occlusion, and which become, under other circumstances, one
of the obstacles to the reduction of certain herniæ."

I therefore advise that strangulated hernia should be
aspirated by means of a needle armed with a previous
vacuum, being convinced that the liquids and gas accumulated in the hernial loop are most frequently the sole
cause that prevent reduction. This plan of puncturing
the intestine is not absolutely new, for in the year 1612,
Pingray spoke of it in his "Epitome Præceptorum Medic.
Chirurgiæ."[||] Mérat relates how A. Paré often found the

* The Treatment of Strangulated Hernia by Aspiration, by
M. Autun. (Thèse de Doctorat, Paris, 1871.)
† The Treatment of Strangulated Hernia, by M. Lecerf. (Thèse
de Doctorat, Paris, 1872.)
‡ The Treatment of Strangulated Hernia by Aspiration. (Thèse
de Paris, Brun-Buisson, 1872.)
§ *Gazette des Hôpitaux*, No. 93, 1872.
|| "Si vero intestinum vento valde inflatum ac refer um esset
uniusque duntaxat flatus impediret quo minus reponi posset, *acu-
pungendum* tunc esset ut flatui via pateret idque citrà periculum."
(Chapter on the Treatment of Strangulated Herniæ.)

good results of an intestinal puncture made by means of a needle. Pierre Low, Garengeot, Sharp, Van Swieten, have had the same idea ; and, more recently, M. Giraldès has spoken of the puncture of the sac first, and afterwards of the intestine, to facilitate reduction, and many surgeons in difficult cases have punctured the intestine when laid bare, and have not had to regret it.

But such a practice had, on the whole, very little value, as it was nowhere general, and was not recommended in any classical work. This operation, of which a vague idea was entertained at various times, but which had not been studied and established, remained, like so many others, a matter of theory or surmise, because the means of execution were wanting, and the plan of plunging a trocar into the middle of a hernial tumour was so little adopted, that M. Nélaton formally rejected it in the following dilemma :—" One of two things : either the opening is very small, and nothing will come out, or it is very large, and the patient is exposed after reduction to an effusion into the abdominal cavity." These words, which condemn the puncture of the intestine, are a sufficient reply to those who pretend that the aspirator was known before my presentation to the Academy. They, moreover, prove that a gap, of which surgeons were conscious, but which they had not filled up, then existed in surgery, and that they often came near to aspiration without discovering it.

The use of the capillary trocar in the treatment of strangulated hernia was then energetically rejected, for its inconvenience and uselessness were understood, whilst aspiration, such as we proposed it, had a new and practical character ; it placed a needle armed with a previous vacuum at our service, it enabled us to slowly traverse the tissues with every chance of success, and to draw out, under cover, by a puncture as fine as that of the exploratory trocar, all that the needle met in its passage—the fluids of the sac, and the fluids and gas of the intestine. I only spoke then from induction, I did not cite my experiments practised on animals, which seemed valueless to me, but I waited for pathological facts which could not be slow to establish the reasonableness of the ideas which I put forth.

In fact, M. Duplouy (of Rochefort) and M. Dolbeau each published a decisive case followed by success. This was the best reply to give to objections that were raised. From that time the harmlessness of the operation was established, and the reduction of hernia by aspiration became an established and demonstrated fact. The patient of M. Duplouy was an old man, æt. 82, suffering from inguinal strangulated hernia. After many fruitless attempts at taxis, aspiration was performed, the hernia was reduced, and the patient was rapidly cured. The operation was performed August 3rd, 1870, at the Rochefort Hospital, and I received a letter from M. Duplouy on the subject; but the case was not published till July 7th, 1871, that is, three months after M. Dolbeau's communication to the Surgical Society, at the meeting of April 5th, 1871. In this communication, so interesting on diverse grounds, M. Dolbeau, who was ignorant of the still unpublished case of M. Duplouy, spoke of a patient under his care in the Beaujon Hospital who had been operated on by aspiration, and he asked for the general adoption of this method in strangulated hernia. I record these facts and dates in detail, and with scrupulous exactness, in order to treat the historic side of this question with complete impartiality.

Since that time numerous cases have been published, but though the path is traced, there is much vagueness and indecision about this new operation, the various stages for it are not exactly defined, and I wish to profit by the abundant materials which we already possess, to establish the state of the question in a more certain manner. This study will embrace three principal questions :—

1st. Is the aspiratory puncture of the intestine in strangulated hernia harmless ? Is it not of a nature to provoke accidents or to compromise the success of other curative, ulterior means, and what is its value as a therapeutical process ?

2nd. In what case and at what time may aspiration be performed in strangulated hernia ?

3rd. What is the mode of operating ?

These are the questions to which we shall have successively to reply.

ARTICLE II.

Of the Harmlessness of Puncture and of Aspiration in Strangulated Hernia.

Is puncture of the hernial intestine harmless, hurtful, or dangerous ? This is too important a question not to claim lengthened discussion, as the answer to it would alone be sufficient to determine the acceptance or rejection of the operation. It is evident that if we could with impunity attempt the reduction of hernia by aspiration, without inducing consecutive accidents, without prejudicing taxis, or without compromising the results of kelotomy, aspiration would of necessity become the most simple and direct auxiliary in strangulated hernia. Taxis would no longer be performed without preliminary aspiration, for it must be evident to all, that it is more easy to reduce an empty flaccid intestinal loop than a tumour distended by fluids and gases. But if the puncture of the hernial sac bring on consecutive ulcerations, if it induce peritoneal accidents, if it expose us to the chance of reducing a perforated intestine ; or, if it be but an inefficacious method of reduction, I see no need for substituting this procedure for those already at the service of surgery. We ought therefore to discuss this question without allowing ourselves to be influenced by the attraction of novelty, but also without leaning to the traditions of the past.

Theories are but of slight assistance in matters such as these ; the physiological experiments which I have tried have not afforded any satisfactory result, for it is not possible to reproduce in animals a strangulated hernia, with all its concomitant conditions. It is, therefore, necessary to keep to the examination of pathological facts ; and from the analyses of these facts, conclusions will be obtained.

I have collected notes of thirty cases of strangulated hernia treated by aspiration, but three of these cases are not suitable to take their place in our table of statistics, since puncture of the sac alone was made, and not puncture of the intestine, so that our cases are reduced to twenty-seven. To facilitate our inquiry, I divide these into three categories.

In the first category are included herniæ which have resisted taxis, and been cured by aspiration alone, without the aid of kelotomy.

In the second category are placed the herniæ for which aspiration has not proved sufficient, but which have been cured by kelotomy subsequently performed.

In the third category are placed the unsuccessful cases of the patients who succumbed to the accidents following kelotomy, aspiration not having been sufficient to induce reduction.

The examination of these twenty-seven cases will furnish us with the elements necessary for forming an opinion as to the innocuousness of aspiration in strangulated hernia.

M

FIRST CATEGORY.

STRANGULATED HERNIÆ WHICH RESISTED TAXIS AND WERE REDUCED BY ASPIRATION.

Cases.	Operators.	Nature of the Disease.	Accidents due to Aspiration.	Result.
I	Duplouy.	Man aged 82. Right inguinal hernia strangulated for four days. Taxis attempted several times without result. Aspiration with needle No. 2. Reduction.	None.	Cure.
II.	Dolbeau.*	Inguinal hernia, strangulated for five days. Aspiration.	—	Reduction.
III.	Dolbeau.	Crural hernia in an old woman. This hernia was primarily strangulated. Aspiration and reduction. Some months later, fresh strangulation. Aspiration and reduction. Finally, a third strangulation, and aspiration performed with equal success.	—	Cure.
IV.	Duplouy.	Strangulated hernia in a young man. Failure of taxis. Aspiration with needle No. 2.	—	—
V.	Cazin.	Strangulated hernia. Failure of taxis. Aspiration.	—	—
VI.	Dieulafoy.	Strangulated umbilical hernia in a woman, aged 50. Five aspirations.	—	—
VII.	Demarquay.	Congenital left inguinal hernia. Inefficacy of taxis with chloroformization. Exhaustion with needle No. 1.	—	—

* This case deserves to be included in this group, for though the patient succumbed to a cardiac affection and asystolism, the hernia was reduced, and the effects of strangulation had disappeared.

Cases.	Operators.	Nature of the Disease.	Accidents due to Aspiration.	Result.
VIII.	Chauveau.	Inguinal hernia in a man of 49. Many fruitless efforts at taxis. Aspiration with No. 2 needle. Reduction.	None.	Cure.
IX.	Chauveau.	Right inguinal hernia in a woman of 75. Two aspirations with No. 2 needle.	—	—
X.	L. Labbé.	Strangulated hernia.	—	—
XI.	Walcher.	Right crural hernia in a woman aged 40. Several useless attempts at taxis. Aspiration and reduction with needle No. 2.	—	—
XII.	Ménard.	Inguinal strangulated hernia in an adult. Repeated attempts at taxis without any results. Aspiration and reduction.	—	—
XIII.	Le Bêle.	Left inguinal hernia. Unsuccessful taxis. One aspiration.	—	—
XIV.	Le Bêle.	Right inguinal hernia. Aspiration.	—	—
XV.	Ollivier.	Strangulated umbilical hernia. One aspiration.	—	—
XVI.	Létiévant.	Inguinal hernia. Efforts at taxis. One aspiration.	—	—
XVII.	Dieulafoy.	Right inguinal hernia. One aspiration.	—	—
XVIII.	Bailly.	Strangulated crural hernia. Aspiration of the uncovered intestine.	—	—
XIX.	Kieter.	Inguinal hernia. Aspiration.	—	—
XX.	Maury.	Strangulated hernia. Aspiration.	—	—

SECOND CATEGORY.

HERNIÆ IN WHICH ASPIRATION WAS INSUFFICIENT. KELOTOMY AND CURE.

Cases.	Operators.	Nature of the Case.	Accidents due to Aspiration.	Result.
I.	Bourdy and Dugué.	Strangulated left inguinal hernia. Two aspirations. No reduction.	None.	Kelotomy and Cure.
II.	Richet.	Left crural hernia. Two aspirations. No reduction.	—	—
III.	Verneuil.	Inguinal hernia. One aspiration of the fluid in the sac; two aspirations in the intestine. No reduction.	—	—
IV.	Terrier.	Left inguinal hernia. Aspiration. No reduction.	—	—

THIRD CATEGORY.

HERNIÆ IN WHICH ASPIRATION WAS INSUFFICIENT. KELOTOMY AND DEATH.

Cases.	Operators.	Nature of the Case.	Accidents due to Aspiration.	Result.
I.	Demarquay.	Crural hernia. Kelotomy; puncture of the exposed intestine.	None.	Death.
II.	Folet.	Inguinal hernia. Aspiration without reduction. Kelotomy.	—	—
III.	Létiévant.	Strangulated hernia. Aspiration; kelotomy.	—	—

In addition to these three categories, we possess three cases which cannot be included in our statistics, since the operation on the sac only was performed, and they do not come within the scope of the method we propose. We here give the summary of these cases, which will be found further on in detail. M. Panas made two attempts at aspiration in strangulated hernia, the one on a woman with crural hernia, in which only the fluid in the sac was removed, the ulcerated intestine was reduced, and the woman died. In the other case the patient was a man with scrotal hernia; the fluid in the sac only was removed, kelotomy became necessary, and the patient died from the results of the operation. M. Fleury reports a series of notes on a case in which several aspirations were performed on a patient who suffered from a large inguinal hernia, irreducible for four days, without being strangulated. Vomiting supervened twice, causing apprehension lest symptoms of strangulation should appear; the patient, tired out by the inefficacy of the treatment, left the hospital. If we examine the twenty-seven cases collected in our three categories, in relation to the innocuousness of aspiratory puncture, we shall not find the slightest misadventure to lay to the charge of the intestinal puncture. Whether the intestine had or had not been reduced, the operators declare that aspiration was always perfectly harmless, and the same conclusion is formulated in the treatises of MM. Autun, Lecerf, and Brun-Buisson. The twenty patients whose cases are recorded in the first category were cured by the help of aspiration alone. Kelotomy became necessary for the four patients in the second category, and the resulting cures proved that the intestinal puncture previously made was perfectly harmless, and in no way endangered the success of the operation. Yet, in the case of M. Verneuil's patient, the intestine was thrice perforated (Case III.); in that of M. Richet (Case II.), the traces of erosion were still visible, but the

punctures were so small, and the little wound made by
the needle was so quickly obliterated, that M. Bourdy
found no trace of it when he performed kelotomy.   M.
Dolbeau's case (Case II.), was also very conclusive, for the
intestinal loop, which had been reduced, and which had
received the punctures, was placed under water and underwent insufflation without giving out the smallest bubble
of air.   The three cases in the third category come under
the head of strangulated hernia, operated on by kelotomy,
and owe their gravity to the consequences of the operation ;
but aspiration is in no way concerned in these accidents.
M. Folet specially insists on the harmlessness of the
intestinal puncture and on the integrity of the intestine,
of which a minute examination was made at the autopsy.
In our twenty-seven notes of cases, therefore, it is not
possible to find a single accident which can be ascribed to
aspiratory puncture, and its harmlessness appears to us
to be definitely demonstrated.

However, M. Fleury records the following case in which
he throws doubts on its harmlessness :—

Several aspirations were performed in a case of hernia
which was only irreducible, and not at all strangulated.
Nothing came away by the needles ; the tumour retained
its size, it became painful, and two attacks of vomiting
supervened.   Now, what does this prove ?   That, without doubt, there was nothing to exhaust in that hernia,
which was only irreducible.   I do not assert that the
manipulation (no doubt complicated with taxis) brought
on the two attacks of vomiting, but, on the other
hand, I see no sufficient reason to ascribe them to the
puncture.   What is certain is, that out of twenty-
seven patients, whose intestine was punctured by the
aspiratory needle, we only have to record in the way of
unpleasant accidents two attacks of vomiting, without
further results, and that in a case where there was specially
no question of strangulation.

Conclusion.—The aspiratory puncture of an intestinal hernial loop, performed by means of the needles No. 1 and No. 2, is completely innocuous. The method may sometimes have proved inefficacious or insufficient, but it has always been harmless.

ARTICLE III.

Of the part played by Aspiratory Puncture in the Treatment of Strangulated Hernia, and of its Value.

The cases which I have collected, and of which I have already spoken, may be summed up as follows : in twenty-seven cases of strangulated hernia not reducible by the other methods, the twenty ranged in the first category have, thanks to aspiration, been reduced without difficulty, whilst attempts at taxis, several times repeated with the aid of chloroform, and performed under the most favourable conditions, had completely failed. In these twenty patients, kelotomy would have been inevitable, if the aspiration of the fluids and the gaseous matters had not afforded means of replacing the difficult and formidable operation by the knife, by a simple puncture.

The reduction of these herniæ was accomplished without any consecutive accidents, and without the least symptoms of peritonitis, and the vomiting was immediately stopped. The intestine resumed its functions, the cure was immediate, notwithstanding that in several of these patients, the conditions were very unfavourable to a successful termination.

One was an old man, aged 82, whose hernia had been strangulated for four days (Duplouy's case). Another was suffering from a congenital inguinal hernia (Demarquay's case), an extremely serious case, since M. Demarquay does not remember having operated with success on a single case of congenital hernia. The patient referred to in Case III. (Dolbeau) showed on three different occasions symptoms of strangulation, and the accidents were thrice averted.

In the woman referred to in Case VI. (Dieulafoy), an umbilical hernia of enormous bulk had to be dealt with. The consequences of the operation were, in every instance, so simple that these twenty patients passed, without transition, from the most serious state to complete cure.

To appreciate the application of aspiration at its just value, it must be taken into consideration that, in most of these cases, taxis had been repeated on different occasions, and by different surgeons, without any result. In Case VII. (Demarquay), taxis had been tried on three different occasions by three surgeons, chloroform had been administered to the patient, and the strangulated hernia had resisted all these means, whilst after aspiration it was reduced without the least effort.

In Case II. (Duplouy), three persons had essayed taxis several times in succession with absolute failure. Aspiration was resorted to, and thenceforward, says the surgeon who records the case, the reduction of the hernia " was nothing but child's play."

In Case XII. (Ménard), we see that seven or eight attempts at taxis were made without any result, when, by the aid of aspiration, reduction was effected without difficulty.

I could accumulate examples, but what I desire to bring into prominence is, that the intervention of aspiration has nothing deceptive about it. It has not been applied to herniæ easily reducible ; on the contrary, we see that it has only been employed as a last resource, and under the least favourable conditions, to the reduction of strangulated hernia of several days' duration, and on patients exhausted by repeated attempts at taxis. Yet, notwithstanding these conditions, so adverse to successful results, aspiration has overcome the strangulation, without difficulty, and without bringing on any accident.

We therefore foresee a great success for this method, when the time arrives for its being employed in a methodical manner.

These facts furthermore prove to us that the presence of the liquids and the gases which distend the intestine, is almost always the true obstacle to the reduction of strangulated hernia ; therefore aspiration is the most rational of all the processes, since it removes the cause, and removes it in a perfectly harmless way.

We will now examine the notes collected in the second category. They relate to four cases. Aspiration was, in the first instance, attempted with these patients, but the issue of gaseous and fluid matter was not sufficient to allow the reduction of the intestine, as other causes of irreducibility existed, such as adhesions (Bourdy and Dugué's case).

The patients, however, recovered after having undergone kelotomy, and the aspiratory puncture in no way jeopardized the result of the operation. With regard to those observations which relate only to the puncture and to the aspiration of the sac, and not to the aspiration of the intestine, they form no part of our statistics. If I mention them here, it is to show the inefficacy of punctures of the sac, and on this subject we cannot do better than repeat the words of M. Dubreuil :—

" These operations prove nothing against the operation proposed by M. Dieulafoy."

We have, therefore, to consider twenty-seven notes of cases, which may be grouped as follows :—

Strangulated herniæ treated by aspiration . 27
Complete success 20
Semi-success 4
Failure 3

This table gives us an average of 85 per cent. of cures in the treatment of strangulated hernia by aspiration, whilst the statistics of hernia operated on by kelotomy, before the discovery of aspiration, only gave 50 per cent. of cures.[*] Thus the difference in favour of aspiration is

[*] Treatise by M. Brun-Buisson, p. 5.

35 per cent.   In other words, out of ten patients suffering from strangulated hernia irreducible by taxis, five were cured ; whilst, at the present time, thanks to the new method, from eight to nine are cured.   Such are the conclusions forced on us by the examination of the facts.

ARTICLE IV.

On the Proper Time for Aspiration in Strangulated Hernia.—New Indication for Taxis.

In what cases and at what moment ought aspiration to be performed in strangulated hernia ?

The accumulation of liquids and gases in the hernial sac being one of the principal obstacles to the reduction of strangulated hernia, the most favourable type for reduction by aspiration would be an enterocele without epiplocele, recently strangulated and free from adhesion.   The nearer the hernia approaches this type, the more chance of success aspiration will have.   But, if the enterocele is complicated with epiplocele, if the strangulation is already of long standing, if the intestinal coats are increased in size, if adhesions exist between the intestine and the sac, which is rare, or between the sac and the ring, which is more frequent, the conditions requisite for reduction by aspiration become less favourable.   Thus, at the first view, the question of treatment would appear to be subordinated to a question of diagnosis, but how is it possible to obtain exact ideas on the anatomical details we have just enumerated ?   The dulness or the resonance of the tumour are very delusive signs ; the dulness due to dropsy of the sac may simulate an epiplocele, whilst the presence of some gases, notwithstanding the predominance of the epiploon, may give rise to the supposition that an enterocele exists.

We shall, therefore, sometimes be exposed to the risk of inserting the needle rather on chance, without knowing with exactness the composition or the state of the tumour; but that is of small moment, since we know that the puncture is *per se* harmless. The worst which can happen is, that the aspiration should not be sufficient; as in the four cases of the second category, but it will not be injurious. If we are thus dogmatic it is because we speak from facts, and not from theories. It cannot be alleged that this harmlessness is due to special skill or special manipulation, since twenty different operators have arrived at the same results. It cannot either be asserted that the success of the method may be imputed to a choice of particularly suitable cases, since amongst the number tabulated we find herniæ of all kinds, umbilical, crural, inguinal, scrotal, and complicated with strangulations, varying from three to five days' duration. Still, we have established the fact that the puncture of the strangulated intestine is, I will not say of an absolute harmlessness, since nothing is absolute in surgery, but so harmless that it may be performed without fear and without danger. The question of seasonableness, therefore, appears to us to be stated in one proposition, and we say aspiration ought to be attempted in all cases of strangulated hernia, whatever they may be, with one exception only; that is, when the case is of a strangulation of sufficiently ancient date to give rise to apprehensions of gangrene or intestinal ulcerations.

Another question presents itself. Should aspiration be performed before or after taxis? Logic indicates that aspiration ought to be tried before any other operation. In fact, our aim in aspirating the liquids and the gases is to place the intestine in the most favourable condition for reduction. The twenty cases of the first category appear to us very significant. Here are twenty patients labouring under strangulated hernia; taxis several times repeated, with the help of chloroform, performed under the most favourable circumstances, gives no result, and it suffices to aspirate some of the gases and a few grammes of liquid to effect the reduction of the hernial loop.

Aspiration, then, is the most direct and most efficacious auxiliary of taxis. It yet remains to be seen if it should not become its indispensable auxiliary. I foresee objections : it will be said that all the herniæ, which until now had been reduced by simple taxis, had done perfectly well without aspiration, and that consequently there is no necessity to make a rule of a method which might only be considered as an exception. That method of reasoning would consist in proposing aspiration when all hope of reduction by taxis is lost.

Thus, given a strangulated hernia: we should begin by making a first attempt at taxis ; then we should administer purgatives ; we should then resume taxis by help of chloroform ; and finally, as a last chance, we should try aspiration. Such is not our opinion. If aspiration brought with it any definite peril, I could understand the propriety of its being reserved for an ultimate or exceptional means. But I ask myself if repeated efforts at taxis, if the delay caused by these fruitless attempts, if the consequent condition of the intestine, do not constitute a state of things more to be dreaded for the patient than the operation of aspiration, which is, on the whole, so harmless.

I am, therefore, of opinion that taxis, whilst retaining its incontestable utility, ought to be relegated to the second rank. The rules laid down so scientifically by M. Gosselin lose nothing of their importance; the method proposed by M. Lannelongue none the less finds its applications ; but, in presence of a strangulated hernia (with the restrictions already laid down), our first care ought to be to perform aspiration without delay, directly the first attempt at taxis has failed, and without fatiguing the intestine and the patient by fresh efforts, which too often lead to delay.

The treatment of a strangulated hernia (before coming to kelotomy) would then comprise three periods : 1st, aspiration ; 2nd, taxis ; 3rd, reduction. We shall go on to examine each of these three periods, and describe the manipulatory operations in each.

ARTICLE V.

Of the Operative Manipulation.—Aspiration.—Taxis.—Reduction.

How, then, should the aspiration of a strangulated hernia be performed ? The choice of the aspirator is immaterial, provided that the instrument creates the previous vacuum thoroughly. This condition is indispensable in the instance we are now considering. As a matter of fact, when we are emptying a pleura or a cyst, the aspiratory force is sufficient, even when the vacuum is imperfect ; but when it is necessary to aspirate the thick and fæculent liquid of a hernial loop through a needle half a millimetre in diameter, the aspiration must be of a very powerful character.

It is quite essential at the moment of operating to assure one's self of the permeability of the needle, a precaution too seldom taken, for the canula of this instrument is so small that a few grains of dust or rust suffice to close up the cavity. It is therefore necessary to pass a stream of water through the needle before the operation ; the omission to do so exposes the operator to the risk of failure from a cause very easily removed.

The aspirator being set, that is to say, the previous vacuum being created, we thrust the needle No. 1 or No. 2 sharply into the part of the tumour selected beforehand. When the needle has passed about a centimetre into the depth of the tissues, that is to say, so soon as the point is no longer in connection with the external air, we turn the corresponding stop-cock of the aspirator, and a vacuum is consequently created in the needle. Thus it is with a vacuum in our hand we slowly pass through the tissues in quest of the liquids and gases.

So soon as these liquids are encountered by the aspiratory needle, they betray their presence by the glass index, and warn us that it is useless to penetrate deeper.

But the operation presents some special features, according as the sac does or does not contain fluid. In the first case, we insert the needle, and we find, at a trifling depth, a liquid of varying colour, of small density, and without any particular smell.

After the aspiration of this liquid, the tumour collapses; but we must on no account perform taxis, for we have not penetrated the intestine. At this stage, percussion may be a good guide in discovering the presence and the direction of the hernial loop; we then direct the needle in search of the intestine, and at the instant we puncture it, we are warned of the fact by the gases and by the liquid which reach the aspirator. If the instrument contained any liquid at the moment it penetrated the intestine, the gases burst forth in bubbles on the surface of the liquid; sometimes they produce a sharp whistle in passing the aspirating needle, but the bubbling is the best sign we possess for recognizing the issue of the gases.

Therefore, at the moment of performing the operation, it is advisable to leave a small quantity of water in the aspirator; thanks to that precaution, we know exactly the instant it reaches the intestine. And when the beads of gas no longer make their appearance on the surface of the liquid, it is because the hernial loop contains no more, or that the aspirator is full of them. This precaution of leaving a few grammes of water in the bottom of the aspirator, is peculiarly advantageous if the needle have not encountered in its passage a sac containing liquid. The intestinal fluid is easily recognizable; it is thick, fæculent, high-coloured, rises slowly, and is sometimes of so firm a consistence, that, when it reaches the aspirator, it preserves the vermicular form it had acquired in the needle.

During the aspiration of the fluid from the intestine, a sudden stop sometimes occurs, on which it is desirable to be enlightened.

At the moment the needle penetrates the hernial loop the gases make their appearance, the intestinal liquid begins to rise into the tube of the aspirator, then everything comes to a standstill. It might then be supposed either that the needle is stopped up, or that the hernial loop contains no more liquid ; but the true reason is, that the gases which have suddenly taken possession of the pump have destroyed the aspiratory power of the vacuum, and the aspirator must be emptied and prepared afresh. The aspiration of the gases and liquids being completed, the question is, should taxis be performed immediately after the aspiration, or should it be deferred ? We believe that there is no reason for waiting. In the majority of cases remarked on, taxis was performed immediately after aspiration, the success of the operation was never endangered, and the intestine was reduced without the supervention of the smallest accident. We need not dwell on the rules of taxis ; it ought to be performed just as if aspiration had never taken place, and one is astonished to see a hernia which had resisted repeated efforts with baths and with chloroform give way before taxis of the most moderate kind.

In all cases the operation is not always so simple, and unforeseen complications must be looked for. Thus it happens that perhaps we have well penetrated into the hernial sac, but do not find the intestine at the first insertion. In this case we must reassure ourselves as to the permeability of the needle, and not fear to make a second puncture in another direction. Experience has taught us that this procedure is unobjectionable, since, amongst other remarks, we have pointed out one case (Verneuil) in which the intestine had been thrice punctured and perforated in several parts without any injury resulting.

To sum up, What is the best mode of proceeding in a case of strangulated hernia? We first commence by performing taxis once, methodically, but without too much effort or too much persistence. If the hernia is not reduced after this first attempt it is useless, it is even injurious, to persist further or to delay, and we must have recourse to aspiration.

Aspiration performed on the patients referred to in our statistics has given results such as cannot be claimed by any other method, notwithstanding that it has almost always been employed as a last resource; under the most unfavourable conditions, for strangulated hernia of several days' duration, and when the patient was exhausted by repeated attempts at taxis. We can thence judge of the success which would be obtained if aspiration were applied methodically, according to the rules we have laid down, when the strangulation was of recent occurrence, and the intestine had not been distressed by ill-timed taxis. But if aspiration, performed according to the precepts we have laid down, does not suffice to reduce the hernia, it is because causes of irreducibility exist, such as adhesions. In such cases division is then necessary, and we believe that kelotomy ought to be performed without any further experiments.

Summary and Conclusion.—The discovery of aspiration has produced notable modifications in the operation for strangulated hernia, and the chances of cure have been almost doubled.

1st. The puncture of an intestinal hernial loop, by means of the needles No. 1 and No. 2 of the aspirator, is perfectly harmless.

2nd. Aspiration ought to be attempted in all cases of strangulated hernia, with one exception only, that is when the long duration of the strangulation gives rise to apprehensions of gangrene or of intestinal ulcerations.

3rd. Aspiration ought to be performed as soon as the

taxis, having been once methodically tried, has failed to afford good results.

4th. The treatment of a strangulated hernia, before reaching the stage of kelotomy, comprises, then, three periods : 1. Aspiration ; 2. Taxis ; 3. Reduction.

ARTICLE VI.

CASES OF THE FIRST CATEGORY.

Strangulated Herniæ which have resisted Taxis, and been reduced by the aid of Aspiration alone.

CASE I.—PUNCTURE OF THE INTESTINE IN STRANGULATED HERNIA (Case reported by M. Dolbeau, read before the *Société de Chirurgie*, on the 5th of April, 1871).

Ten days ago a patient was brought to the Beaujon Hospital, said to be suffering under an inguinal hernia, strangulated from four to five days. I found a hard, painful, and irreducible enterocele on the right side ; the belly was distended. I did not think it advisable to use chloroform, as the patient was in the last stage of a cardiac affection. The general condition was very serious, and believing that the patient could not outlive the day, I would not operate. Besides the cardiac affection and the strangulated hernia, the patient was suffering from ulcerations of the legs, and a false passage in the urethral canal, caused by former applications of the catheter. As the patient was still alive on the following morning, I entertained the idea of puncturing the intestine with Dieulafoy's aspirator. I took the finest of the needles and drove it into the centre of the tumour. Gas, and a fluid with a stercoraceous smell, rose into the tube ; the tumour had subsided, but still remained visible ; moderate taxis reduced the intestine. Two hours after the patient went to the water-closet. He died in the course of the day of his heart affection, without any symptoms of strangulation or

N

of accidents ascribable to the operation.   He was 62 years
old.   The post-mortem examination showed the heart to be
enormously large, filled with clots, and the valves ossified.
The cavity of the abdomen presented no traces of peritonitis ; neither redness, nor false membranes, nor liquid,
only some agglutinated loops of small intestine.   I discovered the loop of small intestine which had been strangulated.   A graze of the serous membrane was found on
the peritoneal surface, but no orifice at the level of the
puncture.   A slow but strong insufflation was performed
under water, but not one bead of air resulted.   The needle
had grazed the serous and eluded the other coats of the
intestine.   I resolved to employ puncture with aspiration
in the first strangulated hernia which should occur in my
hospital practice.   I had felt some doubt as to the reality
of the reduction, because there were two sacs ; the old
one was very thick, and likely to give the impression that
the reduction was not complete.   To sum up, the operation did not produce any accident.

CASE II.—STRANGULATED HERNIA IN A MAN AGED 82—
SUBCUTANEOUS PNEUMATIC ASPIRATION—EASY REDUCTION
—CURE (*Gazette Hebdomadaire* of the 7th July, 1871 :
Correspondence. •By Dr. Duplouy).

To Dr. Dieulafoy.

Sir, and much honoured Colleague,—I have the honour
to make known to you, in all its details, a successful and
novel application of pneumatic aspiration, a process which
has already been of signal service in many cases of hydarthrosis, of ovarian puncture, of tympanitis, and of thoracentesis.   This new application consists of an intestinal
puncture, with aspiration of the gases and liquids,
performed with success on a strangulated hernia, which
had resisted all attempts at taxis.   You may remember
that I had briefly informed you of this important and

unique incident, so far back as the 3rd of August, 1870, reserving to myself the duty of making it the object of a special communication to the Société de Chirurgie so soon as I no longer felt any doubt as to the good or evil results arising from the operation. The preoccupations arising from the war, and the sudden interruptions of our relations with Paris, did not allow me to do so at the right time.

I was gratified to read in the *Gazette Hebdomadaire* (28th of April) of a similar attempt made by Professor Dolbeau on a patient suffering at the same time from strangulated hernia, and heart affection in a very advanced stage. If the patient operated on, *in extremis*, succumbed to the consequences of accidents entirely foreign to the operation, the autopsy gave means of verifying the integrity of the intestinal coats. My observation fully confirms, from the physiological point of view, the harmlessness of the intestinal puncture, which my accomplished colleague was able to demonstrate anatomically. The patient who was operated on did not suffer from the least consecutive accident, notwithstanding his great age, a fact which seems to me calculated to encourage surgeons in this path, and to extend the applications of conservative surgery.

Puncture of the intestine has been more than once proposed in order to facilitate the reduction of strangulated hernia. The sometimes happy, but almost always harmless, results of acupuncture in the treatment of tympanitis bring back the minds of surgeons with almost irresistible force to the very simple idea of removing the obstruction caused by liquids and gases in certain strangulations. But the attempts made in this direction have been so little satisfactory, that M. Nélaton formally condemned them by placing them on the horns of an apparently irrefutable dilemma. "One of two things," said he; "either the opening will be very small and nothing will come out of it;

or it will be larger, when danger will arise, after the reduction, of effusion into the abdominal cavity." With your ingenious instrument it is now possible to appeal from that judgment; it is possible, by a microscopic opening, to aspirate the gases and even the liquids contained in an intestinal loop, and that without the least danger to the peritoneum. I had been greatly struck, whilst reading your paper, with the thought of the services which might be expected from aspiration so performed, in cases of intestinal occlusion, and of the prospects it opens up in certain cases of strangulated hernia, and I was only seeking an opportunity to give them a practical application.

I was called on the 3rd of August, 1870, to a M. G——, a gentleman living at Tonnay, 82 years old, who had laboured for more than twenty years under pulmonary catarrh, and who during the last month had been suffering from a right inguinal hernia, caused by coughing. His constitution was strong, his mind clear, and the natural functions in good order, save a marked tendency to constipation. Since the hernia had appeared, Dr. Bouthet-Desjennetières had been twice called in to replace the intestine in the belly, and advised the use of a truss, which had not been regularly worn. On the 30th of July the tumour again became irreducible, the bulk increased sensibly, action of the bowels ceased, and some colicky pains were felt. M. Gaudin, who was called in two days after the advent of these accidents, attempted simple taxis, and not being successful in it, renewed the attempt in the bath. Dr. Léon, who was called in in my absence, the next morning, had no better success, even with the aid of chloroform. He had previously ordered a purgative and a strong saline injection, which had no effect. The symptoms having become aggravated during the night, I set out, on the morning of the 3rd of August, in company with M. Léon, to visit the patient, prepared to perform the aspiratory operation if necessary, with the enlightened help of our two honourable colleagues. The patient was feeling sharp, shooting pains, starting from the inguinal ring and spreading towards the interior of the abdomen. The belly was slightly distended, and not very painful to palpation. The tongue was slightly dry, the thirst great, but all drinks were constantly rejected from the stomach. The vomited matter had no appearance of fæculence, and the constipation was complete.

The pulse was 86, and rather hard; it presented irregularities which were easily explained by the advanced age of the patient, whose strength was considerably lowered. His countenance was anxious and changed; and the extremities were rather cold.

The tumour, as large as a hen's egg, reached to the bottom of the scrotum; without being very hard, it offered a strongly marked resistance to pressure; it was resonant on percussion, and on pressure gave a very manifest gurgling noise, which indicated the presence of gas and liquids. The skin covering it had kept the natural colour; it was flaccid, containing but little fat, and slipped easily over the surface of the tumour. We evidently had to deal with an enterocele. Dr. Bouthet, who had already had the opportunity of reducing it, had never detected an epiploon. In vain we all essayed, in turns, sustained taxis, endeavouring to drive back the gases and the liquids into the interior of the belly, by a methodical compression, directed from the lower part to the neck.

The hernia, of which the tension was but small, allowed itself to be replaced in the inguinal passage, but it was .impossible to make it clear the internal ring. In presence of this unexpected danger, impressed with the risk of an operation on so old a man, I entertained the idea of aspirating, by a harmless puncture, the liquid and gaseous matters. I employed the 45-gramme aspirator. The needle No. 2 being introduced into the most depending and most prominent part of the tumour, we made a first aspiration, which brought forth nothing but gas, but which, nevertheless, brought on a sufficiently marked relaxation to encourage us to persevere. We left the needle in its place, and resetting the aspirator, we succeeded in extracting a tablespoonful of liquefied fæculent matters, of a brownish-yellow colour and a characteristic odour. A third application produced similar matter in about the same quantity. The tumour was rendered sufficiently pliable to allow the intestinal coats to be rubbed against each other, and the reduction was but child's play. We did not hesitate to do it ; what, in reality, had we to fear from a simple puncture made in the intestine whilst in a state of distention ? Would not the slight graze of the membranes be naturally obliterated by the return of the coats to a flaccid state ? Besides, a purely cutaneous lesion was in question, and it seemed to us that if Velpeau and many others had been able, without much distress of mind, to replace in the belly intestines injured by small perforations after division, we might very well indulge ourselves in the hope that there would be no injurious infiltration into the peritoneum.

The success of the operation surpassed our expectations ; we had restricted ourselves to prescribing some beef-tea, a slight opiate, and on the very evening of the operation, without the aid of any purgative, the patient had a copious motion, the colicky pains were quieted, and from that time to the present—that is, ten months—not the slightest ill effect of the hernia has been felt. I wished to see this interesting case before I transcribed my notes relating to it. I found the patient, with the exception of the weakness due to his catarrhal affection and his advanced age, in a very satisfactory condition. Do not think, my dear colleague, that my gratitude for your valuable instrument leads me so far as to advise its employment in all cases of strangulated hernia. Since the lucky application above recorded, I have met three cases of crural hernia, extremely constricted, of a very contracted volume, seeming to contain little gas and less liquid. I immediately decided on the cutting operation, without attempting aspiration. This method, the indications for which can only be clearly laid down by experience, appears to me to be above all applicable to somewhat large enteroceles, affected by strangulation consecutive either on inflammation or obstruction (if any exist). I have made up my mind not to operate again in cases of this kind without preliminary recourse to this harmless means, and if, by chance, I thought I recognized the presence in the intestines of matters too solid to be easily aspirated, I should not hesitate to soften them with a certain quantity of water injected by the needle of the aspirator.

I end this letter, perhaps already too long, by begging you, my dear colleague, to receive the assurance of my friendship.

Duplouy,
Professor of Surgery at the Naval Medical School
at Rochefort.

Case III.——Strangulated Hernia reduced on Three different Occasions by Means of Aspiration (by M. Dolbeau).——A lady, 63 years old, had suffered for a long time from a reducible crural hernia. This hernia became strangulated, and taxis, performed several times, could not reduce it. Aspiration was practised, reduction was performed without difficulty, and all ill effects averted. But shortly afterwards, the hernia became strangulated again, and it was necessary to have recourse to aspiration, which was practised with success. Finally, some months later, fresh strangulation, and aspiration was employed with an equally happy result.

Case IV.——Strangulated Hernia——Aspiration with

NEEDLE No. 2—REDUCTION (Communication from Professor Duplouy, of Rochefort).—I tried a new application of the aspirator in a case of strangulated hernia. The patient was a young soldier, who was brought into my wards whilst I was giving clinical instruction. He was placed under chloroform, and taxis failed under several hands. I attempted it myself, but without success. I then introduced needle No. 2, and I aspirated, perhaps, some gas ; I say perhaps, because I thought too late of assuring myself of the fact by forcing down the piston under water. I was asking for a little water to insinuate a small quantity into the tumour, when a surgeon, present at the operation, taking advantage of the remarks which I was addressing to my hearers, and of the removal of the needle, which I intended to insert at another point, examined the tumour and perceived a slight gurgling noise, speedily followed by the return of the intestine. I had not touched the hernia since the aspiration, and I had not, in consequence, been able to form a judgment of the difference in the tension of the intestinal coats before and after the operation.

Now should we, in this case, attribute the reduction to a more complete anæsthesia than at the commencement of the operation, or to the extraction of a certain quantity of gas ? It is impossible to be too careful of illusory impressions; but, however it may be, as soon as the aspiration was made, the hernia, which had resisted taxis, was reduced, and no consecutive accident showed itself—a fresh proof of the harmlessness of this mode of operating.

CASE V.—M. Cazin, of Boulogne, performed aspiratory puncture in a large inguinal hernia. The patient was an Englishman, more than sixty years old ; the reduction was complete, and the cure rapid. I have not been. able to get more particulars about it . from

M. Cazin, and regret not having the complete notes he promised me.

CASE VI.—STRANGULATED UMBILICAL HERNIA—FIVE ASPIRATIONS—REDUCTION (BY M. DIEULAFOY).—In the month of October, 1871, I was called in by M. Foucher to see a patient suffering from a strangulated umbilical hernia, which could not be reduced. I found a woman about 45 years old, very stout, with an anxious expression of countenance, and a small and rapid pulse. Hiccup and vomiting had continued since the previous night, and the large hernia had resisted two attempts at taxis. The belly was distended with flatus, and painful. I made five successive punctures into the tumour, somewhat distant from each other, with the needles No. 1 and No. 2. A small quantity of liquid and a large quantity of gas were extracted. As we had taken care to leave some grammes of water in the end of the aspirator, it was easy to see the gases rise to the surface of the liquid. The relief was instantaneous, and the volume of the tumour diminished sensibly. As five punctures had been made, it seemed to us prudent not to irritate the intestine so soon after ; taxis was performed several hours later by M. Souchard, and the hernia was reduced.

CASE VII.—CONGENITAL INGUINAL HERNIA (Case in the practice of M. Demarquay, reported by M. Gerard. *L'Union Médicale*, 13*th June*, 1872).—M. X———, a clerk, 22 years of age, entered a *Maison de Santé* on the 6th of May, after prolonged walking. The evening before he had felt a sharp pain whilst getting into the railway carriage. He put his hand to the fold of the groin and discovered a large tumour, painful to the touch, which he had never previously noticed. Two hours before this he had had a free action of the bowels. The tumour descended into the scrotum and appeared the size of a large hen's egg. The

integuments were rather red and hot; the left testicle was
situated at the lower part of the tumour, with which it
seemed to form one. M. Demarquay diagnosed a congenital left inguinal hernia. The testicles had probably
descended late, for they were small and gathered up near
the rings. The young man did not remember having
noticed them until he was nearly fourteen years old, but
would not positively affirm that they had not descended
before that time. Strong colicky pains ensued during
the night of Sunday, with vomiting, first of alimentary
then of bilious matter. No stools. Monday, same condition. A surgeon, who was called in, discovered a strangulation, performed taxis without any result, and sent the
patient to the *Maison de Santé.* He went in at eleven
o'clock at night, and a gentle and lengthened taxis was essayed (about twenty minutes). The tumour diminished in
size between our hands, but we could not succeed in reducing it. Ice to the belly and a purgative to empty the
lower extremity of the intestine were ordered. On Tuesday
morning M. Demarquay tried taxis under chloroform ; he
did not succeed, and as the general symptoms were very
serious, he decided on kelotomy. The tumour was already
shaved, when he conceived the idea of making an aspiratory
puncture with M. Potain's apparatus, which M. Mathieu
had brought to empty a purulent abscess of the abdomen.
The trocar, No. 1, was inserted perpendicularly into the
tumour, a vacuum having previously been created ; 120
grammes of a blackish-yellow liquid, containing some
particles of fæcal matter, were brought away. Probably
a quantity of gas had also escaped, for the vacuum was
obliged to be re-established before all the liquid could
be evacuated. At a certain moment of the operation
nothing more flowed up ; M. Demarquay then slowly
drew back the trocar about a centimetre. The liquid
then passed afresh into the flask, but this liquid was
much clearer ; it was the contents of the hernial sac.

The hernia became considerably flatter; the trocar was removed. We waited an instant to see if intestinal contraction would effect the reduction, but nothing came of it.

M. Demarquay then wished to assure himself of the state of the tumour. It slipped between his fingers, and was reduced without any effort of taxis. Some graduated compresses, and a spica of the groin were applied over the ring. The patient was ordered to be kept perfectly quiet, to take some spoonfuls of *tisane*, and 10 centigrammes of opium every hour in pills of 1 centigramme. This treatment was adopted by the surgeon of the *Maison de Santé*, who, far from desiring to provoke intestinal contractions, sought on the contrary to calm them during 24, 36 to 38 hours.

Immediately after the reduction, the patient felt relieved, the colicky pains disappeared, the vomiting ceased, the thirst diminished slightly, although it was still great. The pulse, which was small and thready, and marked 120 before puncture, became already stronger and less frequent at two o'clock in the afternoon. In the evening it was 95.

Evening.—The patient had not yet had any action of the bowels; his general condition was very good, and he professed himself cured. The opium pills were still continued.

Wednesday morning, the amelioration still continued; a little beef-tea was allowed to be given. The countenance was no longer drawn, there was no fever, every trace of colic or vomiting had disappeared. Five pills, each containing 1 centigramme of opium, were given, and on Thursday a purgative. The first stool since the operation occurred. After that epoch regular and free action of the bowels took place, with good appetite and easy digestion. On Friday, the 21st of May, fifteen days after the reduction, M. Demarquay showed the patient to the Académie de Médicine.　He took advantage of the opportunity to go and see his relations, and walked more than he ought to have done.　Three days after, an abscess was opened in the scrotum.　Was it the hernial sac which had suppurated?　The patient was discharged on the 31st of May, perfectly cured of this complication.

CASE VIII.—M. CHAUVEAU, of Courtalain, *Journal de Médecine et Chirurgie Pratique*, July, 1872.—STRANGU-LATED INGUINAL HERNIA—ASPIRATION—REDUCTION.—A day-labourer, named Lacroix, had suffered for eight years from a left inguinal hernia, kept back by a truss.

On the 15th June, 1872, this man, whilst employed in some very heavy work, was taken with colic, nausea, and constipation.　At the same time he remarked the presence of a tumour in the left groin.　However, he continued his work, but in the evening, the pains had increased, bilious vomiting had followed the nausea, and occurred several times during the night.　On the morning of the 16th, he sent for me to see his hernia, which he said had passed from the right to the left.　I found a tumour the size of a large egg, pediculated and elastic to the touch; I tried regular taxis for a quarter of an hour, but fruitlessly.　I thought I could delay a little.　Prescription, purgative injection, reclining position, belladonna ointment, and coffee.　Four hours afterwards, the patient became much worse, the constipation continued obstinate, with fæculent vomiting, distention, pain, and fever.　Taxis was again attempted with india-rubber bands, without any result.　Time being precious, I proceeded without delay to puncture the tumour with No. 2 needle of Dieulafoy's apparatus.　Three or four spoonfuls of a liquid tinged with blood and traversed by gases, were aspirated.　An impression had been made on the tumour, but it was not, however, reduced till after taxis of ten minutes' duration.　A few moments afterwards, the bowels acted.　The case progressed quietly, and two days after, the subject of this case, wearing a good truss, resumed his work, having passed at once from the most serious condition to health.

CASE IX. (M. CHAUVEAU) RIGHT INGUINAL HERNIA—ASPIRATION—REDUCTION.—Madame L——, mother of the schoolmaster of Courtalain, aged 75, was attacked by pulmonary catarrh. On the 26th of June, 1872, I was called to see this lady, who, for the last twenty-four hours, had complained of abdominal pain, with constipation and frequent vomiting. In the right inguinal region I found an entero-epiplocele, of which the patient was unaware ; consequently of recent date, and caused by coughing. It was quite irreducible, the belly was distended, fever high, the features were drawn and anxious, and the danger was imminent. A first puncture was made in the centre of the tumour with No. 2 needle, and afforded issue to several grammes of colourless liquid, proceeding from a cystic sac. The needle was taken out and planted in a more depending part. A reddish-brown liquid, disturbed by gases, rose slowly into the body of the pump, and then remained stationary. The collapse of the hernia was very strongly marked, nevertheless the reduction necessitated rather energetic efforts. At the same instant, the patient felt much relieved and the bowels acted.

Like the preceding case, this patient got up two days after, and her health is now in a thoroughly satisfactory condition.

CASE X.—BY M. LABBÉ, PUBLISHED IN THE *Lancet*, OF THE 20TH JULY, 1872—STRANGULATED RIGHT INGUINAL HERNIA—ASPIRATORY PUNCTURE—ISSUE OF LIQUIDS AND GASES — IMMEDIATE REDUCTION — CURE. — The extreme importance which the method of reducing hernia by aspiratory puncture has rapidly acquired in surgical practice, the limited number of facts concerning it hitherto known, and the inducement there is to encourage medical men in following in that path, determine me to publish the following case, which I have had the opportunity of observing.

During the night of the 20th of June, M. D——, a strong and robust man, 70 years of age, after a violent fit of coughing, felt an intense pain in the right inguinal region. It was followed, after some minutes, by nausea and vomiting. Soon, he discovered a large tumour in the right inguinal region.

On the next day, the 21st, at six o'clock in the evening, I saw the patient for the first time in company with his usual medical attendant, who had employed methodical taxis, but without success. I tried taxis myself, but in vain. The nausea and the vomiting continued, the pulse counted 75. Considering that, in this case, the strangulation had only lasted eighteen hours, and that the anatomical lesions were presumably slightly advanced, I did not hesitate to propose puncture with the aspirator, and I introduced No. 2 needle without delay. About 10 grammes of a brownish liquid came away, together with a certain quantity of gas, which I could not exactly estimate. The tumour, which was as large as my fist, collapsed immediately, and a slight pressure, exercised for a minute on the neck of the sac, produced a complete reduction of the hernia. The patient was relieved directly and felt comfortable. During the succeeding hours, from six to eleven, and more especially between eight and eleven, he experienced some nausea, a slight attack of vomiting, then a little fever and a rigor. I administered, as I usually do after the reduction of a hernia by taxis or operation, opium pills, containing 1 centigramme of extract of opium, every two hours, so that 10 or 12 centigrammes may be taken in the course of twenty-four hours, with the object of calming the movements of the intestine.

At eleven o'clock at night, the symptoms before detailed had completely disappeared; and from that time, the patient professed himself perfectly comfortable. On the 22nd of June, the pulse was 60, the aspect normal, the abdomen was still slightly hard above the inguinal region. On the 23rd of June, the patient had three natural stools. There was neither pain nor fever, and the appetite was excellent. Eight days afterwards, the cure, which had declared itself on the third day, was still maintained. At present the patient enjoys excellent health.

CASE XI.—STRANGULATED CRURAL HERNIA, CURED BY ASPIRATORY PUNCTURE WITHOUT REDUCTION (BY DR. WALCHER OF ERSTEIN), *Gazette Médicale de Strasbourg* of the 1st of August, 1872.—On Monday, the 17th of June, M. Walcher was called to see a woman suffering from a right crural hernia, which had been strangulated for two days. Taxis had already been performed; the patient had refused to allow kelotomy. He thus describes the state in which he found the patient :—

" A woman about 40 years old, countenance shrunk, the eyes sunken, forehead covered with a cold sweat, the tongue dry with great thirst, small, rapid, and hard pulse, and continual sickness. She could not swallow any liquid without subsequent regurgitation; nevertheless, she had only had spontaneous vomiting twice since the morning. The belly was much puffed up, and so sensitive that the slightest touch made the woman groan; from time to time colicky pains supervened, making her utter loud cries. The patient had one stool in the night between Saturday and Sunday; it was hard and small, and induced by an injection of decoction of senna; since then nothing had passed. The tumour, situated in the right crural fold, was very painful and as large as a hen's egg; the skin was red and slightly tumefied, the result of taxis. This patient, after I had made my examination, suddenly exclaimed, ' I will not be tortured, I will die quietly; let me alone.' However, I succeeded in persuading her to

allow a little morphia to be injected, so as to calm her.
A centigramme of morphia gave her a little rest, and this
comfort allowed me to speak to her of having another
puncture made in the hernia. She resigned herself to
this fresh puncture. I immediately inserted No. 2 needle
into the tumour, perpendicularly to the skin ; a sensation
of a resistance overcome stopped me : when the tap was
turned, I saw small drops of a sanguineous liquid splashed
over the walls of Dieulafoy's aspirator, and filling the
end of it. More than four teaspoonsfuls of a sanguineous
liquid were removed, and a characteristic smell announced
the presence of intestinal gases. I set the instrument
again, but no more liquid appeared, only gases. After
having set the aspirator a third time, I slowly drew back
the needle to empty the sac, but nothing came.

" As soon as the aspiration was finished, the woman felt
relieved ; she had scarcely felt the puncture. Borborygmi
were heard ; I tried taxis very lightly, but it produced no
effect. The tumour had become smaller by the aspiration.
The belly, still puffed up, had lost its sensitiveness. I applied a coat of collodion over the belly and the tumour. I
had the woman put to bed, keeping the pelvis higher than
her head, ordering her to have a little ice and a few drops
of ether, if the nausea returned. The next day her countenance was calm, her speech less abrupt ; she had slept for
two hours, had no nausea, had been able to swallow a
little beef-tea, and had not felt any colicky pains, although
the belly was still rather painful to pressure. She also
brought up wind. I injected another centigramme of
morphia, and I renewed the coat of collodion. At eight
o'clock she took 40 grammes of castor-oil. At ten o'clock
the bowels had not acted, I therefore gave 20 grammes
of castor-oil, which were vomited. In the evening she
had had six copious stools; she was sitting up in bed,
and asked for food. On examining her, I found the
tumour larger than on the previous day ; by taxis it

became reduced to the size it was after aspiratory puncture. I afterwards learned from the woman that it had not been completely returned for more than a year : the patient wore her truss above it. It was an irreducible hernia. I kept her in bed for six days ; I then allowed her to get up, putting her on a truss with a flat pad, hollowed out to the level of the hernia.

From that time forward, this woman resumed her work in the fields.

M. Walcher proceeds to make this remark, that by aspiratory puncture we may save the life of persons in whom the dangers of operation are aggravated by adhesions which must be destroyed when kelotomy is performed, and which make that operation much more difficult; and also of those persons who shun the operation. M. Walcher goes on to draw this conclusion, that the strangulation must have depended on the gases or liquids which exist in the hernial loop ; since it disappeared, though the hernia was irreducible, as soon as the gases and liquids were taken away. Many surgeons would have termed this an inflamed hernia. This case is very interesting, because it demonstrates the efficacy of aspiratory puncture in irreducible hernia offering appearances of strangulation.

CASE XII.—STRANGULATED HERNIA REDUCED BY ASPIRATION (BY DR. MÉNARD).—On the 28th July, 1872, I was called to Bossuet by M. Oudot, to see a patient suffering from strangulated hernia. The patient, after having worked in the fields part of the preceding day, with his hernia protruding, notwithstanding that he wore the truss which usually kept it up, was taken in the evening with violent pain in the inguinal region. Not being able to reduce the hernia himself, the man sent in great haste to fetch M. Oudot, who made several attempts at taxis without any success. The next day, notwithstanding the use of hip-baths, the pain was equally sharp, the vomiting became very frequent, and taxis, tried several times in the course of the day, remained as unsuccessful as on the evening before.   When I saw the patient, about five o'clock in the afternoon, I found him very much enfeebled—exhausted by incessant vomiting.   A slight attempt at taxis not having been more fortunate than the preceding ones, I had recourse to aspiration with Potain's apparatus.   The finest needle having been introduced, gave outlet to a reddish frothy liquid, mixed with gases, proceeding doubtless from the intestine, and amounting to 70 or 80 grammes.   The hernial tumour diminished immediately. Taxis, performed at once, had no result. I did not persevere, the vomiting ceased, the pain became less acute, and finally the patient fell asleep.   When he awoke, two hours after, the patient pressed a little on the hernia, which went back without the least effort.

M. Oudot and I both felt convinced that we owed this happy and speedy result to aspiration.

CASE XIII.—I owe the communication of the two following cases to the kindness of M. Le Bêle, Head Surgeon to the hospital at Mans :—

In the month of March or April, 1872, X——, a farmer at Tillé (Sarthe), between 35 and 40 years old, came to see me at the hospital with a large strangulated left inguinal hernia.   It was then three o'clock in the day, and since the morning when the strangulation had made its appearance, the patient had made numerous and vain efforts to reduce it.

He assured me that, until then, he had returned the hernia completely every day and without difficulty.   The tumour was the size of a fist ; it was hard at the apex and purplish in colour. I had the patient put to bed, and tried taxis without success.   For a moment I thought of having recourse to anæsthesia by chloroform ; but I thought of what I had recently read in a medical journal, and I resorted to puncture with No. 2 needle of Dieulafoy's aspirator. I made two successive punctures at the centre of the tumour. The first gave no apparent result. Fearing that I had not penetrated into the intestinal cavity, I made a second puncture at 1 or 2 centimetres from the first : this time I obtained a considerable quantity of intestinal mucus, in the shape of a reddish deposit ; the tumour became sensibly less tense, still being somewhat resilient. A careful pressure brought on immediately the return of the intestine, with the usual characteristic sound. The hernia was reduced, and there remained nothing more in the sac. The patient, who had had several attacks of vomiting in the morning, left, free from suffering, and reporting himself cured. He promised to let me know if any accident supervened ; but as I have heard nothing of him, I conclude that everything went on well.

CASE XIV.—INGUINAL HERNIA—ASPIRATION—REDUCTION (LE BÊLE).—Alexander Martin, traveller, from 20 to 25 years of age, came into the Hôtel Dieu Hospital, on the 20th of June, 1872, at ten o'clock in the morning, with a strangulated right inguinal hernia with vomiting. I did not see him until two o'clock in the afternoon. He told me that he usually replaced his hernia easily, but that since the previous day he had not been able to do so. Taxis which I tried after the house surgeon was unsuccessful.

I immediately asked for the aspirator, and after puncture with needle No. 2, followed by several aspirations which did not produce any fluid, I discovered a notable diminution in the size of the tumour. I took away the canula and reduced the hernia without difficulty. I prescribed a purgative injection, seltzer water and beef-tea. On the next day, the 21st of June, I found the patient doing well; he had not vomited, and had had an action of the bowels. He complained of slight pain in the inguinal region and of slight colic. Ordered poultices on the belly, fresh injection, and a draught containing extract of belladonna.

On the 22nd of June he had still some colicky pains, but his bowels acted naturally, and he had taken a little food since the previous night. I ordered him 30 grammes of castor-oil. On the 23rd of June the patient was purged, his appetite had returned, and he was no longer in any pain. He reported himself completely cured and asked to leave the hospital, which he was allowed to do in the course of the evening.

In these two cases, there can be no doubt that the reduction was favoured by the abstraction of the gases, which were aspirated without sound, either at their entrance or exit from the body of the pump.

Case XV.—Strangulated Umbilical Hernia—Aspiration—Cure.—M. Ollivier, of Rouen, sent to the Société de Chirurgie a case of reduction of a large strangulated umbilical hernia, after aspiratory puncture. This case was spoken of at the meeting of the 5th of November, but as I have not been able to procure any details, I confine myself to recording the success of the aspiration.

Case XVI.—Strangulated Inguinal Hernia—Insufficiency of Taxis—Aspiration, Reduction, and Cure (by M. Létiévant of Lyons).—A young man came to me who had been suffering from strangulated inguinal hernia since the night before.

Attempts at taxis had been made without any result, and I decided on aspirating the hernia. I performed the operation with the assistance of M. Valette. Dieulafoy's No. 2 needle was inserted in the tumour and gave outlet to about 40 grammes of somewhat turbid liquid. The tumour collapsed immediately, the needle was removed, and we were able to reduce the hernia with wonderful ease.

CASE XVII.—STRANGULATED RIGHT INGUINAL HERNIA —ASPIRATION—REDUCTION (M. DIEULAFOY).—R——, hall-porter, a man of 53, had suffered for several years from a right inguinal hernia, which he kept in place by means of a truss. Six months ago this hernia showed symptoms of strangulation, and the patient, performing taxis for himself, succeeded, after many trials, in reducing his hernia. This time he tried the same means, but without success. As strangulation had existed for three days, I performed aspiration, without losing time. No. 2 needle was inserted in the tumour, and I extracted more gases than liquid. I then obtained reduction without any difficulty.

CASE XVIII.—STRANGULATED CRURAL HERNIA (M. BAILLY).—At the meeting of the 20th of November last, M. Demarquay made a report to the Société de Chirurgie on an aspiration performed by M. Bailly on a strangulated crural hernia.

M. Bailly first made an incision as if for ordinary kelotomy. Reaching the sac, he punctured it, and aspirated the liquid it contained; he then attempted reduction, believing that he was in an excellent position to perform successful taxis, since the intestine was, as it were, laid bare to his fingers. His efforts, however, were useless. He opened the sac and performed aspiratory puncture of the strangulated loop, which subsided and was easily replaced. This operation is very interesting, inasmuch as it shows us how much more efficacious the aspiratory puncture of the loop is than that of the sac. The latter has no result, the former insures an easy reduction. The efficacy of aspiratory puncture in cases of strangulated hernia is, then, above all, due to the abstraction of the fluids confined in the hernial loop, and it should invariably be made.

CASE XIX.—STRANGULATED INGUINAL HERNIA—ASPIRA-TION—REDUCTION (BY M. KIETER, PROFESSOR OF SURGERY AT ST. PETERSBURGH).—I applied M. Dieulafoy's aspirator in a case of strangulated inguino-scrotal hernia, irreducible by taxis. I abstracted a turbid and ill-smelling liquid and large quantities of gas. Immediately afterwards, I was able to reduce the hernia without the help of chloroform. This case proves the services which may be rendered by the aspiratory method in strangulated hernia.

CASE XX.—This case having appeared at the instant I had finished this Article, I can only give the title : *Strangulated Hernia reduced after Aspiration by Dieulafoy's Apparatus*, presented by M. Maury to the Société de Chirurgie, at the sitting of the 22nd of January, 1878.

ARTICLE VII.

CASES OF THE SECOND CATEGORY.

Strangulated Herniæ not reduced by Aspiration, but reduced and cured after Kelotomy.

CASE I. (BOURDY AND DUGUÉ OF MANS).—LEFT IN-GUINAL HERNIA STRANGULATED FOR FOUR DAYS—ASPIRATION WITH DIEULAFOY'S APPARATUS—REDUCTION NOT EFFECTED — KELOTOMY, FIRM ADHESIONS, REDUCTION—RECOVERY.—A woman, Levrau, aged 38, of a good constitution, called me in in July, 1872, for a colic which had lasted four days. On examination, I felt an enlargement in the left inguinal fold. This woman was completely ignorant of the presence of this tumour, although it was as large as my fist. It was a very much distended inguinal enterocele, resonant and mode-rately sensitive. I attempted reduction several times, but it was impossible. No hiccup, some bilious vomiting, no distention, and no fever were present. I requested my friend and colleague Doctor Dugué to help me in the operation. We decided, by mutual consent, to attempt aspiration, which had succeeded in several hands. Puncture with No. 1 needle. There ensued an issue of 12 grammes of chocolate-coloured liquid, rather thick, with a very characteristic smell, and with abundant gases. The tumour collapsed immediately. The skin being very thin, allowed us to feel the intestine; we attempted reduction, but in vain.

Everything being in order for kelotomy, we performed it with great ease. Very little blood flowed. We searched eagerly for the traces of our puncture, but could not find any whatsoever; not even a bubble of gas, nor a globule of blood. The conjunctive tissue, relaxed and transparent, gave great facilities for observation. The intestine looked healthy, was quite depressed, and held by numerous strong bands, fibrous and shining. One of them, which sprang from the angle of the ring, was as large as a crowquill, and gave a creaking sound as it was divided by the scissors. Many bands sprang from all sorts of situations, and easily explained to us why we had not been successful. A slight division of the neck was also necessary, and the intestine replaced itself with an audible sound. In consequence of the healthy condition of the patient, the wound healed thoroughly after the use of a twisted suture.

Three hours afterwards, there were copious evacuations, induced by 30 grammes of castor-oil and a slight purgative injection. Not the slightest colic supervened, the belly was soft; there was no fever. The wound healed by first intention, four-and-twenty hours later on. Two hours afterwards, the patient ate a good thick cabbage soup, and desired to get up, which she did, without feeling any ill effects.

The nature of the adhesions could not in this case have been suspected, as no indications were presented. Chance alone caused the patient to discover the affection from

which she was suffering. It was possible to attempt
puncture in consequence of the good existing conditions,
notwithstanding the four days which had elapsed, and it
evidently would have succeeded but for the presence of
the bands. It left no trace whatsoever, no liquid was
effused, not a bead of gas was infiltrated, it being easy
to verify these facts from the facilities for examination.
The bands were very fibrous, resembling for the most
part tendons or unyielding aponeuroses. One of them
was specially thick. They were evidently of anterior date
to the strangulation.

CASE II.—SUMMARY OF M. RICHET's CASE (Extracted
from the *Gazette des Hôpitaux* of the 27th July, 1872).—
A woman, left crural hernia of old standing, usually kept
up by a truss; recently strangulated, the size of an
egg, brown and hard. Unsuccessful taxis. Puncture and
aspiration, in the first instance of sanguineous serous fluid.
On inserting the needle a little deeper, an inodorous, clear,
glutinous, stringy liquid was evacuated. No attempts at reduction were made. Seltzer water was prescribed to induce
intestinal contraction, but the tumour, which had become
much smaller since aspiration, was not reduced by its un-
assisted efforts. Kelotomy the next day and recovery.

CASE III. (M. VERNEUIL).—Transactions of the *Société
de Chirurgie* (Meeting of July 31).—A hall-porter, suffering from inguinal hernia, which had descended into the
scrotum, and had been strangulated since two o'clock in
the morning, was brought into my ward at six o'clock in
the evening. The strangulation had lasted sixteen hours.
It was a hernia usually kept up which came down suddenly, and consequently was decidedly strangulated. No
efforts at reduction had been made.

I diagnosed a strangulation at the neck of the sac, and
as the tumour was fluctuating, I performed puncture and
aspiration at the lower part. I took away about 300

grammes of a pink liquid arising from dropsy of the sac. After this evacuation I recognized a medium-sized hernia. I made an effort at reduction, the patient being under chloroform. The liquid being removed, I thought I could reduce, but it was impossible. I then tried a second time puncture and aspiration with Potain's apparatus; nothing came out at first, afterwards a little gas and blood. The tumour did not diminish; I did not know if I had reached the intestine; it is, in fact, difficult to ascertain that. I made a third puncture and reddish blood came out. I stopped at that point and performed taxis, but did not prolong my efforts. I performed kelotomy, and unbound the neck of the sac. The intestine was rather livid, and three perforations were visible on it; one from the second stroke of the trocar, two from the third. The intestine had been thoroughly perforated; a little blood exuded from one of the punctures. I divided the bands freely and tied the epiploon, for the hernia was an entero-epiplocele, and reduced. The patient recovered.

CASE IV. — STRANGULATED CRURAL HERNIA — SUB-CUTANEOUS ASPIRATION—OPERATION—RECOVERY (BY M. TERREIR).—Anastasie Berthault, 46 years of age, entered the hospital of La Pitié, on the 28th of August, 1872. The patient gave the following account of herself. About seventeen years ago, while she was doing some heavy work, she became aware of a swelling in the fold of the right groin. A medical man, sent for immediately, was able to reduce this tumour, and told her that she had a hernia. Since that time, the hernial tumour has frequently reappeared, and, according to the patient's account, the hernia itself was frequently in the habit of coming down. However, when the tumour had protruded for some little time, it became irksome and painful, and these slight troubles disappeared by reduction, which, if the patient be believed, was easy and complete. She has never worn a truss.

On Friday, the 27th of August, towards five o'clock in the evening, the tumour became very painful; attempts at reduction made by the patient were unsuccessful, accidents supervened, vomiting was copious and greenish. A medical man, who was called in, performed taxis after the patient had been for some time in a warm bath, but he could not effect replacement. The patient had a bad night, vomiting continued; she did not pass any solid matters or gases by the anus.

On Thursday morning, the 28th, the patient was brought into the hospital about half-past ten A.M. The general condition was not bad; the face was slightly shrunken, the tongue white, vomiting infrequent and porraceous, the belly was not distended, nor did palpation of the abdominal walls cause pain. The hernia alone was the seat of somewhat acute suffering, aggravated by pressure and attempts at reduction. In the region of the right groin I found a rather large tumour, offering the appearance and of the dimensions of a large egg, with the long diameter parallel to the Fallopian ligament. The size of the hernia, its direction, and its position encroaching on the abdominal walls, made me uncertain as to the diagnosis; however, after a careful examination, I adhered to the notion of a crural hernia.

The tumour was tense, elastic, and resonant to percussion throughout its anterior and external portion, but presenting, on the contrary, little dulness towards the internal portion, on the side of the genito-crural fold. In fine, I felt certain that it contained intestine and epiploon. In addition, the pedicle of the hernia, though deep-seated and difficult to examine, was of such a size that one could almost affirm the presence of a somewhat considerable epiploic mass at that level.

An attempt at taxis without chloroform gave no result. At this stage, taking into account the size of the hernia, its long standing, the absence of all means of retention, finally, the nature of its contents and the slightness of the accidents, I thought I ought to try aspiration. I only had one of Dieulafoy's small aspirators at my command; thus the operation was a little more painful, since I was obliged to set the syringe a certain number of times after each puncture. I made a first puncture on the level of the resonant portion of the tumour, that is to say, above and outward, with No. 1 needle.

I penetrated unquestionably into the intestine, for I aspirated a certain amount of greyish liquid, having entirely the aspect of matters contained in the small intestine. A quarter of a glassful was thus withdrawn, almost inodorous gases issuing forth with the liquid.

The tumour collapsed, and rapidly diminished by nearly one-half; the patient immediately announced her feeling of relief. Still, this amendment in the local symptoms was of short duration; the gases contained in the intestinal loops confined in the abdomen reached the hernial loop with the greatest ease, and distended it with some force. Taking away No. 1 needle, I immediately performed taxis with care, and without using much strength. There was not even the shadow of a reduction; on the contrary, the tumour seemed to be augmented in size and distended by gases. In the afternoon the patient had a warm bath, and the house surgeon immediately tried to perform taxis with the aid of chloroform. Two fresh punctures were likewise made with No. 1 needle. The aspirator became filled with intestinal gases only, and that to all appearance in an incomplete fashion; the tumour scarcely diminished at all, and could not be reduced. Poultices were still applied to the hernia, and it was thought necessary to administer a purgative (jalap and scammony), which was immediately rejected in conjunction with greenish matters. I came back to see the patient about five o'clock in the evening; the symptoms of strangulation had become more decided, the belly had increased in size, there was very strongly marked tympanitis. The patient was feverish, and complained a great deal; I resolved to operate immediately, it being then about four-and-twenty hours after symptoms of strangulation had made their appearance.

The patient was placed under the influence of chloroform. An incision 4 or 5 centimetres long was made on the projecting portion of the tumour, and directed according to its great axis below and inwards. The underlying cellulo-fibrous layers were divided, layer by layer and without hindrance, down to the wall of the sac, which was easily met with. When this wall was divided, a certain quantity of serous liquid exuded, and when the incision was enlarged outwards and inwards, a loop of small intestine, 6 or 8 centimetres long, was seen strongly distended with gases, injected with blood, and surrounded, especially downwards and inwards, by a somewhat voluminous and congested epiploic mass.

In order thoroughly to examine the state of the hernial intestine, I enlarged both the cutaneous incision and the opening of the sac. Not the smallest traces of the punctures made by the needle of the aspirator could be anywhere discovered, and I can testify to having searched for them with care, inasmuch as I expected a different result. The fact has likewise been verified by my colleagues MM. Berger and Richelot. I sought for the neck of the sac; it was very narrow, and appeared to be situated immediately below the crural arch. At this point the intestine appeared almost entirely surrounded by epiploon; however, I was able to divide upwards and outwards by making two small incisions. The release made and the intestine carefully wiped, I used gentle pressure to cause the hernial loop to return, and I observed that it was distended by gases only. The reduction was easy. The epiploon was left out. Extract of opium given. The night was quiet. Gas evacuated by the anus. The following day a little hemorrhage occurred. On the sixth day only, an abundant stool was had after a purgative injection. Perchloride of iron on the epiploon, then two applications of pâte de Canquoin. On the 1st of October the wound was almost cicatrized. On the 21st of October the wound was nearly healed, and the patient soon left the hospital.

ARTICLE VIII.

THIRD CATEGORY.

Strangulated Herniæ not reduced after Aspiration.—Kelotomy.— Death.

CASE I.—STRANGULATED CRURAL HERNIA—KELOTOMY —PUNCTURE OF THE EXPOSED INTESTINE — DIVISION —PERITONITIS — DEATH (Case reported in the hospital practice of M. Demarquay, by his house surgeon, M. Dupuy).—Madame L——, 45 years of age, suffering from strangulated crural hernia, was sent to the municipal *Maison de Santé* to undergo kelotomy. She was placed under M. Demarquay's care on the 14th of November, 1872. Her antecedents were as follows:—Health usually good. Ten years previously, while moving her bed, she used a somewhat violent effort, in consequence of which a hernia formed below the fold of the right groin. The patient took this tumour for a swollen gland, and treated it herself for some time by rubbing; finally, however, thinking that she had a hernia, she went to a truss maker, who put her on a bad truss, which kept the tumour in a very imperfectly reduced condition. She did not have a good apparatus, thoroughly reducing the hernia, until after three years; even then it protruded every evening when the patient removed the bandage. On the 12th November, in consequence of some slight exertion, the tumour protruded more than usual, and it was impossible to return it. Two hours after, Madame L—— was seized with terrible colic, and attacks of vomiting. On the 13th she continued to grow worse, and a medical man was called in. After having tried taxis ineffectually, he ordered an injection of tobacco, which only increased the colic. Two injections of honey were given, and an evacuation of fæces, in the shape of little hard balls, ensued. The vomiting continued frequent. Condition on the 14th of November was as follows :—Face congested, abdomen slightly tense, but very painful. At every instant, acute colic pains, vomiting of bilious matter. At the superior portion of Scarpa's triangle, on the right side, there was a small tumour, resonant at certain points to percussion, but dull at others. The form of the hernia was irregular and lobulated. The integuments which covered it retained their normal aspect. The least pressure on any part of the tumour caused most acute pain. M. Demarquay diagnosed a strangulated crural hernia, and in consequence of the gravity of the general condition, decided on operating there and then.

OPERATION.—The patient being placed under chloroform, M. Demarquay made an incision about 12 centimetres long, from above downwards. The skin and the subcutaneous cellular tissue having been cut through without giving rise to hæmorrhage, the hernial sac was speedily reached. The anterior wall of the sac having been carefully opened, a notable quantity of blackish blood came out, in a somewhat fluid state, on account of its admixture with serous matters. At the upper and internal portion of the sac, M. Demarquay found highly congested epiploon, showing numerous sanguineous extravasations in its tissue.

Outwards and upwards, a small intestinal loop was met with, in a high state of congestion, of a dark violet colour, but without any appearance of gangrene. The intestinal wall was punctured with the small trocar belonging to M. Potain's apparatus; aspiration gave issue to a small quantity of sanguineous liquid. The intestine, which was previously distended, recoiled on itself and shrunk up; but it was easy to see that it was not thoroughly emptied, and that it still contained a certain quantity of matters. M. Demarquay tried, but ineffectually, to reduce the intestinal loop. He then ascertained that it was firmly strangulated in a ring of the *fascia cribriformis*, very superficially situated, and of an almost circular form; this ring was divided at the lower external part. The division produced a flow of blood, and the tissues whence the blood came were seized with the forceps. Then, drawing the epiploic mass upwards and retaining it in that position, reduction was attempted; but again, this time also, these efforts at reduction were ineffectual. It was necessary to make a second division, and then it was possible at last, but not without difficulty, to entirely return the intestinal loop into the abdomen. A pill of 1 centigramme of thebaic extract was administered to the patient every hour. She went on well for three days; 20 grammes of castor-oil were given, as she had not had any action of the bowels. But peritonitis supervened, and she died on the morning of the 19th.

Autopsy.—Intestinal loops strongly distended by gases, redness and intense vascularity of the two peritoneal coats. In the vicinity of the pelvis the intestinal loops were agglutinated by false membranes, the cavity was filled with a sero-sanguineous, reddish effusion, containing floculi of thick yellowish pus. In the right iliac fossa, the lesions were more distinct, the false membranes agglutinating the intestine were thicker. At this level it was easy to recognize the intestinal loop, which was originally strangulated. It belonged to the small intestine, and showed, in a surface of 12 centimetres, the following lesions:—The diameter of that portion was notably contracted, while the neighbouring intestinal loops were, on the contrary, strongly distended by gases. In front, a

blackish ring was remarked, an evident trace of strangulation.   The tissue of the intestinal wall had a bluish-
black look; it was infiltrated with blood and plastic
lymph, consequently rigid, and inextensible.   The tissue
was nevertheless solid, and did not contain softened or
perforated points.   It was easy to verify the absence
of perforation by injecting water into that portion of the
intestine.   Finally, there existed intense congestion of
the intestine, without gangrene.   The epiploon, which
invaded the crural canal, was highly congested and full
of sanguineous extravasations.

CASE II.—STRANGULATED INGUINAL HERNIA—TAXIS—
ASPIRATORY PUNCTURE (NOT FOLLOWED BY ATTEMPTS AT
REDUCTION)—KELOTOMY—CŒCAL HERNIA—PERITONITIS
—DEATH—AUTOPSY (BY DR. FOLET OF LILLE).—On the
4th of last July, a man, of about 30 years old, came into
hospital, having a large inguinal hernia of the right side,
which he had kept up for several years by means of a
truss.   When he took off the truss, the hernia protruded
easily, and was generally returned in the same manner.
Several times, however, the reduction was difficult.   He
often went into a hospital to have his hernia reduced,
when it had protruded for four-and-twenty or forty-
eight hours, without his being able to return it himself.
The last time this occurred was about a year ago, symptoms of strangulation appeared, and taxis was attempted
several times, with the help of chloroform, without
results.   Operation for strangulated hernia was about to
be performed by M. Parise; the invalid was already under
chloroform for the purpose, when a last attempt being
made before cutting, the hernia returned.   Even this
lesson did not suffice to convince this unfortunate man
of the necessity of his never walking or working without wearing a truss.   In the last days of the month of
June, the spring of the truss he wore being broken, he

neglected to provide himself with another. The hernia came down and resisted all efforts to reduce it. Very acute pains made themselves felt in the hernial portion, and the patient could not make two steps without being bent double. Constipation and vomiting soon came on. This state of things had lasted more than two days when the patient came into the hospital. The hernia was a large inguino-scrotal one, as large as one's fist; it was somewhat painful to the touch, distended by gases, and gave a tympanitic sound. I first tried taxis without chloroform, the patient being placed on his back with the muscles completely relaxed. After some minutes consumed in vain efforts, I gave chloroform and endeavoured, for about a quarter of an hour, to replace this voluminous hernia by gently compressing it at the level of the neck, so as to make it repass gradually by the ring. I arrived at no result. Finally, I tried a band of india-rubber rolled round the hernia, so as to exercise a powerful compression from the bottom towards the neck. No success. I allowed the patient to come to. I had some ice applied over the tumour, and prescribed small pieces of ice to swallow, to quiet the vomiting, and also purgative injections. During the day, I begged my friend M. Castiaux, who was at Lille, to come the next day to the hospital, provided with his apparatus for aspiratory puncture. On the morning of the 5th, nothing was changed in the state of the patient; he had had more vomiting, and no action of the bowels. The tumour was still painful, and the skin covering it rather red, the evident result of the attempts at taxis. The hernia being still distended by gases and probably fluids, I saw indications of a necessity to remove the fluid and the gases by means of a very fine hollow needle, placed in communication with a pneumatic apparatus. M. Castiaux agreed with me, and without delay, we performed a puncture with No. 1 needle, in the middle portion of the anterior surface of the hernia.

P

A vacuum having been created in the receiver, and the needle adjusted to the connecting tube, we saw, as soon as the tap was opened, a liquid rush up into the receiver, the appearance and odour of which left no doubt as to its stercoraceous nature. When a few minutes had elapsed, the flow having ceased, without any sensible diminution in the size of the tumour, a second capillary puncture inside the first was made. It did not give issue to any liquid or gas ; in all probability, we had come upon the perihernial, cellular tissue.

A third puncture was made on the same vertical line as the first, but higher up.

This gave issue to a large quantity of gases and stercoraceous liquid. When the outflow ceased the receiver contained from 75 to 100 grammes of liquid, and the tumour was reduced to about half the original size. The question now was whether I should try to reduce. I might have been able to do so without using too much effort. I own that, like M. Richet, I dared not press and work up an intestine which had just been the seat of two or three punctures. It is true that it is asserted that the solutions of continuity, made with a capillary needle, only consist in a sort of pushing aside of the tissues, which return to their places as soon as the instrument is withdrawn, and stop the orifice so thoroughly that it cannot give exit to any liquid or even gas. Notwithstanding, I was not yet convinced that these intestinal acupunctures, however capillary they might be, would not allow a certain quantity of intestinal liquid to well out under the influence of the efforts at taxis, and which would give rise to serious results in the peritoneum. This mode of treatment had not been practised sufficiently often to relieve me of all fears on that point. I also found that M. Castiaux, who, having performed a large number of pneumatic punctures, ought consequently to have been bolder in the matter than I was, adhered to the opinion that it was better to leave the emptied hernia, in the hope of seeing it return spontaneously under the influence of intestinal excitants. I therefore had ice placed again on the hernia, and I prescribed several glasses of *lemonade Rogé*, and purgative injections. The patient had a bad day, no reduction occurred, the vomiting continued, and the pains again made their appearance. The next morning the hernia was as large as it was the day before. The skin of its anterior surface was intensely red, the slightest palpation gave great pain. Pulse rapid and small, and drawn countenance. I considered operation to be urgent, and performed it immediately. The intestine which presented itself was the cæcum in its entirety, with its vermiform appendage. We examined the intestine with care, and found no other indications of the punctures of the preceding day than a sort of small white elevation, which appeared to us to be a trace of one of the punctures. At another point a small, violet, coloured spot was visible. The intestine was intact at the level of the constriction. The patient died of peritonitis five days after operation.

AUTOPSY.—Lesions of acute peritonitis. The cæcum, the first part of the ascending colon, and the terminating part of the ileum, were removed and carefully examined.

The only possible trace found, of the two punctures, was a sort of small bluish-black swelling on the anterior surface of the cæcum, and it did not appear certain to me that this was indubitably the cicatrix of one of the two acupunctures. Insufflated under water, the intestine, although much distended, did not allow any air-bubbles to pass, the wall was perfectly intact, and the cæcum remained perfectly inflated.

ARTICLE IX.

CASES OF STRANGULATED HERNIA IN WHICH ASPIRATION OF THE SAC ONLY WAS PERFORMED.*

Large Strangulated Hernia.—Puncture of the Sac only.—Kelotomy.—Extra-Abdominal Volvulus.—Death (Case reported by M. Vallat, House Surgeon to M. Panas).

A man named Junker, 50 years of age, entered M. Panas' ward in the St. Louis Hospital, on the 21st July, 1872, for a right inguinal hernia which had been irreducible for about ten hours. This patient usually wore a truss to retain his hernia, which was very large, and had made its appearance thirty years previously. But for some short time back he had neglected that precaution, and on the 21st, after breakfast, he was taken with violent colic, whilst at the same time the distended scrotum became the seat of violent pain. He vainly tried to reduce his hernia, and a medical man who was called in was not more successful; in the evening he had rigors and vomiting, and he was then taken to the hospital, where the house surgeon performed taxis under chloroform, but without any result. Prescriptions for the night:—Ice on the tumour, purgative injection, and ice taken internally. When visited next day the patient was in a most alarming state, vomiting, distinctly fæcaloid, continued almost without intermission. The belly was inflated and painful, the countenance shrunk, the skin icy cold, and the pulse scarcely perceptible. The inguino-scrotal tumour was as large as two fists; hard and dull throughout the whole extent. Fluctuation was

---

* These cases, as we have already stated, should not be included in our statistics, since puncture of the sac only was performed.

distinct, the skin was affected by a very perceptible redness; finally, the testicle, which was recognizable by its
special sensitiveness, occupied the top of the tumour.
The puncture of the sac alone, performed by the aspirator,
gave outlet to 175 grammes of sanguino-serous matters.
Taxis was again essayed with chloroform, but without
result. It was then decided to operate. An incision
following the long axis of the tumour, and about 8 centimetres long, gave access to the sac, the hard and
resisting wall of which was divided on the grooved
sound. The intestine then appeared. It was of a
bluish red, and had not formed any adhesions with the
internal surface of the sac, the smooth whitish look of
which reminded one of fibrous tissue. The hernial loop
did not measure less than 15 centimetres ; it was turned
round on itself like a figure of 8, and formed a tumour as
large as one's fist. The inguinal ring was, however, perfectly free, and sufficiently dilated to allow the finger to
move freely around the intestine. The latter, after having
been untwisted, was replaced in the abdomen, but not
without difficulty, in consequence of the size of the ring
itself, and the enormous bulk of the hernial loop, which
had a tendency to protrude again, whilst it was being
reduced. Treatment—simple dressings, mercurial inunc-
tions.

On the 21st, in the evening, there was no improvement ;
the pulse was 100. Temp. 38·6 C.

On the morning of the 23rd the vomiting continued.
Temp. 38 C. Death took place at seven o'clock in the
evening. No autopsy could be obtained.

CASE II.—STRANGULATED HERNIA—ASPIRATION OF THE
LIQUID IN THE SAC (BY DR. AGUILLON OF RIOM)—KELO-
TOMY—RECOVERY.—A single woman, 35 years of age, had
suffered from a right crural hernia for five or six years,
which she often reduced herself, but of which, from motives

of delicacy, she had never spoken to any one. This hernia had been brought on by trying to lift a bundle of linen.

One evening last July, about six o'clock, symptoms of strangulation showed themselves suddenly, without any apparent cause.

They did not wish to disturb my father, who was confined to his bed by an attack of rheumatism. Two other surgeons who were called in employed taxis and all the usual means without success. The next morning, at seven o'clock, my father was informed of the uneasiness felt on her account; not being able to rise, he thought of trying an aspiratory puncture. I went to see the patient, provided with M. Potain's instrument. At that time the tumour was the size of a large hen's egg, hard and painful.

Puncture was performed by means of the capillary trocar, and gave issue to about 50 grammes of sanguino-serous fluid without gases.

The tumour immediately went down to the size of a walnut. It gave to the touch the distinct impression of a very hard intestinal loop. It was impossible for us to reduce it. We then saw that the trocar had only penetrated the sac. The somewhat uncertain results of the punctures hitherto performed, the difficulty of introducing the trocar into this small and deep-seated intestinal loop, made us reject the notion of a fresh puncture. We decided on performing kelotomy. My father succeeded in overcoming his pains, and reaching the patient's house, where he performed the operation at three o'clock in the evening. When the intestine was exposed, we saw, as we had supposed, that the sac alone had been punctured. No trace of puncture existed on the intestinal loop of which I have before spoken, but a graze, about a centimetre long, showed that the trocar had passed over it. Another portion of intestine, smaller than the first, and situated above it, was strangulated by the *fascia cribri-*

formis. Would a second puncture, performed over the main strangulation, have induced simultaneous reduction of these two portions of intestine was the question to be resolved. However that may have been, the patient recovered perfectly.

CASE III.—PUNCTURE OF THE SAC—KELOTOMY—DEATH. —Adrienne Marchais, artificial flower maker, æt. 30, came into the St. Louis Hospital at ten o'clock in the evening of the 16th July, 1871, under the care of M. Tillaux, for a strangulated hernia of the right side. The patient exhibited drawn features, pallor, hollow eyes, and distorted countenance.

The pulse was small and thready, marking 92 beats to the minute. The accident took place forty hours before admission to hospital, and the patient had had no subsequent action of the bowels. But hiccup and vomiting had set in since the previous night; the last mentioned having been composed of alimentary matters and bile. The tumour was the size of a hen's egg; it was hard, and very painful on the slightest pressure. It was the starting point of very acute colic, which preceded and brought on the fits of vomiting. The belly was painful, but very little distended. Before the patient came into hospital, taxis had been thrice unsuccessfully performed. M. Lebail, the house surgeon, tried it a fourth time, the patient having previously taken chloroform. He did not obtain any reduction. Then judging kelotomy urgent, he sent to fetch M. Tillaux. In his absence M. Panas was called in. He came at half-past ten—that is, more than forty hours after the appearance of the strangulation. The patient being placed under chloroform, M. Panas, after having in vain attempted reduction by a lengthened taxis, decided on operating. However, before proceeding to operate, it was agreed to try to obtain reduction by the aid of M. Dieulafoy's aspirator. The capillary needle was introduced into the tumour, but instead of penetrating in the first instance into the cavity of the intestinal loop, so as to withdraw the gases and the liquids which distended it, it took a wrong direction and found its way into the hernial sac.   About 120 grammes of clear yellowish liquid were quickly removed from it.   When this evacuation of the liquid in the sac was completed, the canula was withdrawn, and reduction by taxis essayed.   Reduction was effected with great ease.   The patient passed the remainder of the night quietly enough ; she had a copious evacuation the next morning, induced by a purgative injection.   Her face was less drawn, and her pulse 84.   The 18th passed tolerably well.   Beef-tea, a draught containing 15 drops of tincture of opium, and poultices on the belly were ordered. The night from the 18th to the 19th was good.   In the morning of the 19th, while the surgeon was going his rounds, the patient suddenly uttered a great and loud cry. She was immediately taken with acute colicky pains, rigors and unconquerable fits of vomiting of greenish and porraceous matters.   The pulse was small, hard, and thready, at 112.   The countenance was shrunken, the belly painful and distended.   The patient died three hours after, no doubt from peritonitis through perforation.   An autopsy could not be made.

CHAPTER IX.

OF THE PART PLAYED BY ASPIRATION IN INTESTINAL OCCLUSION AND IN INTESTINAL PNEUMATOSIS.

THE successes obtained by aspiration in the treatment of strangulated hernia would appear to indicate that this method might prove of equal utility in those intestinal disorders which have so much analogy with strangulated hernia.

I am not, however, in possession of sufficient data to write a chapter on this subject. In principle, experience has shown us that we may, without danger, puncture the intestine with No. 1 needle, and aspirate the gases which accumulate in such great abundance in gastro-intestinal pneumatosis and typhoid fever. Immediate relief is afforded to the patient by this proceeding, and the intestinal puncture may be repeated several times in the same day without any inconvenience. As to intestinal occlusion, it is so variable a disorder, in its nature and causes, that the utility of aspiration will depend on the circumstances of each case. Dr. Cazin, of Boulogne, obtained the cure of an intestinal occlusion by aspiration, proving that the obstruction was calculated to give way easily. He may have been dealing with a volvulus or an invagination, but, when the obstacle is caused by a tumour, a cancer, or by cicatricial bands, it is evident that aspiration would be powerless to effect a cure. The important fact is, that aspiratory punctures performed with Nos. 1 and 2 needles are as harmless in tympanitis, in gastro-intestinal pneumatosis, and in intestinal occlusion, as in strangulated

hernia.   I have employed them in two cases of intestinal
occlusion in which I have withdrawn gases and liquids to
the great relief of the patient, and without any consecutive ill effects.

M. Demarquay recently spoke, at the Société de Chirurgie, respecting the innocuousness and usefulness of this
process, in reference to a woman on whom he was about
to perform gastrotomy.

M. Douaud has employed aspiration in a case of intestinal occlusion, without the slightest accident having been
brought on by the aspiratory punctures.

PART III.

ON ASPIRATION OF THE SEROUS CAVITIES.

CHAPTER I.

ON THE TREATMENT OF EFFUSIONS INTO THE PERICARDIUM BY ASPIRATION.

Summary :—Article I.: History.—Description of the Method.—Article II.: Harmlessness of Aspiratory Puncture.—Puncture of the Heart.—Choice of the Place of the Puncture.—Experiments on the Dead Body.—Article III.: Description of the Operation.—Article IV.: Value of the Method and Remarks on it.—Article V.: Cases.

ARTICLE I.

History.—Description of the Method.

THE treatises which have been published on paracentesis of the pericardium, show that those surgeons who have performed this operation have always had two preoccupying ideas with regard to it ; one, to avoid the heart, and the other, to facilitate the outflow of the liquid contained within the serous membranes. The presence of the heart makes the operation a very delicate one, and although the indications obtained by percussion and auscultation are of the most precise kind, we still experience great repugnance in plunging the trocar into the pericardium, we hesitate before coming to a decision, we apply blisters, we administer purgatives, and, in a word, we try by every method to gain time and avoid operating. If we act thus, it is because, notwithstanding the extreme precision arrived at by clinical methods of investigation, it would still be possible to find some instances in which the diagnosis had been at fault.

Trousseau relates two facts of this kind, which I borrow from his clinical lectures. The first occurred in Vigla's wards at the Hôtel Dieu. It relates to a young man who came into the hospital in a state of dyspnœa approaching to asphyxia, and unable to give any account of himself. The patient bore the cicatrices of a recent application of leeches over the precordial region, and the expression of the face as well as external appearances testified to a recent illness. Examining the man as thoroughly as his condition allowed, Vigla found the lungs exempt from appreciable lesions, but there was extensive dulness at the region of the heart, complete absence of pulsation, no sounds, either normal or abnormal, with extreme frequency and smallness of the pulse.

The diagnosis of all those who saw the patient was : considerable effusion of fluid into the pericardium of recent date and inflammatory origin. The imminence of certain death made prompt and decided action indispensable, and paracentesis alone seeming to meet the symptoms, Roux was requested to perform it. Roux proceeded with great caution, employing incision in preference to puncture. The event proved that he had done wisely in so acting. When the thorax was opened and the surgeon had come upon the pericardium, he felt, and caused the assistants to feel, the heart, which beat immediately under the finger plunged into the wound, without the smallest fluctuation being recognizable. The operation was suspended, in expectation of that death which no skill could avert. At the autopsy a phenomenal dilatation (to use

Vigla's expression) was found, with attenuation of the walls of the heart; there were no valvular lesions, nor any serous matter in the pericardium.

The following circumstance occurred at the Hôtel Dieu hospital, in M. Trousseau's wards. The patient was a young woman attacked by dyspnœa, with œdema of the lower extremities and weakness of the pulse. For a long time this patient had suffered from palpitation of the heart, and her affection was of a complicated character. The great dulness of the præcordial region, the indistinct and, as it were, distant beat, a blowing murmur, of a grating character, heard during the systole and at the base, and prolonged through the vessels of the neck, the smallness of the pulse—all these signs warranted the conclusion that there was a serous effusion into the pericardium, and also a contraction of the aortic orifice. M. Barth, who saw the patient, shared this opinion. The patient improved a little, and left the hospital, but she came in again a few days afterwards, suffering from the same symptoms, but in a much more marked degree. She died two days after.

The autopsy demonstrated the existence of pericarditis, with considerable hypertrophy of the heart; the latter affection alone accounted for the great extent of the dulness in the præcordial region. The quantity of serum was not considerable. It is evident that cases of this kind, however rare they may be, have been so much the less favourable to paracentesis of the pericardium, because no method of performing the operation, at the same time easy of execution and satisfactory in result, is yet known. Thus this operation, though brought forward at various periods modified by the hands of skilful operators, and patronized by the most illustrious names, has never been thoroughly accepted, and is only included amongst the category of exceptional operations. In this it differs from paracentesis of the chest, which has become so rapidly popular. The reason is, that the apprehensions and dangers peculiar to the two operations are by no means identical. In the latter, the diagnosis is more simple, a single insertion of the trocar into an intercostal space constitutes the whole of the operation, and the liquid accumulated in the pleura issues forth abundantly as soon as an outlet is open to it. ' In paracentesis of the pericardium, on the contrary, we must reckon on difficulties and on accidents ; many precautions must be taken in order to penetrate into the cardiac envelope ; the operator must possess skill and some boldness ; he must be careful of the pleura, lest he produce pneumo-thorax ; he must avoid the mammary artery for fear of hæmorrhage ; he must, above all, dread any wound to the heart likely to bring on syncope and death ; and when these dangers have been avoided, when the liquid is reached, it flows badly, and only comes forth imperfectly and with great difficulty. If, to these considerations, we add the fact that paracentesis of the pericardium, performed under these unfavourable circumstances, has given but indifferent results, it is easy to comprehend why this operation has hitherto only enjoyed a limited reputation, and why it is only performed in the most exceptional cases. Since Riolan, who was the first to conceive the idea of penetrating into the pericardium, and Schuh, who put the plan into execution, many methods have been recommended, but none of them have yet arrived at rendering the manipulative process practical and easy. It is not my intention to here retrace the history of this operation, which, besides, has been so exhaustively treated by my venerated teacher, Trousseau. I shall content myself with passing in review the different methods which have been extolled, and the indications which they have endeavoured to realize, before describing the operation I propose.

Laennec recommends penetrating into the pericardium, after having trepanned the sternum above the xyphoid appendage.

Schuh chooses the intercostal space, comprised between the third and fourth rib, immediately outside the left edge of the sternum.

Heger perforates the space comprised between the fifth and sixth rib, 5½ centimetres outside the sternum.

Larrey penetrates between the fifth and sixth rib.

Trousseau, following the example of Aran and Fobert, chooses the fifth intercostal space; but, instead of at once performing puncture with the trocar, he, for safety's sake, recommends incising with the bistoury the different layers from the skin to the pericardium, with as much care as if the operator was dealing with a strangulated hernia.

This first stage of the operation being terminated, the next consists in penetrating between two cartilages as close as possible to the sternum, and as the cartilages touch each other at this point, they are moved by means of a spatula, or, if necessary, some portions are taken away. By this method the finger, introduced into the wound, takes simultaneous note of the absence of cardiac pulsation and of the tension of the pericardium by the liquid, and it is at this instant that Trousseau advises puncture to be made with the trocar.

This wise and prudent method is the one which has won most favour, but at this point, when we have penetrated into the pericardium, a real difficulty arises; and that is, how to promote the outflow of the liquid. The patient, at the moment of operation, is in a state bordering on asphyxia; he is lying flat or slightly raised by pillows, and it is not easy to change his position. Therefore, on reperusing the different cases of paracentesis of the pericardium, we see that, in the majority of cases, the liquid flows incompletely, it issues in driblets, infiltrates between the lips of the wound and falls partially into the pleura; for the reason, that the opening of the pericardium occupies a necessarily defective situation, and one little favourable to the flow. This is the reason why Larrey thought it preferable to make the puncture between the edge of the xyphoid appendage and the cartilage of the eighth rib on the left side, so as to attack the pericardium in the most depending position. In order to remedy the same inconveniences, use has, in several cases, been made of sounds allowed to remain for a long time in the pericardial cavity ; and Trousseau even tried unsuccessfully to remove the liquid by adapting a syringe to the end of a hollow sound. This expedient, however, not having proved successful, he goes so far as to say " that it is useless to try the different methods which have been recommended to expedite this evacuation, the use of aspirating pumps not affording any assistance, and complicating the process of operation in a very troublesome manner."

These words of Trousseau prove how far we were from the aspiratory method some years ago ; they also show that in this instance, as in many others, we were very near to it without perceiving it. It was felt deeply that there existed a chasm in medicine which no one knew how to fill up, and when the evacuation of a liquid was concerned, the use of pyulca and syringes was resorted to without giving a thought to the pneumatic machine and the previous vacuum, which was soon to give to us the aspirator. It is an undeniable fact, that at the moment of coming to a decision, and of evacuating an effusion of the pericardium, the dilemma presented itself, whether to perform simple puncture of the pericardium by means of a trocar, and to run the chance, in case of mistake, of transfixing the heart ; or to undertake incision by the bistoury—a very delicate and difficult operation to execute, and but little satisfactory in result. In the face of such an alternative, active intervention was generally avoided, temporising was resorted to, the operation was eluded by means of leeches or blisters, and it must be conceded, that data were wanting to arrive at the true value of a therapeutic method which was only employed under such unfavourable conditions.

Matters were in this state when I proposed in my communication to the Academy of Medicine at the meeting of the 2nd of November, 1869, to apply to effusions into the pericardium, the method of aspiration which I had extended to the treatment of all the pathological fluids. The method I pointed out seemed to me to unite all the conditions sought for by those who had occupied themselves with this question, that is to say : harmlessness of the operation, and complete and easy issue of the fluid. It was thenceforth possible to penetrate into the pericardium without fear or difficulty, by means of an extremely fine needle carrying a vacuum with it and intended to aspirate the fluid as soon as it met with it in its passage. For the difficult or delicate operation proposed by Aran, Jobert, and Trousseau, I substituted a simple puncture, neither necessitating special skill nor exceptional surgical attainments. Clinical observation was not backward in confirming the ideas which I had brought forward. On the 28th of January, 1870, Dr. Ponroy, then dresser to the Hôtel Dieu, performed aspiration in M. Frémy's ward on a patient attacked by purulent effusion into the pericardium, and the patient was cured. I shall report this interesting case further on, as well as those which followed it, but I wish first to explain the operation I propose in all its details.

ARTICLE II.

HARMLESSNESS OF ASPIRATORY PUNCTURE.

Puncture of the Heart.—Place to be chosen for the Puncture.—
Experiments on the Dead Body.

The harmlessness of the operation, and the facility in extracting the fluid are the conditions fulfilled by aspiratory puncture, as we shall endeavour to show.

Q

In the case of an effusion into the pericardium, we use, for performing aspiration, a needle measuring the third of a millimetre in diameter, and three times as small as the old-fashioned capillary trocar. The aspirator being prepared, that is to say, the previous vacuum being created, the needle is inserted into the tissues in search of the pericardial effusion. Supposing the misfortune of an error in diagnosis, the worst which can happen is that the needle may meet with the heart instead of meeting the fluid; the operator expecting to find an effusion, finds cardiac hypertrophy, a very uncommon mistake, but a possible one, since it has been made, as we have already stated, by clever and experienced men. Now what happens in such a case? Let us go through the different stages of the operation in detail. No. 1 needle inserted into the previously indicated intercostal space, is slowly pushed forward in search of the supposed fluid, and the operator carefully superintends its progress through the tissues, expecting with impatience the jet of fluid which would confirm his diagnosis. But the fluid does not make its appearance, and the needle, driven down more deeply, is soon seized with oscillatory, cardiographic movements, which very plainly show that the heart is reached. It remains to be proved that this puncture is not dangerous, and if the exploration is well conducted it ought to be unattended by danger.

In the search for fluids in the pericardium, more than in any other situation, it is necessary to proceed methodically. As soon as the needle has been introduced into the tissues, it must be pushed very slowly indeed, in the direction of the fluid, with the certainty that, after a passage of from 3 to 6 centimetres, it must meet with either the fluid or the heart. If it encounters the fluid, the latter immediately betrays its presence by traversing the crystal index, and indicates to us that it is useless to go further; if it meets the heart, at the moment it has pricked that organ, and before penetrating deeply, it is seized with a rhythmic movement, almost isochronous with the arterial pulsations, in a word—cardiographic, which shows us that the heart is reached.

Warned immediately of the error of the diagnosis, the needle is removed.

The puncture of the organ is so superficial and the needle is so fine, that these two circumstances alone would suffice to explain the harmlessness of the cardiac lesion. MM. Legros and Onimus have demonstrated that electro-puncture of the heart can be performed with impunity, and M. Steiner, continuing the experiments on the subject of the treatment of syncope during chloroformization, came to the same conclusion.

The diameter of the No. 1 aspiratory needle being the same as that of the acupuncture needle, it results that it enjoys the same harmlessness.

There exists an additional reason which should increase our security in the contingency of puncture of the heart, following on a mistake in diagnosis; it is that when an error is made as to the existence of an effusion into the pericardium, the error may be imputed to exceptional hypertrophy of the heart, and as the puncture (in consequence of the place chosen for it) touches the organ in the left ventricle and towards the apex, it follows that all the conditions of thickness are united, and that the puncture is so much the more insignificant from its encountering a hypertrophied cardiac muscle.

If the puncture touched the auricles, if the needle were as bulky as the old-fashioned capillary trocar, if the ventricle were perforated as far as the interior of its cavity, the conditions would be very different, and the danger would become very serious; but all these fears are removed, the auricle is never touched, the ventricle is scarcely pierced to the fourth part of its thickness; and if we add to that the fineness of the needle and the ventricular

Q 2

hypertrophy, we shall have collected all the causes which make the exploration of the pericardium harmless, even when there is an error of diagnosis. A needle with so small a diameter would be powerless to allow the fluid of the pericardium to pass, were it not in connection with the powerful force given to us by the aspirator. By aspiration, however, whatever may be the nature of the fluid, whether hematic or purulent, it is withdrawn with the greatest ease, so that the two difficulties of the problem, harmlessness of the operation and easy extraction of the fluid, so often sought for, seem to us to have at last found their solution.

The manipulatory part of the operation is therefore modified and singularly simplified by this new method, and in order to formulate it in all its details and to establish the different stages in the operation of paracentesis of the pericardium, I undertook a series of experiments on the dead body, of which the following summary gives the details.

First Experiment.

Performed on the body of an adult female of middle size. The sterno-thoracic plastron being removed and the pericardium carefully treated, I injected some water into the interior of the pericardial sac by means of No. 1 needle of the rack aspirator. The injection was slowly increased to 750 grammes, after which I took the dimensions of the pericardium thus distended :—

From the base to the apex . . 14 centimetres.
Transverse diameter . . . 16 centimetres.

The apex descended below the sixth rib, and the maximum of the transverse diameter coincided with the fourth intercostal space.

At this depth there is an indentation in the lung.

Second Experiment.

This was performed with the aid of M. Bougon, house-surgeon, on the dead body of a powerful man. The sterno-thoracic plastron being removed, I injected 950 grammes into the pericardium.

Professor Sappey, who was present at the experiments, was astonished at the elasticity and the capacity of the pericardium. Measurement gave us the following results :—

From the base to the apex . . . 17 centimetres.
Transverse diameter . . . 16 centimetres.

The maximum of the transverse diameter coincided with the fourth intercostal space and overlapped the left edge of the sternum 7 centimetres.

Third Experiment.

Performed on the dead body of a young man. The sterno-thoracic plastron being removed, the lungs were first insufflated so as to show their relations with the pericardium distended by fluid. I injected 900 grammes, and I found the dimensions of the pericardium to be—

From the base to the apex · . 16 centimetres.
Transverse diameter . . . 16 centimetres.

The pericardium overlapped the left edge of the sternum 9 centimetres; the maximum of the transverse diameter corresponded with the fourth intercostal space, and the lung was deeply indented at that point, in the form of a crescent. Other experiments, slightly varied, and undertaken with the same object, have afforded me analogous results, and enable me to formulate the following conclusions :—

1st. In a well-grown adult, the pericardium is able to contain a quantity of fluid amounting in exceptional cases to 1,000 or 1,200 grammes.

2nd. Whatever the degree of repletion of the pericardium may be, the maximum limit of the transverse diameter coincides with the fourth intercostal space, or with the fifth rib.

3rd. On this level, the pericardium is not covered •over by the lung ; on the contrary, the lung forms an indentation, a sort of crescent-shaped notch, which retains its form, even when the lung is insufflated. This notch is so situated that it coincides with the maximum point of the transverse diameter of the distended pericardium, and consequently leaves the way free for the aspiratory needle.

4th. The injected pericardium overlaps the left edge of the sternum to an extent varying from 7 to 12 centimetres.

5th. According to these experiments, the place· chosen for the puncture should be in the fourth or fifth intercostal space, and 6 centimetres outside the left edge of the sternum. These limits, however, are not absolute, they are susceptible of some modifications according to the particular conformation of the patient. We shall return to this question when describing the method of operation.

ARTICLE III.

Method of Operation in Aspiratory Puncture for Effusions into the Pericardium.

When about to perform paracentesis of the pericardium by aspiration, our first care ought to be to determine the situation to be chosen for the puncture. I have just demonstrated by experiments made on the dead body, that the maximum transverse diameter of the distended pericardium is in relation with the fourth and sometimes with the fifth intercostal division, and on the same plane; the lung is the seat of a notch which allows one to reach the pericardium several centimetres outside the left edge of the sternum. The operator may then take his choice of the fourth or fifth intercostal spaces, and if the fifth space appears to me to be preferable to the fourth, it is because it is nearer to the apex of the heart, and corresponds with a more depending situation of the fluid. Therefore by making the puncture in the fifth space, at 5 or 6 centimetres beyond the left edge of the sternum, the lung is avoided, and the operator need not trouble himself about the internal mammary artery, which is only a few millimetres distant from the edge of the sternum. Besides, if even, in an exceptional case, the aspiratory needle should encounter the lung in its progress, the inconvenience would be of the most trifling character, for these fine wounds of the organs are by no means formidable; but we shall have to descant more largely on this subject, when we study the treatment of pleurisy. The situation selected for puncture being then determined on, it is carefully marked in ink or pencil, and the operation is proceeded with.

The patient is slightly raised in bed by means of pillows, and if he be nervous, the annoyance of the puncture may be spared him by applying local anæsthesia by Richardson's instrument. If there is doubt about the diagnosis, it is better to use No. 1 needle to make the puncture; if the diagnosis is absolutely certain, it is better to use No. 2 needle.

I cannot too strongly recommend the operator to make sure of the permeability of the needle. Its calibre is so small, that a few grains of dust or rust are sufficient to block up the canal, and in operating with an obliterated needle, we run the risk of not recognizing the presence of the fluid and of puncturing the heart. It is therefore

imperative to pass a silver wire and a thread of water
through the needle, so as to make certain that it is
permeable. The aspirator being then set, that is, the
previous vacuum having been created, the needle is
introduced at the point decided on. When it has passed
through about a centimetre of the thickness of the tissues,
that is to say as soon as the opening situated at its
extremity is no longer in connection with the external air,
the corresponding tap of the aspirator is opened, and a
vacuum is made in the needle, which then becomes aspiratory. Thus we advance, vacuum in hand, in search of the
effusion.

It is necessary to be very precise in the direction given
to the needle. It ought not to be driven perpendicularly ;
on the contrary, it must be directed obliquely upwards
and inwards, and this movement must be carried on with
extreme slowness, watching attentively for the moment
when the fluid shall appear in the crystal index of the
aspirator. Thanks to the previous vacuum, the exact
moment the effusion is met with is known, and the
operator is not exposed to the danger of overrunning the
goal and puncturing the heart. As soon as the fluid is
reached, it flows into the aspirator, and the operation is
finished in a few minutes. If the flow stops suddenly,
and it is supposed that an obstructive body has stuck
in the needle, it suffices to give a reverse stroke of the
piston, to drive back the obstructing body, and aspiration is continued. In proportion as the fluid diminishes
in the pericardium, the heart draws nearer to the
needle. Theoretically one would be inclined to suppose
that a wound of the heart might be the consequence,
but practically one sees that it is not so ; besides,
according as the liquid flows, it suffices to move the
needle slightly backwards and forwards so as to place it
in a position nearly parallel to the ventricle. After the
fluid is evacuated the needle is withdrawn, leaving so

delicate a puncture that it is scarcely possible to find the traces of it on the skin, and the operation is finished without any need of the slightest dressing. The operation is thus shown to be of the greatest simplicity; fixing on the intercostal space alone may present some difficulty. In fact, the anasarca in certain patients, of which Case I. is an example, is so great that it is difficult to count the ribs through the thickened and infiltrated tissues.

There is then a risk of taking one space for another, and so far the evil would not be great; but a more grave consequence is the risk of passing through a costal cartilage, thus causing a round piece of cartilage to pass into the needle, and completely close up the orifice.

This error is the more easily explicable, as the costal cartilages converge at this point, and circumscribe only very incomplete spaces. In such a case, where the patient is suffering from anasarca, it is necessary, by means of continued pressure or repeated frictions, to induce local disappearance of the œdema, to enable one to find the intercostal space, and thus to avoid the danger which we have just pointed out.

If the pericardial effusion shows fresh tendencies towards forming again, we can without the slightest inconvenience renew the aspiration several times, making the incisions at the same point. If it is deemed necessary to make an injection, it is easy to do it there and then, without displacing the needle, by means of an aspiratory-injector. The injection can be measured, left *in situ*, or removed to the last drop at the pleasure of the operator. Thanks to this new instrument, we work protected from the air, and we know exactly the quantity of liquid introduced and taken away, because the aspirator is graduated. Aspiration and injection are performed one after another with the same facility and by the same mechanism. Without a single drop diverging from its true destination, the aspiratory needle lends itself, without displacement, to both uses, and the narrow conduit which serves to remove the pathological, also serves to introduce the modifying liquid. In a case of chronic pericarditis, with formation of purulent fluid, we think the indication would be to leave *in situ* a trocar analogous to the thoracic trocar,* so as to apply to the serous membrane the method of aspirations and successive washings, which give such good results in the treatment of chronic collections of fluid.

ARTICLE IV.

Value of the Method and Criticism.

Paracentesis of the pericardium by aspiration, as I have just described it, seems to me to realize a progress over the methods of operation which have been extolled since the time of Riolan to the present.

For puncture made with the trocar, full of uncertainty and danger, for incision with the bistoury, a difficult and little-practised operation, I substitute a simple needle prick, which does not necessitate boldness, nor special anatomical knowledge, nor particular surgical dexterity. For the imperfect and difficult flow of the pericardial fluid ; for the infiltration of that fluid into the lips of the wound and the pleura ; for the introduction of sounds, allowed to remain several hours, I substitute a powerful aspiratory force, capable of drawing the thickest fluid through a needle only half a millimetre in diameter.

The operation is now performed, subcutaneously, without pain to the patient, and without apprehension for the operator, who no longer has to contend with the serious preoccupations of a possible error in diagnosis,

* See Treatment of Chronic Pleurisy.

and who no longer has to dread the division of a vessel, the opening of the pleura, or the wounding of the lung.

The extraction of the fluids of the pericardium is incontestably one of the most useful applications of the aspiratory method. This formerly difficult operation is no longer exclusively confided to the skill of the surgeon—it enters the domain of medicine, enlarges the sphere of so-called medical operations, and is adapted to all capabilities, a consideration of some importance in the country, and in small towns or villages, where surgical skill is less commonly to be met with than medical knowledge.

Nowadays, paracentesis of the pericardium will be as simple to perform as paracentesis of the chest. The same reasons will not exist for avoiding interference, and for delaying to the last. Action will be taken in good time, and the operation, performed under the most favourable conditions, will give results which will allow it to be estimated at its true value. Such is the part played by the aspiratory needle in effusions into the pericardium. Whether it relate to fluids accumulated in the pleura, in the liver, in an articulation, or in the bladder, the means employed are always the same. · The mission of aspiration is to create a therapeutic unit by fusing into one the different methods which, before its advent, addressed themselves to the treatment of pathological fluids.

CASE I.—PERICARDITIS—EFFUSION OF SERO-PURULENT FLUID—PUNCTURE WITH M. DIEULAFOY'S INSTRUMENT—CURE (*Gazette des Hôpitaux,* 21 June, 1870).

(Case recorded by M. Ponroy, dresser to M. Frémy at the Hôtel Dieu.)

James R——, aged 21, a bricklayer, of robust appearance, had never been laid up, and had never suffered from articular pain. He came into hospital on the 28th of February, 1870, complaining of spots of pain on both sides of his chest, and suffering from fever, cough, depression, and slight oppression. Auscultation revealed mucous râles, and a slight blowing sound at the back of both lungs. His affection had originated a fortnight previously.

We diagnosed bronchitis with pneumonic spots in process of resolution. Two blisters and an antimonial draught got the better of this in five days.

Convalescence, at first decided, soon seemed to become but slowly confirmed, and finally retrogression set in. The pulse became higher, the tongue dry, there was much depression, and the belly became slightly distended.

The original symptoms did not, however, reappear in the breast, and in the difficulty we found in making a diagnosis, we held fast to the idea of enteric fever in the prodromic period, and waited for further evidence.

This preconceived notion unfortunately had the result of attracting our attention too particularly to the abdominal organs, and very probably caused us to misconstrue the true lesion which was developing itself. In fact, the series of enteric symptoms were not apparent.

The pulse had become small, the depression persistent, without having arrived at prostration. No epistaxis, no diarrhœa; the patient ate a little, and got up to go to the water-closet. He complained, however, of sleepless nights, was slightly oppressed, and showed a slightly cyanotic colour.

Whatever might have been the reason, we did not discover the true lesion until the 10th of March, after examination of the thorax. We found ourselves in presence of a considerable pericardial effusion, and of a pleuritic effusion occupying the base only of the left pleura. The other local symptoms of the effusion into the pericardium were arching of the superficial region, characteristic and decided dulness with loss of elasticity.

On auscultation, the heart sounds were muffled, distant but regular, their maximum of intensity was audible at a point situated well above the base of dulness. Treatment, a blister, a diuretic, julep, extract of rhatany. The following days, the symptoms, both general and local, grew in intensity, the cyanotic tint of the face grew deeper, the cellular tissue became infiltrated with serum ; thirst became excessive, the patient lost his appetite, had entirely sleepless nights, perhaps owing to the difficulty of breathing, which became more and more pronounced. We examined the urine several times ; it was not albuminous.

On the 28th of March, slight diarrhœa set in, which lasted until the 3rd of April, when it ceased without special treatment. Finally, after having applied five blisters on the cardiac region, without being able to arrest the progress of these symptoms, it became necessary to think of puncture. The state of the patient on the 7th of April, the day on which the operation was performed, was as follows :—

He was lying on his left side, indifferent to everything about him, with anasarca so considerable as to double the size of the lower members ; his eyelids were closed, his eyes dull, and dyspnœa was intense. The skin was very pale, the lips bluish, the pulse thready, giving 116 pulsations. We had never observed syncope, even at this period of the malady. Considerable arching at the region of the heart ; pressure caused pain at the level of the fifth and sixth ribs.

The dulness extended towards the right, 6 centimetres beyond the median line of the sternum ; downwards, it had passed the diaphragm and descended below the xyphoid appendage ; on the left, it passed into the lung-dulness. It will be remembered that we had pointed out a slight effusion at the base of the left lung, the effusion had increased with the pericarditis, it now occupied the inferior half of the backward portion of the left pleura. On auscultation, we found the heart sounds sensibly diminished, but they were not stifled as the intensity of the other symptoms would have led us to believe. At the base of the left lung, there was an absence of vesicular murmur, and a diminution of thoracic vibrations ; at the superior portion mucous râles ; no respiration, no ægophony. The right lung acted well and presented no signs of lesion. Notwithstanding the gravity of the general symptoms, a tongue as dry as a chip, and excessive thirst, there was no diarrhœa. From this description it will be evident that our sole remaining hope was in puncture. It was performed on the 7th of April with M. Dieulafoy's aspiratory instrument. We regret that our limits prevent us from giving a description of this apparatus. We shall only be able to say as much as is necessary for the right understanding of the matter. We employed a needle measuring a millimetre in diameter, that is to say, rather smaller than an ordinary capillary trocar. This needle is deeply bevelled at the lower part, an arrangement which allows it to penetrate without the need of an internal stiletto. It is provided at the top with an adjustment which can be put in direct communication with the mouth of a glass aspirator, in which a vacuum has been previously made. Thanks to the extent of the dulness, and above all owing to the perfection of the instruments, the puncture presented but little difficulty. The anasarca, however, was so great that we found it impossible to reckon the intercostal spaces, though the integuments thickened to the extent of several centimetres. We chose a situation 1 centimetre above the base of the dulness, and about 6 centimetres to the left of the median line of the sternum. At the depth to which we had penetrated, the costal cartilages correspond to the false ribs. They only circumscribe imperfect spaces ; independent at their external part, these cartilages converge, unite with each other at an acute angle, and are inserted at the same point of the sternum. We inserted the canula inclined from below upwards, imparting a rotatory movement to it; it penetrated easily, without meeting with more resistance at one point than the other, and disappeared under the tegument to the depth of 6 or 7 centimetres. A little liquid came in driblets out of the external extremity; we were in the pericardium. Then applying the syringe directly over the canula, we made the aspiration.

This puncture produced almost 800 grammes of fluid, opaque and of a yellowish-white colour; in a word, a perfectly purulent fluid. Rather discouraged by the purulent appearance of the fluid, and judging in advance that in consequence of the general condition, the operation would be useless, we gave up the idea of making an injection. The fluid ceased to flow. We took away the canula, and were not a little surprised to see the lower end stopped up by a little circlet of cartilage not less than a centimetre long, and which had become fixed in the opening as in a cutting drill. We had passed through a costal cartilage, and the flux of liquid was owing to the presence of an opening which fortunately for this case was placed at the side of the canula. The opening was itself half obturated by the upper part of the cartilage. The patient did not feel immediate relief, the dyspnœa and exhaustion persisted; the pulse, however, was rather better. Though the dulness was still present, it was less extended; it scarcely passed beyond the left edge of the sternum. The loss of elasticity was less complete. On the left the dulness of the pericardium was blended with that of the pleura. On auscultation, the heart sounds were manifestly louder, whilst the original signs of pleurisy were present at the base of the lungs. The next day the improvement was decided, the dyspnœa was less, the anasarca diminished; the patient showed some signs of appetite, but on the other hand he was tormented by paroxysms of coughing, and the pulse was still at 116. On the next day, the 8th of April, the anasarca had still further diminished; the cough was persistent, with vomiting of food during the fits. The pulse was at 95 in the morning, 108 in the evening. We found a differ-ence of two degrees between the morning and evening temperature taken in the axilla. Auscultation showed no friction sounds. The first sound was reduplicated at the base. The pleurisy, with all its symptoms, still persisted.

The ensuing days we seemed to be witnessing the resurrection of our patient. The anasarca was inclined to disappear, the dyspnœa, the cough ceased, thirst diminished, and sleep was good. On the 10th of April, slight epistaxis; the patient was put on ordinary diet, at his own request. He got up on the 18th. The anasarca was reduced to a small amount of perimalleolar œdema. Of all the symptoms of pericarditis there only re-mained a very limited dulness. The acute stage was past, but had made way for a chronic stage, which we could see would be long before it progressed to recovery. The patient was very emaciated, very anæmic. The least exertion exhausted him, the colour of his face was that of a man in whom hematosis is ill-performed. His lips were blue. The pulse, which gave 80 beats in the morning, rose to 100 in the evening. Profuse sweats came on in the night. It became a question to what this state of marasmus, which was greatly prolonged without ameliora-tion after the cure of the pericarditis, was due. Had the patient tubercles in the lungs, or was pus forming some-where, or did the symptoms point to a heart changed in its elements ? Or did not the pleurisy, the fluid of which was being slowly reabsorbed to organize itself into false membranes, suffice to explain these symptoms of exhaus-tion and slow asphyxia. We adhered to the last idea, for the reason that we found no lesions elsewhere than in the pleura. In fact, with regard to the heart, there were no signs of adhesion or hypertrophy, only a simple prolongation of the first bruit at the base. With regard to the lungs, we had never been able to detect any symptom of tubercle of the apices, whilst on the contrary the effusion into the left pleura gave us the following indications :—

In proportion as the fluid became reabsorbed, and the vesicular murmur became audible over a larger area, we perceived the dulness preserving the same extent, and we heard a more considerable pleuritic friction develope itself at the points abandoned by the fluid. From time to time the cough and the painful spots reappeared, and disappeared after the application of blisters. In a word, we were witnessing the manufacture of false membranes in the left pleura, and the pleura was full of them when the patient left us on the 27th of May to go to Vincennes.

Before he left, he was still emaciated and cyanotic, his nails had become hypocratic. In the evening, his ancles showed œdema, at the same time the pulse rose, sweating came on and continued through the night. Sleep, however, was moderately regular, and the appetite so large that the patient could eat three portions. His digestion was good, and there was no diarrhœa. We were able to make the following summary of the case: Cure after a puncture of a considerable sero-purulent effusion into the pericardium.

CASE II.—PERICARDITIS AND PLEURISY—ASPIRATION (BY DR. CHAILLOU OF TOURNY).—I was called in to see a patient attacked by effusion into the pericardium, the diagnosis of which was not, however, absolutely certain. The appearance of the patient did not recall to my mind the asystolism which terminates cardiac affections. A man still young, lividly pale, was partly recumbent, partly supported by pillows. His breathing was laboured, he was trying to find an easy position. His hands were cold and blue, and the pulse was irrecognizable. If I had had a sphygmograph I should have obtained a death-curve. The cardiac shock was no longer perceptible. The pericardial arching was strongly pronounced, and dulness extended over a large area. The two physicians who were present agreed with me that the death of the patient was imminent. I rejected the idea of a valvular affection, and I had no trouble in demonstrating the existence of an effusion into the pericardium. Examination of the patient also enabled us to discover another effusion into the pleura of the left side. It was evident that no medical means could relieve the patient. The intervention of surgery could alone give some respite and keep off impending dissolution.

I therefore proposed to make use of the aspirator, first to empty the pleura in order to isolate the dulness of the heart, then to puncture the pericardium.

The puncture of the pleura was made with Dieulafoy's needle No. 2; and gave a litre and a half of slightly pinkish, serous matter. The puncture of the pericardium, made with the same needle, gave issue to 625 grammes (carefully weighed) of a dull, brownish-red, serous fluid, differing greatly from pure blood.

These 625 grammes flowed slowly, notwithstanding the aspiration. But in proportion as the fluid collected in its appointed receptacle, the pulse regained its normal strength, the far-off heart sounds seemed to draw nearer, and the cardiac movement became perceptible. Immediately after aspiration the face and hands regained their colour.

Three hours after the operation, the hands were sufficiently warm, and the face more than usually flushed. The patient could sleep, which he had not been able to do for many days. From this time forward the improvement was progressive. But I was called in again ten days afterwards. The pleuritic effusion had reappeared. As to the pericardial effusion, it seemed also to be in process of reproduction, but not in sufficient abundance to necessitate a fresh puncture of the pericardium. I took away a litre and a quarter of fluid, and I made a small iodized injection. The first drops of this injection produced sharp pain, so I did not persevere.

The patient, in addition to an incessant cough, expectorated sputa, resembling those of the second stage of pulmonary phthisis.

Four days afterwards, the patient died, with symptoms of pulmonary congestion, and without any fresh appearance of the pericardial effusion.

CASE III.—PERICARDITIS AND PLEURISY—ASPIRATION—PULMONARY PHTHISIS—DEATH (DR. CHAIROU, SURGEON TO THE ASYLUM AT VÉSINET).—François Thomirel, a soldier, 27 years of age, without any hereditary diathesis, entered the asylum at Vesinet on the 31st of July, under the care of Dr. Fleury. The patient had been seized with oppression and cough in the month of June of the same year, which had obliged him in the first instance to go for a fortnight into the hospital of Versailles.

The man was very much emaciated; and considerable ascites and œdema of the scrotum and of the lower limbs were remarked. His breathing was greatly oppressed, there were fifty-five to sixty inspirations per minute; the voice was weak and muffled, with incessant anxiety. Several veritable asphyxial crises occurred during the day. Auscultation showed fine hissing and mucous râles in the two lungs and ægophony of the left side; the heart sounds were weak and distant. Percussion showed absolute dulness on the left side to within two centimetres of the right edge of the sternum, and descending as far as four centimetres above the umbilicus. The diagnosis gave the following results: 1. A pleuritic effusion on the left. 2. A hydropericardium.

R 2

On the 2nd of September, in consequence of the constantly increasing danger, M. Chairou performed thoracentesis in the situation decided on, in the presence of Drs. Maugras, Fleury, and Alibrand, with No. 2 needle of Dieulafoy's aspirator. 1,430 grammes of dark, yellow fluid were removed. The heart, examined immediately after the operation, did not appear modified in its relations. The two following days, the general condition not being ameliorated, and the pericardial dulness being the same, aspiratory puncture of the pericardium was performed.

The operation was performed on the 4th of September by means of needle No. 2. The puncture was made in the fifth intercostal space, 2 centimetres outside the nipple. The needle was directed from before backwards, and from without inwards, and it met with the fluid after traversing 6 centimetres. The operation lasted thirty minutes, and 995 grammes of reddish, serous fluid were evacuated. The patient felt immense relief; he was able to sleep for some hours, respiration became regular, and the next day he was walking about the galleries. But the œdema did not diminish, fresh attacks of asphyxia took place on the 6th and 7th of September. The pericardial dulness also remained unaltered in extent, and it was evident that the fluid was accumulating afresh in the pericardium. Nevertheless, there was an improvement from the 8th, lasting nearly a fortnight, but this improvement was not maintained; the patient coughed and became thinner, completely lost his appetite, his strength diminished rapidly, and death took place on the 25th of October, six weeks after the puncture of the pericardium. This interesting case was read by M. Chairou at the Academy of Medicine, and amongst the very circumstantial details reported of the autopsy, it is particularly to be noted that the heart was hypertrophied, and that the lungs were loaded with tubercles.

CHAPTER II.

THE DIAGNOSIS AND TREATMENT OF ACUTE AND CHRONIC
EFFUSIONS INTO THE PLEURA BY ASPIRATION.

Summary: Article I.: History.—Exposition of the Method.—Article
II.: Function of Aspiration in the Diagnosis of Effusions
into the Pleura.—Uncertainty of Diagnosis.—Insufficiency of
the Symptoms.—Description of the Operation.—Puncture of
the Lung and of its Harmlessness.—Article III.: Treatment
of Acute Pleurisy.—Article IV.: Treatment of Purulent
Pleurisy and Pneumothorax. — Article V.: Value of and
Remarks on the Method.

ARTICLE I.

History.—Exposition of the Method.

Two men above all others have contributed to make known
and to popularize the treatment of acute and chronic
effusions into the pleura : Trousseau, who was, so to speak,
the inventor of thoracentesis ; and M. Potain, who, by
inventing an ingenious syphon system, has shown us the
results which may be expected, in purulent pleurisy, from
frequently repeated washings.

The methods employed up to the present time seemed
to suffice for our therapeutic needs, when I proposed to
substitute aspiration for them, and the new method was
applied for the first time to the diagnosis and treatment
of effusions into the pleura in January, 1870, in the wards
of M. Axenfeld, whose house surgeon I had the honour to
be. A patient suffering from acute pleurisy had been
admitted into the Beaujon Hospital, with an enormous effusion situated in the left side. The indication was urgent,

the heart was greatly displaced, and I performed thoracentesis by means of the aspirator. The operation was of the most simple description. I evacuated eighteen hundred grammes of fluid. The patient did not have a single fit of coughing, the outflow did not stop for an instant, and some days afterwards, the man was able to leave the hospital in perfect health. In a short time, I collected a certain number of cases of the same kind, I made the new method known in my first memoir on aspiration, and I described it in detail in an article published in the *Gazette des Hôpitaux* of the 18th April, 1870, entitled " Diagnosis and Treatment by Aspiration of Effusions into the Pleura." Thenceforward the impulse was given, the trocar and gold-beater's skin were destined to fall into oblivion, and aspiration was about to become the classic method of thoracentesis. If I recall these facts and dates, it is because they have been somewhat overlooked in a recent academic discussion. It is true that at the same period they were recalled to the memory of the *Société Médicale des Hôpitaux* by Dr. Libermann, who, after examination and study of the subject, settled the question of priority once for all, in terms which admit of no doubt.*

"Let us be clear," said M. Libermann, "on this method of aspiration, for it is obtaining such extension, that it is desirable to determine clearly its origin and to discuss its value. In all epochs, the notion of facilitating the outflow of the fluids of the pleura by means of instruments destined to draw these fluids out has been entertained. M. Bouchut, in a lately published work, treats the historical side of the question with his customary erudition. He describes to us the method employed by Galen in the operation for empyema, that is to say the introduction into the chest of a long

* Report of the meeting of the *Société de Médicine des Hôpitaux*, May 10th, 1872.

canula on which was fixed a syringe destined to draw out the pus. Galen had given to this instrument the name of pyulcon. In the 17th century, suction of the chest, performed by means of different kinds of pyulca, was very much in vogue; witness the description given by Scultet in 1640. The same instruments have again made their appearance in a nearly analogous form in our times. I would specially mention M. J. Guérin's instrument, composed of a syringe and a flattened, capacious trocar. These different instruments have fallen into oblivion, of which proof is afforded by the fact that they are nowhere mentioned by the recent writers who speak of thoracentesis. One proceeding alone was everywhere described and everywhere employed, the evacuation of the fluid by means of trocars of varying dimensions, from Reybard's large canula to M. Blachez' capillary trocar.

"Matters were in this state when we saw, a short time since, the history of thoracentesis enter on a new phase. Cases in which operation had been performed by means of a certain method of aspiration came in upon us by hundreds from France and from abroad. It was a veritable infatuation. Now in what does thoracentesis by aspiration as it is nowadays performed consist, and what is its true value?

" To my mind, it does not only consist in the perfecting of methods fallen into disuse, it does not only consist in a simple modification of the action of an instrument, but it may be said that we are at this moment in possession of new instruments, which have received the name of aspirators from M. Dieulafoy, and which allow aspiration to be raised to a method which leaves suction as practised by the ancient authors far in the background.

" The novelty of our present aspirators does not only lie in the powerful vacuum and the extreme fineness of the needle, but in the application of the previous vacuum, which is so valuable a resource in therapeutics. It is this principle which differentiates our aspirators (a genuine French discovery) from the instruments which preceded them, and we were not a little surprised when M. Broca came to the Academy to claim priority for a trocar of M. Van den Corput, whilst I could not see the smallest analogy between the two instruments."

In a communication made by M. Potain to the *Société de Médicine des Hôpitaux,*[*] he, studying the same question from historical and clinical points of view, gave a similar judgment, and did me the honour to attribute the priority of this new method to me. I quote his words literally. "Thoracentesis is now no more than a pin-prick, which M. Dieulafoy has incontestably the honour of having been the first to perform."

Dr. Ligerot arrived at the same conclusions in his inaugural thesis, so that it appears to me that this question, which it is useless to discuss farther, is definitively decided.

It is aspiration as it has been here described, and as I laid it before the Academy of Medicine (meeting of the 2nd of November, 1869), which I am about to examine in its application to effusions into the pleura. It seems to me that the diversity of opinions which are pronounced at the present time, on the value of this method, proceeds from a confusion which it is important to dispel, and the discussion threatens to be sterile if we do not understand one another from the first.

Notwithstanding the quantity of data we already possess with regard to the new method—perhaps even on account of that abundance—the question is far from being decided.

Information reaching me from abroad, and my own observation, lead me to believe that goldbeater's skin and the trocar have already made way for the aspiratory needle, that puncture is replaced by aspiration, and the question of

---

[*] Meeting of the 10th of May, 1872. De l'utilité des Trocarts capillaires dans la Thoracentèse.

the treatment of acute and chronic effusions into the pleura completely opened up afresh. This new method has largely occupied the Parisian Academy of Medicine, it is discussed in the different scientific societies, employed in the hospitals, and every day forms a subject for clinical lectures, theses, and numberless publications.

Three years have sufficed to work these changes, and by casting a glance over the entire medical press, both of France and of other countries, it is easy to convince oneself that men's minds are drawn into a fresh channel.*

But will not this infatuation, which is usually a concomitant of all novelties, be followed by reaction ? And is aspiration in regard to pleural effusions a real advance on the former methods ? This question we shall proceed to

* Du Diagnostic et du Traitement des Epanchements de la Plèvre par Aspiration. Dieulafoy. *Gazette des Hôpitaux.* Ap. 18th, 1870.

Deu serose Pleurits operative Behandlung, by Dr. Rasmussen, Dec., 1870.

De la Thoracenthèse par Aspiration, dans la Pleurésie purulente et dans l'Hydro-pneumothorax. Bouchut. Paris, 1871.

Société de Médicine des Hôpitaux. A communication made by M. Potain on the Utility of Capillary Trocars and of Aspiration in Thoracentesis. Meeting of May 10th, 1872.

Société de Médicine des Hôpitaux. De la Thoracentèse par Aspiration Meeting of July 12th, 1872.

Académie de Médecine. Empyème et Thoracentèse par Aspiration. Meeting of July 13th, 1872, and following meetings.

Berliner Klinische Wochenshrift. Nos. 6, 7, 8. 1872.

" Etude et Critique de l'Ouvrage de M. Woillez " by M. Blachez. *Gazette Hebdomadaire.* Feb. 2nd, 1872.

Observations de Pleurésie traitée par Aspiration. Chaillou. *Gazette des Hôpitaux.* May, 1872.

La jeune et la veille Thoracenthèse. Bouchut. *Gazette des Hôpitaux,* July, 1872.

Resumé sur la Thoracentèse ; thèse de doctorat. Lejerot. Paris, 1872.

Du Diagnostic et du Traitement des Epanchements de la Plèvre par Aspiration. Dieulafoy. *Bulletin de Thérapeutique,* 1872.

Usages de l'Aspirateur de M. Dieulafoy en Russie. Report of Dr. de Kieter, Professor of Clinical Surgery at St. Petersburg.

examine. In this, as in everything else, the first impulse
was to rebel against the new method; and inevitable
theory proceeded to play its part in demonstrating the
inefficacy and the uselessness of aspiration. It was put
forward how the needle might wound the lung and cause
accidents, and how the strength of the vacuum might
bring on pulmonary hæmorrhage and tear the false membranes. These reasonings were disguised under an
appearance of logic, and the question was entangled
in this dilemma :—if the needle be too fine, the pus will
not pass ; if it be capacious, wherefore reject the ordinary
trocar, and of what good are such innovations ? But no
theories prevented cases from arriving in abundance from
all sides, and it is by means of these numerous facts that
we shall be enabled to reply to every one of the objections
which have been made, and that we shall establish the
worth of aspiration, 1st, as a means of diagnosis, 2nd, as
a means of treatment.

ARTICLE II.

PART PLAYED BY ASPIRATION IN THE DIAGNOSIS OF EFFUSIONS INTO THE PLEURA.

Uncertainty of the Diagnosis.—Insufficiency of the Symptoms.—
Description of the Operation.—Puncture of the Lung and its
Harmlessness.

Pleurisy is a disease full of surprises. When it is
clearly acute, and when the typical symptoms are all
present, its diagnosis is of unparalleled simplicity.
Dulness, absence of thoracic vibrations, and ægophony,
constitute a triad of symptoms which never deceive, and
which enable us to plunge a large trocar into the chest
without apprehension or danger.

But these signs are often absent, or so altered in
character, that considerable effusion may only arouse

slight suspicion, and pass unperceived. Above all, in interlobar pleurisy the progress is insidious, and the symptoms slightly marked; as a matter of fact, the effusion is developed and becomes encysted in the depth of the organ; it is not peripheral, it is central, the lung conceals and surrounds it so effectually that the too often unrecognized disease terminates by a vomica or by a pneumothorax.

Under other conditions, the symptoms of an effusion are recognized in a pleura which does not contain any fluid, a phenomenon sometimes noticed when thoracenthesis is performed; the patient is examined at the moment the fluid is withdrawn (*sic*), and the signs of effusion are yet so evident that we should willingly believe in its presence if we had not proofs to the contrary. What is occurring in such a case ? It is probable that very slight modifications of the pleura suffice to change the normal conditions of auscultation and percussion; a thin layer of fluid interposed between the lung and the thorax, or still more, the imbibition of the serous membrane, and its thickening consequent on the presence of an exudation, are the causes of the phenomena pointed out. I am the more ready to believe this, as in certain patients attacked by pleuro-pneumonia in whom the effusion was reduced to very small proportions, it sufficed to aspirate the 30 or 40 grammes of fluid which separated the pleura from the lung, to cause the ægophony to disappear. Certain signs of pleurisy are then independent of the abundance of fluid effused, and show themselves, provided that an insignificant quantity of fluid intervene to change the relations existing between the pleura and the lung.

Although it will not be new to any one to find that the diagnosis of a pleuritic effusion may be surrounded by the greatest difficulties, we wish to offer some cases in proof of the fact. The following is a summary :—

1. The developement of the thorax of the affected side may be wanting with an effusion of 1,600 grammes. (Case reported by Dr. Brochin. *Gazette des Hôpitaux,* 26th March, 1870.)

A woman, under the care of M. Axenfeld, at the Beaujon Hospital, presented on examination the whole assemblage of the clearest signs of a pleuritic effusion. It was a typical case, not one sign was wanting, but we deceived ourselves, there was one absent, or rather contradictory; we refer to the comparative capacity of the two sides of the chest. The effusion had taken place on the left side, and it was the right side of the chest which showed a larger capacity than the left. A hint may here be given to those who give exaggerated value to certain signs taken singly. Aspiration was performed, 1,600 grammes of serous matter removed, and the patient recovered rapidly.

2. Thoracic vibrations may be preserved and even exaggerated with an effusion of 900 grammes. (Case communicated by M. Blain, house surgeon to M. Hérard.)

A young man of 18 was suddenly taken, six weeks previously, with a general feeling of illness, accompanied by shiverings, fever, and pain in the back. The cough was not severe, and ceased completely after a fortnight. The patient, feeling better, took a two-hours' walk, but returned very much fatigued, with a painful spot under the left nipple. On coming into the hospital the young man still complained of the same pain, and had a slight access of fever every night. There was no dyspnœa, sleep was good, appetite as usual, and the bowels regular. Respiration was so easy that the patient sat up in bed without difficulty, and would have got up had he been allowed to do so.

Percussion showed normal resonance of the left side, and absolute dulness of the right, from the apex to the base of the lung. Auscultation revealed normal respiration on the left side, but a considerable weakening of the vesicular murmur of the right side, with some sub-crepitant *râles,* imitating friction sounds, and situated particularly below the spine of the scapula. There was no ægophony, but slight muffled breathing. Thoracic vibrations existed as clearly on the right side as on the left; they were perhaps even slightly increased on the right side. It is true that this anomaly was sufficient greatly to obscure the diagnosis. Recourse was had to M. Dieulafoy's aspirator, and 900 grammes of fluid were taken away from the right side of the chest. The patient went out of the hospital shortly afterwards cured.

3. Resonance partly preserved may coincide with an effusion of 2,000 grammes. (*Gazette des Hôpitaux,* 28th April, 1870.)

In the course of the month of January, M. Matice, physician to the Beaujon Hospital, requested that the thoracic cavity of a patient in his ward should be explored by means of an aspirator. The case was sufficiently doubtful to make it very satisfactory to acquire certainty as to the presence of an effusion before deciding on thoracentesis. M. Axenfeld examined the patient, and he found so marked an absence of characteristic signs at the back of the chest, that if he had not pushed the examination further, it would have thrown doubt on the presence of a collection. It was only in the right axilla that he found a somewhat extended dulness, varying a little according to the position of the invalid, and accompanied by a slight ægophony. The liver appeared lowered. With such scanty indications there was reason to accede to the idea of an effusion, but there was no reason to believe there was any ground for thoracentesis. I performed aspiration, and the almost doubtful effusion did not cease flowing until 2,000 grammes of slightly purulent fluid had been removed. By the side of these cases, where the most typical signs, developement of the thorax, disappearance of the vibrations, and dulness, were wanting, we could cite instances in which the assemblage of these signs was due to the existence of some disease other than effusion. I remember, amongst others, a cancer of the left lung, on which Dr. Dechambre did me the honour to consult me ; a cancer which offered all the signs of a thoracic effusion. Aspiration performed, first by me, and a fortnight later by Dr. Hénocque, demonstrated that there was not the smallest quantity of fluid. Professor Sée told me, some days before, that after having verified the symptoms of an effusion into the pleura, he had decided on aspiration. The operation was performed with the assistance of M. Choyau, but the aspiratory needle was introduced into the thorax three times in vain ; a few drops of blood proved that the lung was touched, and demonstrated at the same time that there was no fluid there.

Dr. Martineau lately informed me of an analogous fact. He found symptoms of an effusion into the pleura in a woman, he performed aspiratory puncture with the help of M. Bouilly, house surgeon, but he found no fluid.

I could multiply these examples ; indeed I have just verified a fresh one under M. Tardieu's care at the Hôtel Dieu. We made several aspiratory punctures on a patient who showed indubitable symptoms of effusion into the pleura, and these multiple punctures demonstrated to us that fluid did not exist.

It is certain, from a clinical point of view, that on the one side it is possible to find effusions which are not accompanied by characteristic symptoms, and on the other to observe these symptoms without the existence of any effusion ; therefore puncture of the pleura for the evacuation of fluid, the presence of which seems doubtful, or exists only in small quantities, is looked upon as rash and useless. Thoracentesis is reserved for undoubted cases, and it must be granted that difficulties stand in the way of forming a judgment about a means to which recoursè is only had for want of a better, and as a last resource. What an amount of hesitation in difficult cases, how many paintings with tincture of iodine, how many blisters destined to favour the absorption of the effusion, do we sometimes see! Are these different means, which we say openly are sometimes rather abused, always the result of a therapeutic conviction? are they not sometimes inspired by the prudence and uncertainty which are the consequences of our powerlessness to ascertain the diagnosis? I do not think it out of place to make such an avowal here. The signs of pleurisy are not always sufficient to incontestably establish its diagnosis; ægophony, inspiration, diminution of thoracic vibrations, the amplitude of the affected side, all these symptoms may be wanting. We suspect pleurisy, and we often are in doubt as to the quantity of the effusion; it is then that we dwell with so much complaisance on an idea which seems to reconcile the treatment and the indecision in which we find ourselves; and we say, we must have here a pleurisy with false membranes. This does not absolutely exclude the presence of fluid, but it is a reason which one is glad of, in order to avoid thoracentesis. The problem may, then, be stated in these terms :—How can a means of diagnosis be found which shall be completely harmless and absolutely certain? This problem appears to me to be solved by aspiration, and it is here that the importance of the previous vacuum shows itself, to which I do not fear to refer so often, for it constitutes one of the most salient characteristics of the method. Let us imagine a difficult case, in which we want to assure ourselves as to the existence of an effusion into the pleura. How shall we proceed? The aspirator being set, that is to say the vacuum being made, we introduce, into the intercostal space chosen, No. 1 needle, which is extremely fine. The needle has scarcely pierced a centimetre through the thickness of the tissue, that is to say as soon as the openings situated at its extremity are hidden, when we open the corresponding tap of the aspirator, and the vacuum is consequently made in the needle, which becomes aspiratory. It is therefore with a vacuum in hand that we proceed in search of the effusion ; the moment the aspiratory needle encounters the fluid, the latter rushes into the aspirator, and the diagnosis is complete. Thanks to this operation, we are certain not to go beyond the layer of fluid, which is of importance if it is not very deep. We have supposed, for the due description of this operation, an effusion into the pleura respecting the presence of which we are undecided, but the opposite case may occur, that is to say, when we believe in the existence of fluid which really does not exist. We more rarely commit the last-mentioned error, it is more usual to doubt the presence of fluid actually existing than to diagnose a non-existing collection. The process of investigation is, however, the same ; we introduce the needle, after having assured ourselves of its permeability. We drive it into the depth of the tissues, but the expected fluid does not make its appearance. We then penetrate deeper ; the patient complains of a sensation of pain ; some drops of blood spurt into the aspirator, it is evident that we have punctured the lung, and we become certain that the pleura contains no fluid, at least at the level of the exploration. What is to be thought of the wound of the organ, and what are its consequences ? This important question deserves to claim our attention, for that alone would be enough to cause the method we describe to be received or rejected. I have been witness to the puncturing of the lung several times, and I have never seen any accident supervene under any circumstances. I have thoroughly convinced myself that punctures performed with No. 1 needle are harmless, and experiments on animals have given me the same

results. When we puncture a congested lung (as in the first period of pneumonia), we may, by leaving the needle *in situ*, aspirate a few grammes of blood, perform a true blood-letting of the organ, and this local blood-letting may bring decided relief, and diminish the pain in the side.

Some patients, though in very rare instances, throw up sanguineous sputa after the puncture; this happened after the exploration which I had to perform at the house of one of the most eminent professors of our faculty, but with the exception of this unimportant occurrence, I have never seen the smallest complication supervene. In 1870, Dr. Brochin, witnessing these punctures of the lung in a case difficult to diagnose, and struck by their harmlessness, published the case I report from the *Gazette des Hôpitaux.* " A woman under the care of M. Axenfeld had been suffering from catarrhal affections; she also had a catarrhal angina, complicated with complete aphonia. Examination of the chest disclosed a notable difference between the two sides. The right side showed normal resonance throughout; the left side, on the contrary, was dull from the base for at least two-thirds or three-fourths of its height. Loud breathing was heard nearly throughout the whole extent of the dulness. There was no expectoration the character of which would aid in the diagnosis. There was complete loss of voice, and consequent impossibility of appreciating these modifications by auscultation. It was a question whether we had to deal with an effusion, or a pneumonia accompanied by hepatization. The question was not easy to solve, but aspiration was at hand to remove our doubts.

" It will be asked, how we could have contemplated plunging a trocar into the chest, at the risk of penetrating the lung? Doubtless the imprudence would have been great if an ordinary trocar had been used; but with the

s

needle adapted to the aspirator, we could proceed with perfect safety. The needle was inserted in three different places at three separate times, and each time we satisfied ourselves that there was not a single drop of serous matter. A few drops of spumous blood alone appeared in the transparent barrel of the aspirator. No doubt any longer existed, the diagnosis was confirmed. It must be added that no other inconvenience resulted to the patient from this exploration than the sensation of three pricks of a pin."

Since that time, I have very often introduced the aspiratory needle into the lung without ever having had to repent so doing. If, however, the innocuousness of these punctures of the lung be not allowed, the process of exploration which I have just described is inadmissible. The operator ought to introduce the needle boldly, without hesitation, with the conviction that the organ will be punctured if he be mistaken about the presence of the fluid, and with the intention of penetrating several centimetres deep if he desire to confirm the diagnosis thoroughly. This immunity enjoyed by the puncture may be explained in two ways; firstly, by the smallness of the needle; and secondly, by the state of the lung, which is rarely in the physiological condition at the time it undergoes exploration, so that the puncture is so much the more harmless, that the needle penetrates a more compact and condensed tissue. We are not as yet quite accustomed to the aspiratory needle. It must be handled with confidence, if we wish to attain the advantages to be expected from it. To fear or to hesitate is to fall back into the state of doubt which appertained to the use of the old exploratory trocar.

In certain interlobar pleurisies, which are completely surrounded on all sides by the lung, the puncture of the organ is not only an accidental fact, it is a necessary act; if a first exploration does not suffice, a second and third may be performed, with the certainty that if the pleura contains fluid, it ought to well up into the aspirator.

CONCLUSIONS.—The following conclusions may be drawn from this examination :—

1. Thanks to aspiration, a certain diagnosis can always be obtained of thoracic effusions, and pleural or pulmonary cysts and abscesses.

2. Information is at the same time obtained respecting the seat, the existence, and the nature of the fluid.

3. Exploration ought to be performed with No. 1 or No. 2 needle, prepared with the previous vacuum.

4. The symptoms which announce the puncture of the lung are pain, the aspiration of a few drops of blood, and, but very rarely, the ejection of sanguineous sputa.

5. The puncture of the lung by the aspiratory needle is an insignificant accident, and is even, in a case of mistake, the only means of establishing the diagnosis with certainty.

ARTICLE III.

Treatment of Acute Pleurisy by Aspiration.

PARAGRAPH I.—THE TIME FOR THORACENTESIS— THE METHOD OF ASPIRATION IN THORACENTESIS.—The first question to solve, when the operation for thoracentesis, by any method whatever, is proposed, is to know what is the most opportune moment for giving issue to the fluid. We are told, and with justice, that the fluid is formed during the acute or febrile period of pleurisy, and it is added, that it is preferable not to remove it until it is completely collected. The proposition thus formulated leaves something to be desired, for the period of formation is as variable as its duration, and the fluid may attain so large a developement from the fourth or fifth day before the abatement of the fever, that it would be imprudent to defer thoracentesis. On the other hand, decidedly acute pleurisy may be unaccompanied by any fluid secretion, this is dry pleurisy; whilst another, almost latent, and, so to say, apyretic, will engender an enormous effusion. The acuteness of the fever and the epoch of defervescence are consequently insufficient signs in determining the opportuneness of thoracentesis.

We should be equally wrong in relying on the deceitful appearances of respiration, for we see patients in whom effusions of several pints do not cause any dyspnœa, a fact which does not, however, prevent the effusion from determining displacement of the heart, torsion of the great vessels, thrombosis of the pulmonary artery, and becoming, through these different mechanical actions, a cause of syncope and death.

I have often heard Trousseau relate facts of this kind, and I have seen one instance in M. Grisolles' wards. M. Blachez has reported some on the authority given by autopsy, and it would not be difficult to collect a certain number of similar examples. Undue delay in evacuating the fluid, reliance on the deceptive appearances of the respiration, and putting off to the morrow an operation which should have been previously performed, exposes the patient to the danger of sudden death by syncope.

It follows, then, that general indications, such as the amount of fever and the state of respiration, are insufficient and unfaithful guides when the question of determining the time and the opportuneness of thoracentesis is in debate. Less variable signs must be sought elsewhere, and the indications for the operation seem to us to rest on the examination of local signs, that is to say on the presence and on the quantity of fluid effused into the pleura.

M. Moutard-Martin, being his remarks on numerous

cases, has demonstrated that thoracentesis performed during the febrile period of pleurisy has no injurious influence on the ulterior progress of the effusion, and may even lower the temperature of the patient. In any case, it is not urgent to wait for the abatement of the fever, and there is every advantage in not deferring the operation, as the fluid accumulated in the pleura can only have a bad influence. It plays the part of a foreign body, interferes with the action of the lung, and narrows the field of hematosis. Consequently, good reasons exist for ridding the patient of it, without persisting too far in the frequently long and useless phase of blisters and paintings with iodine.

Let us, however, guard ourselves from falling into a contrary-extreme ; we do not assert that the fluid should be removed from the chest so soon and in proportion as it is produced, we must have regard to the conditions under which the disease is developed, and take into consideration not only the pleurisy but the pleuritic.* However, we think that in the great majority of cases, it is necessary to operate early, without waiting until the effusion shall have attained large proportions, and this opinion appears to us capable of being summarized and formulated in the two following propositions :—

1. The degree of fever and the state of respiration are insufficient and delusive guides in the question of the opportuneness of thoracentesis.

2. Thoracentesis ought to be based on the estimate of the quantity of fluid contained in the pleura, which ought not to be allowed to accumulate in adults above five or six hundred grammes.

We know that even this estimate is difficult to determine even approximately ; we may, in many cases, be deceived by

* See the remarkable chapter that M. Peter has devoted to the treatment of pleurisy and pleuritic patients, *Clinique Médicale*, **Paris, 1873.**

several hundreds of grammes, but it is to be remarked that the mistake always leans towards a lower estimate than really exists, and when the fluid of pleurisy is estimated at twelve hundred grammes, it is seldom that fourteen or sixteen hundred are not found. Consequently it is better to rely on a rough estimate ; and in presence of an effusion which in the adult rises above the inferior angle of the scapula, we shall always be below the truth in diagnosing an effusion of five hundred grammes, and we ought to perform thoracentesis. The worst which can happen is that the liquid will be less abundant than had been supposed, but where would be the evil in such a case ? That some hesitation should be felt when only the trocar and gold-beater's skin were available, is very comprehensible ; thoracentesis was not then undertaken without absolute necessity. Many surgeons delayed by the help of iodine and blisters ; perhaps they expected to gain time ; and it was only when the pleura was thoroughly filled, the lung compressed, and the organs displaced, that the decision was taken, from the pressure of necessity, to give issue to several pints of liquid. Then the lung, suddenly freed from compression, expanded in jerks, the patient was seized with long and fatiguing fits of coughing, but notwithstanding these unfavourable conditions, recovery rapidly ensued, so rational and beneficial is the operation of thoracentesis. But at the present day we have not the same reasons for hesitating and waiting, for we are in possession of instruments which have greatly simplified the process of operation. The aspiratory needle is so harmless, it can be handled with so much facility, that we can perform aspiration of a relatively minute effusion without the smallest inconvenience, and resume the operation on fresh occasions, always with the same harmlessness. The process of operation does not, therefore, deserve to be taken into consideration, and our decision ought no longer to rest on anything but clinical indications. The operation being determined on, how is the manipulatory part of the aspiratory puncture accomplished ? In the old-fashioned proceedings the place for puncture was fixed in the fifth or sixth intercostal space, at the level of the axillary region ; this choice was made by an excess of caution, so as to keep away from the surrounding organs. It appears to us preferable to make the puncture much lower, and to traverse the pleura in the eighth or ninth intercostal space on the prolongation of the inferior angle of the scapula, so as to attack the fluid in its most depending parts. The aspirator being set, that is to say the previous vacuum being created, the index finger of the left hand limits the intercostal space on which the puncture ought to strike, and serves as a conductor to the aspiratory needle, which is driven sharply into the tissues.

Then, the corresponding tap of the aspirator being opened, the needle, which carries the vacuum within it, is slowly driven forward till the fluid traversing the glass index indicates that the effusion is reached. The patient can be operated on either sitting up or in bed ; the position is but of secondary importance, for the fluid, solicited by an unvarying force, flows out in an equal and continuous manner ; and the lung not being subjected to a sudden dilatation as in the old-fashioned thoracentesis, fits of coughing are scarcely ever observed, and respiration is established uniformly and without shocks. If the effusion does not exceed twelve or fifteen hundred grammes, it is evacuated at once, but if the pleura contain two or three litres of fluid, it is preferable to make two sittings and to recommence the aspiration on the next day, or the one following that, so as not to deprive the lung of the force which compressed it, and oblige it to resume the functions it had lost too suddenly.

For performing thoracentesis, I always use No. 2 needle, and although its diameter is very small, the aspiration, which quickens the flow, allows a litre of liquid to be withdrawn in a few minutes. It is useless—nay, it is even injurious—to employ a needle of a greater diameter, or a more capacious trocar, for then the flow becomes too rapid, and we consequently lose the benefit of aspiration. The object of aspiration is to remove the fluid by means of an extremely fine puncture, but if this puncture be made larger, the aspirator becomes useless; it even does us the ill office of accelerating the issue of the liquid and the dilatation of the lung too much. We must not, therefore, make use of a diameter greater than that possessed by No. 2 needle, if we wish to obtain all the benefit expected from aspiration, and if this condition be observed, the outflow of the fluid is moderate, and the patient does not suffer from paroxysms of cough, fatigue, or syncope. Many have asked themselves if the lung does not run the chance of being wounded by the point of the needle, and notwithstanding that practice has demonstrated the unfounded nature of this apprehension, some operators, with an excess of precaution, replace the needle by a trocar possessing the double inconvenience of suppressing the previous vacuum, and of imparting too great a rapidity to the outflow. On the hypothesis of a wound of the lung, Dr. Castiaux invented a special trocar, in which the point could be made to disappear directly the instrument had penetrated to the fluid collection. This trocar, in addition to its excessive bulk, does not appear to us to be of any utility, for it does not respond to any therapeutic indication, and it complicates the manipulatory part of the operation, which all our efforts tend to simplify. Wounding of the lung by the needle, at the moment when the fluid flows out, only rests on theory. Similar hypotheses had been enunciated when I proposed to apply aspiration to cases of retention of urine and strangulated hernia; it was asked if the opposing walls of the bladder, or the intestine, would not advance to meet the needle; experience has demonstrated that there is no ground for these fears. I have seen, or I have practised myself, some hundreds of operations for thoracentesis by aspiration, and I have never discovered pulmonary lesions any more than other observers.

The organ, in its movement of expansion, does not follow the retreat of the fluid so closely as to be pierced by the needle. It may touch it, but no harm results therefrom; and in support of what I advance, I cannot do better than cite the authoritatively-expressed opinion of M. Blachez *:—

"M. Dieulafoy's aspiratory instruments enable the pleura to be relieved of the fluid it contains, with a facility and promptitude which cannot be claimed by any medical means. We have ourselves made thirty punctures with the aspiratory needles. We have obtained such results that we shall not in future hesitate to have recourse to this mode of treatment as soon as the chest contains a notable quantity of fluid. The pain is trifling, and may be obviated if necessary. In order to empty the chest rapidly, the needle is placed in communication with the barrel of a syringe capable of holding about 150 grammes, and which fills itself in a few minutes. We have never seen the needle cause the slightest accident; in fact, there is nothing easier than to slightly lower the point, so as to make it nearly parallel with the thoracic wall, if there be any fear of puncturing the lung at the end of the operation. This accident, which we much dreaded at the commencement of our practice of this operation, never occurred, or at least never revealed itself by any appreciable sign. In young and vigorous subjects a single puncture may suffice, and we have seen patients fit to leave the hospital eight days after they had come in with

* *Gazette Hebdomadaire*, February 2, 1872, p. 72.

formidable effusions.   If the effusion reproduces itself, a
fresh puncture is performed.   Most frequently the fluid
reappears in diminished quantity, and is spontaneously
absorbed.   Thus all the annoyances and inconveniences
of treatment by purgatives and blisters are avoided."

No. 2 needle is then the proper instrument for thoracentesis by aspiration ; wounding the lung by expansion
of the organ at the moment when the fluid is withdrawn
is not at all to be dreaded.   It is enough slowly to withdraw the needle as the liquid flows away, or slightly
to alter the position of the point so as to make it parallel
with the thoracic wall.

It sometimes happens that towards the end of the
flow the fluid assumes a pinkish tint, which indicates
the mixture of a few drops of blood ; this appearance
supervenes also in thoracentesis by the old methods.   It
is better to stop the flow when it is observed, so much
the more that it is unimportant to leave a few grammes
of fluid in the pleura, whilst it might be injurious to
push the aspiration too far.

PARAGRAPH II. — VALUE AND CRITICISM OF THE
METHOD.—Thoracentesis, as I have just described it, no
longer merits the name even of an operation ; it is a simple
puncture, innocent, unimportant, within the capabilities of
all practitioners, exacting neither skill, courage, nor special
surgical knowledge.   We have no longer to dread either an
error of diagnosis, or wounding of the lung, or penetration of air into the pleura ; we need no longer trouble
ourselves, particularly in the case of children, about the
dimensions of the intercostal space, nor the size of the
trocar.   The pain is *nil*, and the lesion of the tissues so
trifling, that when the operation is terminated the traces
of the puncture are scarcely visible on the skin, and that
if, as in purulent pleurisy, the fluid is re-secreted several

times, the puncture can be renewed every day without the slightest annoyance.

Nevertheless, theories have not been wanting to demonstrate that thoracentesis by aspiration is an injurious and dangerous proceeding, and very inferior to the methods previously employed. It has been said that the needle is so fine that the issue of the liquid is too slow, and consequently the operation is too long, a quarter of an hour being needed to empty an effusion with the needle, which would be evacuated in ten minutes by the trocar. We reply to this objection, that this is entirely to the benefit of the patient, for it is the slowness of the flow which allows the lung to expand without jerking, and without causing fits of coughing ; the objection is even to the advantage of the operator, for if he lose a few minutes through the length of time taken by the flow, he regains them fully from the moment that he has no longer to occupy himself with the preparations for the operation, the arrangement of the gold-beaters' skin, and the working of the trocar.

Other objections have been made to aspiration ; it has been asked if it is not likely to produce purulence in the fluid. This objection does not, however, specially apply to aspiration, for some observers have made it with regard to simple thoracentesis, they having remarked, that premature evacuation of the fluid in pleurisy might impart a purulent character to the reproduction of the fluid. I do not wish to deny the fact ; but I have never observed it, and even if it has occurred, it is allowable to question if it were not a coincidence, rather than a relation between cause and effect.

Aspiration has also been reproached with accelerating the dilatation of the lung too violently, and with causing, according to circumstances, rents, congestion, and hæmorrhage ; but these theories cannot keep their ground against the accumulated experience of every day. I have never observed these accidents, nor have I ever seen them pointed out by others ; and Professor Béhier, in his clinical lectures at the Hôtel Dieu, has summed up the question in terms which tell entirely in favour of the argument I maintain.

He says, " I must own that these objections leave my conscience perfectly easy. You have seen that aspiration has been performed a certain number of times in our wards, with different instruments ; and that nothing, absolutely nothing, I will not say resembling, but even analogous to, the serious troubles which have been lately formulated as probable, have been anywhere observed. Nothing on the part of the lung. Often even the cough, so usually observed after thoracentesis of large effusions by Reybard's process, the cough, I repeat, has been completely absent. As to the serous oozing, said to be caused by aspiration, you were able on two of our latest operations, to judge of the emptiness of that accusation. In fact, when the flow of serum had stopped, we continued aspiration in our instrument, even increasing it ; and though we have remained waiting for a considerable time, no fresh sanguineous or serous fluid made its appearance. These accusations are entirely theoretical, veritable *à priori* objections, the consequences of the false and exaggerated idea conceived of aspiration, its powers and its consequences."

We must not therefore blame aspiration with being injurious because it is too active ; but we should blame the operator who employs aspiration without understanding it. It is not enough to have in one's hand an aspiratory needle and a powerful force ; it is above all necessary to learn how to use it, how to select the diameter of a needle, and to adapt it to the case ; not to evacuate the effusion at a single operation if it be too abundant ; and to increase, or arrest the power in proper season, these are the conditions essential to success. It is, in a word, necessary to know how to handle the vacuum, and then we perceive all the advantages which can be realized by this method.

If an aspirator, placed in communication with a collection of fluid, was necessarily obliged to exhaust all its power at once, and without there being any possibility of arresting its effects, then I should comprehend how its working might be objected to. Then, it is true, a strong aspiration, carried too far, and continued too long, in the interior of the pleura, might occasion accidents, such as hæmorrhage, rents, &c. But such need not be the case; the operator suspends the aspiration at his will; it is enough to turn the tap of the aspirator, as we tighten the brake of a machine, to dispose of the amount of vacuum required; it is given, taken away, distributed, according to circumstances. We employ it according to our own idea, in such a manner that all objections to it fall to the ground. Aspiration constitutes an improvement so much the more real on other methods of thoracentesis, that it has all its advantages without having any of its inconveniences.

To sum up : thoracentesis is no longer an operation, it is a prick of a needle, which obviates at once pain and danger, and which enables us to cause several litres of fluid to pass through an opening so minute that, when the needle is removed, it is scarcely possible to find the trace of it on the skin.

ARTICLE IV.

Treatment of Chronic Pleurisy and Purulent Pleurisy by Aspiration.

PARAGRAPH I.—THE PART PLAYED BY REPEATED ASPIRATIONS, WITHOUT IRRITANT INJECTIONS—CASES.— Purulence is not always a sign of chronicity, and it is not very uncommon to see acute effusions suddenly assume the purulent character.

But whatever may be the origin of this morbid state, whether it be connected with tubercle, which is of frequent occurrence ; whether it be consecutive to an injury, or to a primarily simple effusion ; whether it be referable to a generally serious condition, such as the puerperal state, or Bright's disease, the therapeutic indications are unvarying ; they may be epitomized in these two propositions : evacuate the fluid, and prevent its formation.

Purulence implies the idea of tenacity, and as a fact, while the fluid of simple pleurisy but rarely reproduces itself when it has been allowed vent, the fluid of purulent pleurisy, on the contrary, reappears with astonishing rapidity. This effusion is generally accompanied by the formation of false membranes, which fix the lung driven back by the fluid, and confirm the unnatural position of that organ. Then the flattened lung, bound round with false membranes, finishes by undergoing a true carnification ; it loses its structure, its physiological properties, and the possibility of regaining its normal position in the thorax.

In other circumstances, the process is so rapid and the purulence is the result of so acute an inflammatory process, that pleural and pulmonary ulcerations result, after which the patient is attacked by pneumothorax. I have recently seen two examples of this, one in a man fifty years old, who had become pleuritic during the course of diabetes ; the other in a young girl, in whom pleurisy, at first hæmorrhagic, rapidly became purulent.

It is therefore of importance not to defer direct intervention in purulent pleurisy, and if the signs revealed by percussion and auscultation are not sufficient to enlighten us in a difficult case, we must hasten to confirm the diagnosis of the affection by means of aspiration, and commence the treatment without delay. The question then arises, what mode of treatment should we employ ? The variety of the methods would be a cause of hesitation.

The discussion which recently arose at the Academy of Medicine, has not done much to clear up the matter; all the therapeutic means were passed in review. Simple puncture of the chest, extraction of the pus by means of syringes and syphons, drainage, irritant injections, the operation for empyema, all these methods were brought forward; each of them found warm defenders; but as there is not one of them which, though having given good results, has not serious drawbacks, it follows that the question is still undecided, and we feel some difficulty when it becomes necessary to make a choice. On the occasion to which we refer, the question of aspiration was raised, but documents respecting the new method were wanting, and it was too frequently confounded with extraction of pus, by the help of syringes or instruments with a very imperfect vacuum, methods which are perhaps useful under certain circumstances, but which, to avoid confusion, ought to be separated from the method by aspiration.

It then becomes necessary to place the question on its true ground, by placing aspiration on its right footing, by ascertaining what services it can render us in the treatment of purulent pleurisy, and by fixing the extent to which it ought to be associated with the different treatments which have been so much extolled. I have, however, been preceded in this path by M. Bouchut, who, in a recent very remarkable work, has shown what results can be obtained by repeated aspirations; and by M. Hérard, who has, at the Academy, summed up the question, as regards purulent pleurisy, with remarkable ability. Our own opinion on the subject is as follows : A purulent pleurisy being in question, what proceedings should we take ? Ought we to employ aspiration at once ? In what case ought we to perform simple aspiration, and when ought we to associate medicated injections with it ? We must examine these different propositions. Let us suppose, for argument's sake, a purulent effusion, without for the moment troubling ourselves about the nature of the cause which gave rise to it. Our first care is to give issue to the fluid, for which purpose the manipulatory part of the operation is the same as I have just described for simple pleurisy. The facility of the operation, the fineness of the needle, and the harmlessness of the puncture, allow us to renew the aspiration several times, until the fluid is completely exhausted. Here again, as in hydarthrosis, and in hydatic cysts of the liver, observation often decides in favour of that therapeutic law which I am endeavouring to popularize, viz.: when a fluid, whatever may be its nature, accumulates in a serous cavity, or in an organ, and when that cavity or organ is accessible, without danger to the patient, to our means of investigation, our first care ought to be to remove the fluid ; if it forms again, we must again withdraw it, and so on for several times if necessary, so as to exhaust the serous matter by a perfectly mechanical and absolutely inoffensive means, before thinking of modifying the secretion by irritant and sometimes dangerous agents. We must, therefore, aspirate the purulent effusion, then aspirate it again as soon as it reappears, three times a week if necessary, a course of action which has no inconveniences, since we work subcutaneously and with a needle which makes an unimportant wound.

Patients willingly undergo this operation, which gives scarcely any pain; and even this amount may be completely annihilated if the seat of the proposed puncture be rendered anæsthetic by the use of a few grammes of pulverized ether. As to irritant injections of alcohol, or tincture of iodine, they are not yet necessary ; we shall see later on when there is need to employ them.

CASE I.—PURULENT PLEURISY—TWO ASPIRATIONS— CURE (AXENFELD).—A man 35 years old, entered the

Beaujon Hospital, under the care of M. Axenfeld, with all the signs of pleurisy in the left side of the chest. The progress of the malady had not been decidedly acute, and the first appearance dated back about two months. Aspiration, performed with No. 2 needle, gave issue to 750 grammes of purulent fluid. This purulence of the fluid did not seem connected with any cause other than phlegmasia of the serous membrane, and there was no occasion to refer it to tubercle. Five days after the operation the fluid began to form again; a fresh aspiration was made, and 300 grammes of pus were taken away. Shortly after the patient went out cured, without necessity for further intervention.

Case II.—Purulent Pleurisy—Thirty-three Aspirations—Cure. (This case is taken from M. Bouchut's memoir.)—During convalescence, after a mild attack of typhoid fever, a child was attacked by acute purulent pleurisy of considerable extent. Aspiration was performed, and at first the effusion was emptied once, then two or three times a week. As the puncture of the capillary trocar did not leave any trace, what had been commenced from necessity was continued purposely. But the pus reproduced itself with disheartening rapidity, and the cavity of the pleura became filled in three days.

M. Bouchut then tried, by means of the aspirator, to inject pure tincture of iodine into the pleura ; this was done on three separate occasions, but did not seem to prevent the pus from reforming with rapidity. The injections of tincture of iodine were suspended ; aspiratory punctures alone were continued, and after six months the quantity of pus diminished. Finally recovery took place. Whilst this local treatment was going on the child was placed on an excellent system of diet, consisting of raw meat, beer, and alcohol.

T

Case III. — Simple Pleurisy, advancing to the Purulent Stage, cured by Two Aspirations. (This case is taken from M. Bouchut's memoir.)—A little girl, of four years old, was attacked with pleurisy in the left side of the chest, accompanied by considerable effusion. M. Bouchut, not wishing to wait for the effect of internal medication, and without using the usual revulsives, performed aspiration by means of the finest needle of the aspirator. 500 grammes were removed, but three days afterwards, the effusion being reproduced, a fresh aspiration was made. This time the fluid was thicker, and slightly purulent. The child was a long time recovering, but at the end of some weeks regained her strength, and left cured without any contraction of the chest. This had not yet reached the condition of purulent pleurisy, with effusion of phlegmonous pus; but a few days' delay in the second puncture would have brought about this unpleasant result. So regarded, it is a case of the greatest interest, as showing us the value of direct intervention, and of the means employed.

It is a fact that this method succeeds better with children than with adults.

Case IV.—(Extracted from a Report by M. De Kieter, of St. Petersburg.)—A patient having come into the Military Hospital of Kieff, with all the symptoms of effusion into the pleura, aspiration was performed by means of Dieulafoy's instrument. A first operation gave issue to a large quantity of pus. Some days later a second aspiration was performed, with the same result. These two operations sufficed to cure the patient.

Case V.—Acute Costal and Diaphragmatic Pleurisy —Purulent Effusion—Six Aspirations—Consecutive Deviation of the Thorax — Rectification by the Application of a Layer of Collodion on the

HEALTHY SIDE—CURE. (Case published in the *Gazette des Hôpitaux,* 11th June, 1872.)

I here give the summary of this case, reported by M. Labadie-Lagrave, house surgeon to M. Bouchut:—

A child of seven years old came into M. Bouchut's ward for pleurisy, with effusion into the left side of the chest. A first aspiration was made in the axillary line at the level of the nipple, and gave issue to 300 grammes of a thick, purulent, greenish-yellow, inodorous fluid. A second aspiration was made on the 2nd of February, when 60 grammes of greenish creamy pus were again removed. The vesicular murmur was then audible from above downwards. On the 7th the heart was pushed back to the right, and downwards under the sternum. The respiratory murmur reappeared under the clavicle. On the 8th a third aspiration was performed, and 30 grammes of pus removed. On the 15th, a fourth aspiration was performed on the same level as the others; about 100 grammes of pus were removed. On the 25th, a fifth aspiration; 300 grammes of thick inodorous pus. On the 3rd of March a sixth and last aspiration was made, when nearly 200 grammes of fluid were removed. On the 8th of April an abortive aspiration was performed; the thorax was drawn in on the affected side. To overcome this deformity, a band of collodion was applied on the right side of the chest. On the 13th the child was quite straightened, and went out on the 13th of May, completely cured.

Remarks.—In the case of this child suffering from acute pleurisy with purulent effusion, thoracentesis by means of M. Dieulafoy's aspirator, six times repeated, enabled us to cure the evil without opening the chest, and without causing wounds or consecutive fistulas. Such is the bearing of this uncommon incident in the history of purulent pleurisy. In fact, we know that after puncture by ordinary thoracentesis, the purulent effusion is again secreted; and frequently, after two or three punctures, the pus filters into one of the openings which becomes fistulous, and the air penetrating into the interior of the pleura, brings on putrescence of the pus.

To these cases others might be added, amongst them that of M. Bucquoy, quoted by M. Hérard, and in which the cure took place after 18 aspirations.

These cases are very instructive; they show that the source of the fluid may often be dried up by aspirating a purulent effusion as often as it forms, which is done without any inconvenience, since we act subcutaneously and with a needle which makes but a slight puncture. Irritant injections with tincture of iodine and alcohol need only to be employed when the fluid resists mechanical exhaustion, or when the progress of the disease gives reason by its acuteness or by its character to fear a fatal termination or the occurrence of pneumothorax. The cases of M. Bouchut bear upon purulent effusions in infancy, and we know that in children this disease is cured more quickly and more thoroughly than in adults. We must not therefore draw deductions relating to all ages, and exaggerate the value of repeated aspiration without injections; for it is sometimes useful, especially in the adult, as we have said, to apply to them another kind of treatment.

PARAGRAPH II.—WASHING AND INJECTIONS OF THE PLEURA IN PURULENT PLEURISY—THE THORACIC TROCAR, ITS USES AND APPLICATION.—Thus far we have spoken of purulent pleurisy in which there is no difficulty in evacuating the pus; but we are sometimes confronted with more complicated cases: in one the issue of the fluid is obstructed by the presence of false membranes, or by the detritus of the pleura or lung, as is seen in effusions consecutive to traumatism in certain interlobar pleurisies, and in gangrene of the pleura, sometimes the pus is reproduced with such obstinacy that aspiration often repeated does not succeed in drying up its source, and under similar circumstances, simple aspiration performed by means of fine needles does not fulfil the indications, the idea of employing larger openings naturally suggests itself here. Is this the right occasion for suggesting the operation for empyema ? Not yet ; between the simple puncture made with the aspiratory needle and the large incision for empyema there is an intermediate phase, and under these conditions a sound should be introduced into the pleura and left there, or one of the special trocars that I have had constructed for this purpose, in order to practise frequent washing out followed by injection ; and for this purpose the ingenious syphon of my learned master, M. Potain, is useful. M. Potain may be considered as the creator of this method, which consists in washing out the pleura several times a day, and modifying its surface by means of appropriate liquids. In order to arrive at this result he devised a system of syphons, simple and easy to manage, and which allows the patient himself to perform the washing out of his thoracic cavity, and in many cases I have witnessed cures obtained by this excellent proceeding. If washing out of the pleura and injections, practised by means of the aspiratory injectors, appear to us preferable to the cleansing and injection made by means of the syphon, it is in truth only a very slight modification, consisting in some details inherent in the mode of operating. The fluid of purulent pleurisy, which is thick, and often loaded with false membranes, and which hangs about the anfractuosities and pockets of the pleura, can only be put in motion by a sufficient force ; now the force of aspiration given by a syphon, the length of which only measures the space which separates the patient's bed from the floor, is five or six times less than the force given by an aspiratory apparatus. Moreover, the projective force applied to the fluid to be injected is almost nil in the syphon, whilst it acquires a certain energy when the injection is thrown in by means of the piston of an aspirator. The consequence is that, without detracting from the success of the washing of the pleura by the syphon, experience has shown us that the morbid cavity is better cleansed in its anfractuosities and sloping parts when the injection is set in motion by an aspiratory apparatus.

This proceeding will be developed more in detail in the following cases.

CASE VI.—PURULENT TRAUMATIC PLEURISY—MULTIPLE ASPIRATIONS—TUBE *in situ*—WASHING AND INJECTION BY MEANS OF THE RACK ASPIRATOR—EFFECTS OF THE DEVIATION OF THE CATAMENIAL PERIOD—RECOVERY—(DIEULAFOY).—On May 28th, 1871, at the time that the Versailles army took possession of the Madeleine quarter, a young girl, æt. 22, who from curiosity had mounted on to the roof of the house, received a ball in the middle of the chest. It entered at the left, sixth, intercostal space, a little external to the heart, and made its exit not far from the vertebral column. It was probable that the lung was not traversed, as the patient had no hemoptysis, but it was doubtless grazed by the ball, and the pleura was injured; for, whilst the wounds made by the projectile were healing, fever was set up, and from the second day pleurisy showed itself in the left side. Dr. Linas did me the honour of calling me in consultation to the patient. There was considerable dyspnœa, forty inspirations a minute and 130 pulsations; as physical signs we observed a considerable deviation of the heart, which beat under the right nipple, a very marked skodic bruit under the left clavicle, with an absence of vibrations, no souffle nor ægophony. In the presence of these evident signs of a traumatic effusion, we decided, with the consent of Dr. Linas, to aspirate the fluid, and the puncture was made by means of the No. 2 needle in the sixth intercostal space near to the wound made by the entrance of the projectile. But aspiration only drew out pure blood, which made us conclude that we had pierced the lung, and that that organ had undergone adhesions at the level of the wound.

A fresh puncture was made further back, and we drew off a litre of inodorous fluid, strongly coloured by blood, and which held a remarkable quantity of leucocytes in suspension. The evening of the operation the girl had menstruated scantily.

June 1st.—The amelioration which followed this operation was of short duration; and, the effusion being reproduced, a fresh aspiration gave issue to 500 grammes of purulent fluid of an offensive odour.

June 5th.—The oppression was considerable, the fever acute, and the third aspiration was made with needle No. 2, but the pus was drawn out with difficulty, the needle was often obliterated, and it was evident that pieces of false membranes or gangrenous portions of the pleura prevented the issue of the fluid. What were we to do? Have recourse to the operation for empyema, and make a large incision? It did not seem to us necessary to adopt as yet this extreme decision, so a middle course was followed. An india-rubber tube, with resisting walls, 15 centimetres in length, and 5 millimetres in diameter, was introduced into the pleura and maintained *in situ* by means of collodion and tapes. This tube, when put into communication with the rack aspirator, which is much more convenient under these circumstances than the notched aspirator, enabled us to draw off a great quantity of fluid. But instead of using the previous vacuum, the piston was gradually raised so as to regulate the force of aspiration, and by these means the cavity could be gently handled, and the clots of blood and detritus of false membranes which floated in the pus extracted.

When the tube became clogged, an inverse-stroke of the piston pushed the obstructing body back into the thoracic cavity, where it was subsequently broken up. We were thus able to draw out the pus, and at last to wash out the cavity, twice a day with water mixed with a thousandth part of thymic acid. After the second day of this treatment there was great improvement; sleep returned, and the fever diminished in intensity, but the cough was still frequent. Our patient's diet was broth, fowl, and Bordeaux; for internal treatment morphia draught and extract of bark. This treatment and the washings with thymic acid were regularly continued, and the morbid cavity of the pleura sensibly diminished every day. This was easily ascertained by means of the aspirator, which being graduated, the number of grammes of fluid injected or aspirated could be exactly seen.

June 28*th.*—Matters were going on excellently when the patient was taken with violent shivering fits, and had two attacks of fever in the same day; her face was changed, her body covered with sweat, and these symptoms made us fear the commencement of purulent infection. A gramme of sulphate of quinine was administered. The fluid aspirated was thin and sanguineous. The next day a fresh access of fever declared itself, and the quantity of blood drawn from the pleura was greater than before. After two days of alarming symptoms and reasonable fears, improvement set in, and Dr. Linas and I had no doubt that the sole cause of these accidents was the deviation of the catamenia; the normal monthly hæmorrhage being defective, the young girl menstruated by the pleura.

The washings and injections were continued twice a day, and thymic acid and iodide of potassium were alternately used as the modifying fluid; the appetite was good, the morbid cavity of the pleura was almost entirely filled up, and we were thinking of withdrawing the tube when new accidents occurred.

July 15*th.*—The patient was attacked by fits of violent coughing, and with fever and pain in the left side of the chest. Auscultation discovered the fine râles of pneumonia in the back and upper part of the right lung, and in the back and middle part of the left lung a slight souffle with ægophony : this souffle was more pronounced the next day. We had evidently to face new difficulties, pneumonia in the right, pleurisy in the left lung, and in three days we lost the benefit of six weeks' treatment. The next day we decided to puncture at the level of this new effusion. I first sought for the fluid with No. 2 aspirating needle, and drew off 100 grammes of a purulent fluid, and so thick that I did not hesitate, at once, to introduce into the thoracic cavity the india-rubber tube that we had used to exhaust the first effusion.

This new cavity was washed out twice a day, and such a rapid improvement followed, that we allowed ourselves to hope that recovery was this time near at hand ; sleep was excellent, and the patient was beginning to get up for some hours in the day, when, on the 25th of July, fresh shivering fits occurred, fresh access of fever, with hæmorrhage by the pleura and slight hemoptysis. There could be no doubt that we were again in the presence of a deviation of the catamenia, and for two days we drew off almost pure blood from the pleura ; the accidents then improved, and the amelioration continued its course.

August 10*th.*—The purulent source was dried up, the patient got up, the tube was withdrawn, and two months later this young girl was completely cured, without thoracic fistula, without the slightest pain in the side, or the least difficulty of breathing.

It is now eighteen months since this case occurred, and there has been no relapse.

Reflections.—This case plainly indicates the course to be followed when successive capillary aspirations do not lead to good results. Before deciding on the operation for empyema, recourse must be had to a mixed method, which consists in introducing a resisting tube into the pleural cavity, so that it can be washed out and cleansed many times a day. A rack aspirator allows of the operation being done easily and with the greatest precision. The force of aspiration can be better regulated by the subsequent vacuum than by the previous vacuum. If the thoracic tube becomes blocked up, an inverse stroke of the piston will push the obstructing body into the pleura, and the operation is continued. It is easy to exactly gauge the progress of improvement, for it can be known to within a few grammes what is the capacity of the cavity, and to what extent it diminishes every day.

Critical Examination of the Process.—This process is, however, not exempt from drawbacks, and the gutta-percha or india-rubber tube is the defective part. The walls of this tube ought to be firm, otherwise they become flattened together under the influence of aspiration or from the pressure of the ribs ; but to be firm, these walls should be of a certain thickness, which makes the tube a larger size. It follows, then, that the thoracic opening must be very large, and that the tube, which is very difficult to keep *in situ*, helps by its movements to cause ulceration of the integuments, and from all this a very incomplete obliteration of the pleural cavity results, and penetration of the air into the cavity, the issue of the fluid across the edges of the wound, and often serious accidents, without reckoning the formation of a fistula difficult to cure. This is not all, if an india-rubber tube be used for iodine injections. The deterioration of the tube exposes us to other dangers. In a case of M. Bucquoy's, in which an india-rubber tube was made use of for injecting tincture of iodine into the chest, it underwent such alteratons that it could only be extracted by a long and painful operation. Dr. Dujardin-Beaumetz performed some experiments which led to the following conclusions : Firstly, that pus has no action on an india-rubber tube. Secondly, amongst modifying injections, tincture of iodine seems the only one that alters in any important degree the texture and properties of this tube. Thirdly, these changes are—a very considerable increase of the diameter, to almost a third more than the original size of the tube ; an extreme brittleness, with hardening of the material, and complete loss of elasticity. The external surface of the tube becomes striated, rough, and irregular. Fourthly, that these changes are caused when the solution contains at least 3½ grammes of tincture of iodine in 100 of water. Fifthly, these changes are brought about so rapidly that, forty-eight hours after contact with the fluid, they have already become very marked. Sixthly, vulcanization does not at all prevent the action of tincture of iodine. Seventhly, these changes seem to be caused by the combination of certain molecules of the india-rubber

DIEULAFOY'S THORACIC TROCAR.

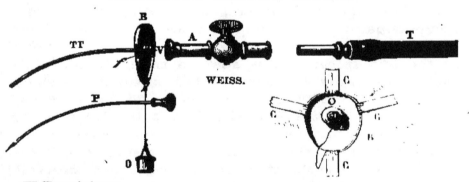

TT Thoracic trocar.
B The shield of the trocar with openings, C, to allow tapes to pass.
P Needle of the trocar.
A The intermediate fittings, putting the aspirator into communication with the trocar.
T Tube of the aspirator.
O Obturator.
V Screw by means of which the obturator is fitted to the intermediate parts.
CC The trocar viewed in front and placed.

with the iodine (iodide of caoutchine). It is with the view of remedying these various inconveniences, the exaggerated size of the tube, the thoracic ulcerations and consecutive fistulas, the penetration of the air, and the alteration of the tubes, that I have made some thoracic trocars which seem to me free from these defects. The following is a description of them.

The volume of these trocars is not greater than that of the aspiratory needles Nos. 2 and 3, and this size varies according to the size of the patient; they have none of the inconveniences of india-rubber and gutta-percha tubes, they undergo no change by contact with liquids, and their manner of closing renders the access of the external air impossible. They are fixed in the thorax without the slightest difficulty by means of tapes passing through the openings of the shield, and a few drops of collodion, and their small calibre makes their introduction so easy, that by often removing them in the course of treatment ulcerations and fistulas may be prevented. Finally, the projection which they make on the surface of the skin is so minute that it causes the patient neither pain nor discomfort, and he can get up, walk, and continue his occupations whilst carrying a trocar in his chest for weeks and months.

The thoracic trocar can be adapted in length and size to the patient under treatment. The mode of operating is very simple: the trocar introduced and fixed in the pleura is closed by the obturator O; at the moment of performing aspiration or injection, the obturator is unscrewed and replaced by the intermediate fitting A (care being taken to close the stop-cock of the latter), which is put into communication with the tube of the aspirator T, so that the cleansing and injection of the pleura can be effected with the greatest ease, protected from the air.

The play of the piston of the aspirator allows of the fluid being injected with the amount of force judged necessary; the injection is regulated, withdrawn from the pleura, or allowed to remain, at the will of the operator. When the operation is over, the intermediate fitting is replaced by the obturator, which screws into the shield.

I made use of the thoracic trocar in the following case.

CHRONIC HÆMORRHAGIC AND PURULENT PLEURISY— PNEUMOTHORAX — APPLICATION OF THE THORACIC TROCAR—WASHINGS AND INJECTIONS OF THE PLEURA (DIEULAFOY).—On July 20th, 1872, I was called by my esteemed friend, Dr. Veillard, to a young girl suffering from chronic pleurisy of the left side. Mlle. B—— had been seized eight months previously with acute pleurisy, and had shown all the signs of an effusion in the left side of the chest. Although she had not enjoyed very robust health, nothing had ever occurred to lead any one to suppose the existence of tubercle. The pleurisy had been submitted to a treatment in which blisters had played the principal part ; but the effusion not being absorbed, and the general symptoms increasing in intensity, thoracentesis was decided on. The operation, performed May 15, gave issue to three litres of fluid deeply coloured with blood, without the cause of the hæmorrhagic pleurisy being discovered. The relief was immediate, but of short duration ; in fact, a few days after the operation the fluid began to be reproduced, the appetite was gone, the nights were bad, and every evening the patient experienced a slight access of fever, followed by profuse sweats.

When I saw her I found her general condition very serious, and examination of the chest enabled me to discover an effusion which both Dr. Veillard and myself estimated at about two litres.

On the 30th of August, I performed aspiration with needle No. 2, and I stopped after having drawn off a litre of a very sanguineous fluid. I did not draw off all the fluid at the first stroke, being unwilling to submit a pleura which seemed so much disposed to hæmorrhage to too active a process of aspiration. The patient was much relieved, which is usual after thoracentesis, and on the

2nd of September I again drew off a litre of fluid of the same appearance and bad odour.

September 4th.——I drew off a litre of sanguineous fluid with a very decided odour of maceration.

September 6th.——The same result.

September 9th.——A fresh aspiration; the fluid was less red, it had a greyish tint, and on examination it showed a large quantity of pus globules; purulent pleurisy was taking the place of hæmorrhagic pleurisy.

Repeated aspirations did not aid us much in this case; the benefit given by the issue of the fluid was very fleeting, the effusion was reproduced with great rapidity, the patient was not able to digest any food, the emaciation became extreme, and the temperature was very high; and thus establishing a thoracic tube *in situ* became a question discussed by Dr. Veillard and myself. But our resolution was not taken soon enough, for on the 14th of September a violent pain declared itself in the left side, accompanied with much dyspnœa, and by auscultation we discovered amphoric respiration, which plainly showed the approach of an attack of pneumothorax. The night was passed very badly, 50 inspirations and 130 pulsations could be counted a minute, and the condition of the patient seemed to us so alarming that we hesitated to operate. However, as only an insignificant puncture was needed after all, the thoracic trocar No. 1 was inserted into the seventh intercostal space, and fixed by means of tapes and collodion, and thus two washings and two injections could be performed a day. The fluid drawn off had a gangrenous odour, the washings were with lukewarm water containing carbolic acid, and the injections were composed of water 400 grammes, sulphate of zinc 4 grammes. Twice a day 100 grammes of this solution were injected, and the washings and injections were continued the next and the following days. Under the influence of this treatment the patient improved rapidly, and from the first week the change was remarkable, the offensive odour of the fluid disappeared, the purulence became less, and the gravity of the general symptoms sensibly improved. For diet, Mlle. B—— took milk, eggs, and wine, which she digested perfectly well.

The cavity of the pleura filled up but very slowly, for after a month of this treatment the same quantity of fluid could be injected. However, towards the 15th of October, the lung began to perform its functions, the patient regained strength, she ate with a good appetite, and was able to get up and walk a few steps in her room.

In November, Mlle. B—— began to go out, from that time the washing and injection of an evening were discontinued, and done but once a day, in the morning. The fluid still preserved its purulent nature, but air passed through a good half of the diseased lung, and the cavity of the pleura was considerably diminished.

To-day, the 20th of January, we went to see our patient. Her condition was very satisfactory, she was able to go out and to attend to her occupation. The pleural cavity did not admit more than 30 or 40 grammes of fluid, the thoracic trocar remained still *in situ*, and the sister of Mlle. B—— washed out the cavity and injected the fluid every morning by means of a rack aspirator.

Reflections.—Here we had to contend with chronic hæmorrhagic and purulent pleurisy, against which repeated aspirations were of no avail. We were wrong in waiting so long before modifying the treatment, and we instituted the repeated washings and injections at the time when the patient was almost dying, and was suffering from pneumothorax. After a few days, the amelioration was already manifest, and it has continued until the present time, and if the patient is not yet completely cured, it is because months are required for a lung which has been so badly treated to regain its original position and normal function.

The thoracic trocar, left *in situ* for five consecutive months, caused no accident, no ulceration, and its volume is so slight that on the day on which it will be withdrawn the little wound will commence to cicatrize rapidly without leaving any fistula.

PARAGRAPH III.—PLEURISY WITH PNEUMOTHORAX—DRESSING OF THE PLEURA—WASHINGS AND INJECTIONS —EMPYEMA.—When pleurisy is complicated by pneumothorax what course must we follow, and what service can the method just described render us? One condition appears to us to be above all other considerations, that is the etiological question; and our first care should be to discover if the patient is suffering from tubercle or not. If the pneumothorax is depending on tubercle it is almost useless to undertake treatment, but if tubercle is not implicated in the developement of the symptoms, the pleurisy must be treated as if the pneumothorax did not exist.

The thoracic trocar being in its place, the washing out of the pleura and the injection of an appropriate fluid, such as a strong solution of sulphate of zinc, is performed two or three times a day, so as in the first place to obtain the cicatrization of the pulmonary ulceration, and 'in the second the gradual contraction of the cavity.

The treatment of purulent pleurisy, with or without pneumothorax, by the means of washings and injections, is of the same kind as the treatment which I applied to suppurating cysts and abscesses of the liver, by means of the hepatic trocar. When the thoracic trocar is fixed, we begin by drawing off a part of the fluid contained in the pleura, say 150 grammes, replacing it immediately by 120 grammes of the injected fluid, and this is repeated five, six, ten times in succession, until the morbid cavity is cleansed, and thus the pathological fluid is gradually replaced by a modifying fluid. It is an insensible substitution. This process of successive washings with small quantities of fluid is preferable to that mode of injection which consisted in withdrawing at one stroke the whole of the pathological fluid, and replacing it by an undetermined quantity of injection. Here we proceed slowly, we know to within a few grammes what is the volume of the fluid put into motion, we can regulate the force and the quantity of the fluid aspirated and injected, and when this cleansing of the pleura is finished, a modifying fluid, a veritable collyrium, is introduced and left in the cavity.

By this process, the pleura is washed twice a day, and with as much precision as an external suppurating wound, for the modifying fluid reaches every part. Under the influence of this treatment, the general and local symptoms improve, the purulent secretion gives place to a reparatory proliferation, the lung, by its slow and progressive movement of expansion, regains what it lost in the thorax, the cavity gradually fills up and contracts, which contraction of the morbid cavity the operator can see every day.

The thoracic trocar can be more or less voluminous and more or less long, according to the patient. If during treatment the little wound made by the trocar shows a tendency to ulceration, the instrument can be taken out as often as is considered necessary.

The amelioration which follows this treatment is soon seen ; from the third or fourth day, that is to say, after a small number of washings, the state of the pleura alters, and the intensity of the general symptoms decreases. But if the improvement is not so rapid, if the false membranes and the gangrenous débris of the serous membrane of the lung are so large that they prevent the flow of the pus, or the cleansing of the pleura, then intercostal incision must be performed without delay, for it offers the

U

patient the only chance of recovery. We are not very much disposed to favour the large incisions for empyema, but we think that this operation should be reserved for particular cases, such as gangrene of the pleura, interlobar pleurisy, hydatids of the lung, and when the other means that we have described have failed.

SUMMARY AND CONCLUSION.——In the presence of purulent pleurisy, this is, we believe, the treatment to be employed.

1st. To practise successive aspirations, without access of air and often repeated, by means of needle No. 2 or 3. This practice has been already very successful, especially with children.

2ndly. If these oft-repeated aspirations have no good result, we think it advisable, without waiting too long, especially with an adult, to pass on to the intermediate phase——that is, to cleanse the pleura two or three times a day by means of appropriate washings and injections, veritable collyria, and this procedure is rendered easy by connecting the thoracic trocar with an aspiratory-injector.

3rdly. This latter process is applicable to cases where effusion is complicated with pneumothorax, provided always that the pneumothorax is not of a tuberculous nature.

4thly. In case these different methods are not successful, the operation for empyema must be performed without hesitation or delay.

We have thus explained, as we understand it, the treatment of purulent pleurisy. This disease, the prognosis of which has been considered so serious, seems to us to have lost a part of its gravity since we have possessed this new means of overcoming it.

The cause of the disease governs the course to be pursued, and enables us to clearly separate into two large classes purulent effusions of the pleura. Is the pleurisy, or is it not, of the tubercular character ? If it is due to tubercle, we do not think it possible, in the present state of science, to find successful treatment for it ; but if it is not tubercular, though it be already far advanced, accompanied with false membranes and even with pneumothorax, our opinion is that purulent pleurisy is curable in the great majority of cases.

———————————

CHAPTER III.

TREATMENT OF HYDARTHROSIS AND EFFUSIONS INTO THE KNEE BY ASPIRATION.

Summary.—Article I.: History.—Explanation of the Method.—Harmlessness of Aspiratory Punctures.—Possibility of the Cause of Accidents existing in the manner of Operating.—Article II.: Treatment of Hydarthrosis by Aspiration.—Cases.—Duration of the Treatment.—Value and Criticism of the Process.—Mode of Operating.—Article III.: Treatment of Hematic Effusions of the Knee by Aspiration.—Cases.—Article IV.: Treatment of Purulent Effusions of the Knee by Aspiration.—Cases.

ARTICLE I.

History.—Harmlessness of Aspiratory Punctures.—Possibility of the Cause of Accidents existing in the manner of Operating.

It is curious to see with what facility certain therapeutical ideas, alternately found good and bad, are successively admitted and abandoned. When we read the works which the master-minds of the last generation left us, Velpeau and Bonnet of Lyons, we observe the good results which puncture and iodine injections produced in their hands in certain cases of hydarthrosis of the knee, and we ask ourselves if it is not from a rather timid prudence that we generally prefer the interminable and unsatisfactory treatment of the blister and painting with iodine.

Iodine painting and the blister, which have been so abused, seem to us as little favourable to the suppression of fluid in hydarthrosis, as they are useless to absorb the effusion in pleurisy. This plan is most frequently treatment by expectation thinly disguised, and it is not always exempt from pain and accidents. How many patients has one seen suffering with an effusion of the chest or knee after their third, fourth, or fifth blister, with a large surface of the skin denuded of its epidermis, exposed to the chances of suppuration, cystitis, or erysipelas, without this mode of treatment having shown any advantages which might serve to excuse it. If the puncture of the joint, followed by the injection of irritant substances, is a process which is not generally followed, it is because, together with incontestable good results, there are cases in which the remedy has proved worse than the disease. It is enough to read the twenty-four cases collected by M. Boinet,* and published by Roux, Velpeau, Bérard, &c., to be convinced that iodine injections very often cause intense inflammatory accidents, sharp reaction, violent pain, so much so that, in order to remedy the tension and rapid swelling of the articulation, it becomes necessary to employ energetic antiphlogistic treatment. It is thus seen how this method, which is far from always triumphing over the disease, has fallen into discredit, and it is, with reason, reserved for exceptional cases, or for old-standing hydarthroses which have resisted the usual methods of treatment.

As to the simple puncture of the joint which on several occasions has been tried without success by various surgeons, Boyer, Denonvilliers, Malgaigne, &c., it has been completely laid aside, for want of the means to practise it perfectly, both the ordinary trocar and the

* Traité d'iodothérapie.

large trocar of M. J. Guérin offering but insufficient
guarantees : and if an articular puncture was performed
with these instruments, great care was taken not to
operate many times in succession on the same articulation.   If after the first or second puncture the effusion
was observed to be reproduced, it can be well understood
how the observers, fearing the indefinite reproduction of
the fluid, occupied themselves in seeking elsewhere than
in the simple puncture of the joint for a therapeutical
means.   The result of this was that all surgical
interference was proscribed, and that acute or sub-acute
effusions into the knee, of a serous, hematic, or purulent
nature, as well as hydarthrosis of traumatic, blennorrhagic, or rheumatic origin were submitted till now to one
uniform treatment, which was slow in its action, insufficient in its results, and which can be comprised in two
words—revulsives and compression.

I have therefore proposed to apply aspiration to articular
effusions, and at my presentation to the Academy of
Medicine (at the meeting of November 2nd, 1869) I said
that it was possible " to aspirate articular collections by
means of a capillary needle armed with a previous vacuum
without the fear of introducing a single bubble of air,
and without the minute puncture causing the accidents
of traumatism."

This was the first time that this process was discussed.
In the course of the year 1869, I had experimented at the
Necker Hospital, of which I had the honour of being the
house surgeon, and I described these experiments in a
paper published in 1870, and again I gave in the *Gazette
Hebdomadaire* of November 10, 1871, a detailed account
of the indications, counter-indications, and the modes of
operating, in applying the aspiratory method to the treatment of hydarthrosis.

From the commencement, Professor Gosselin, by patron-

izing this operation,* had ensured its success.   Dr. Aubry
made it the subject of his inaugural thesis,† and foreign
journals, in Denmark,‡ England,§ and Russia, ‖ reproduced
the articles published in Paris, described their own cases,
and showed that this mode of operation was adopted in
other countries.   On this account I trust I may be allowed
to thank my learned colleagues, MM. De Kieter and
Yanovitch-Tschaïnsky (of St. Petersburg), Bilroth and
de Mosetig (of Vienna), Rasmussen (of Copenhagen), and
Dr. James Little (of New York), who have contributed so
much by their influence to the popularization of this
new method.

In spite, however, of the number of documents gathered
from all parts, and the numerous successes that have been
registered, many surgeons still doubt the harmlessness of
the aspiratory puncture in the knee, and this question
of harmlessness has just been raised at the Surgical
Society of Paris in relation to a case reported by Dr.
Dubreuil.   Consequently, before judging of the value of
aspiratory punctures as a curative means in hydarthrosis,
our first care must be to discuss its harmlessness.

Articular wounds, even those apparently most simple,
have always given rise to serious fears.   Examples are not
rare of persons in whom insignificant wounds of the knee-
joint have been the beginning of serious accidents, and

* *Gazette des Hôpitaux,* January 8th, 1870.
† The Treatment of Effusions into the Knee by Aspiration.
Thèse de Paris, 1871.
‡ Hydartrus, behandlet med aspiration.   Hospitals-ridende.
Copenhagen, December, 1871.
§ Observations illustrative of the Use of Dieulafoy's Aspirator.
By Dr. Laffan, Physician to the Union Hospital, Cashel.   March,
1872.
Illustrations of the Surgical Uses of the Aspirator, by T. Jessop,
in the *British Medical Journal,* December, 1872.
‖ Applications et usages de l'aspirateur de M. Dieulafoy en
Russie, rapport de M. de Kieter, professeur émérite de clinique
chirurgicale à Saint-Pétersbourg.   December, 1872.

facts of this kind explain the repugnance that some surgeons feel in plunging any instrument into the joint, even an aspiratory needle. As theory has never convinced any one, I might speak for a long while of the tolerance of the synovial membrane in the pathological state, and the extreme fineness of the needles, without bringing over to my side those who doubt, whilst if I appeal to clinical facts, absolute and incontestable proofs, I hope to succeed in making them share my convictions, and to establish the harmlessness of aspiratory punctures in the treatment of effusions into the knee-joint. After solving this first part of the problem, we will proceed to discuss the value of aspiration as a means of treatment.

To exactly estimate the harmlessness of aspiratory punctures, it is enough to attentively examine all the cases which have been treated after this method; to review the cases in which the operation has been innocent, and the cases in which it has caused accidents, and from the conscientious examination of these facts, to draw the conclusions which they necessarily impose on one. By adding together the cases that have been published or communicated to me on this subject, we arrive at a total of more than 150 aspiratory punctures performed on the knee for effusions of different kinds.

We have divided these cases into two categories; in the first are the operations which have caused no accidents; in the second are the failures, or rather the cases of puncture followed by accidents.

The cases of the first category are united in the following table; it can be seen that they relate to effusions of every kind, serous, hematic, and purulent, of a blennorrhagic, traumatic, and rheumatic nature.

FIRST CATEGORY.

ASPIRATORY PUNCTURES OF THE KNEE-JOINT, HAVING CAUSED NO ACCIDENT.

No. of Cases.	Authors.	Disease.	No. of Punctures.	Accidents.
I.	Dieulafoy.	Simple hydarthrosis.	1	None.
II.	Gosselin.	Hydarthrosis with a foreign body.	1	—
III.	Gosselin.	Purulent hydarthrosis.	1	—
IV.	Dieulafoy.	Traumatic ,,	3	—
V.	Dieulafoy.	Purulent ,,	7	—
VI.	Faucher.	Acute ,,	1	—
VII.	L. Labbé.	,, ,,	1	—
VIII.	Horteloup.	Traumatic hydarthrosis, sanguineous effusion.	• 2	—
IX.	Tillaux.	Traumatic hydarthrosis, sanguineous effusion.	2	—
X.	Duplouy.	Hydarthrosis.	1	—
XI.	Gosselin.	Purulent hydarthrosis.	1	—
XII.	Chairou.	Simple ,,	2	—
XIII.	Duplouy.	,, ,,	1	—
XIV.	Dieulafoy.	Double ,,	30	—
XV.	Phelippeaux.	,, ,,	2	—
XVI.	Chairou.	Chronic ,,	4	—
XVII.	Dieulafoy.	Rheumatic ,,	3	—
XVIII.	L. Labbé.	Double ,,	2	—
XIX.	Axenfeld.	Traumatic ,,	3	—
XX.	Aubry.	Traumatic hydarthrosis, sanguineous effusion.	1	—
XXI.	Aubry.	Traumatic hydarthrosis, sanguineous effusion.	1	—
XXII.	Laboulbène.	Blennorrhagic hydarthrosis.	2	—
XXIII.	Désormeaux.	Traumatic hydarthrosis.	2	—
XXIV.	Vergely.	,, ,,	2	—
XXV.	De Kieter.	,, ,,	1	—
XXVI.	Ball.	Blennorrhagic ,,	2	—
XXVII.	Dieulafoy.	Simple ,,	1	—
XXVIII.	Chairou.	Rheumatic ,,	1	—
XXIX.	Chaillou.	,, ,,	1	—
XXX.	Chaillou.	,, ,,	1	—
XXXI.	Gosselin.	,, ,,	2	—
XXXII.	L. Labbé.	Traumatic hydarthrosis, hematic effusion.	1	—
XXXIII.	Tillaux.	Hydarthrosis.	2	—
XXXIV.	Dieulafoy.	Double blennorrhagic hydarthrosis.	2	—

No. of Cases.	Authors.	Disease.	No. of Punctures.	Accidents.
XXXV.	Le Bèle.	Blennorrhagic arthritis.	3	None.
XXXVI.	Le Bèle.	Simple hydarthrosis.	3	—
XXXVII.	Le Bèle.	Traumatic arthritis.	1	—
XXXVIII.	Dieulafoy.	Double blennorrhagic hydarthrosis.	2	—
XXXIX.	Dieulafoy.	Hematic effusion of the knee-joint.	4	—
XL.	Ménard.	Purulent effusion.	2	—
XLI.	Savreux-la-Chapelle.	Hydarthrosis.	1	—
XLII.	Després.	Chronic hydarthrosis.	2	—
XLIII.	Douaud.	Rheumatic ,,	1	—
XLIV.	Dieulafoy.	Rupture of the patella ligament, serous effusion.	1	—
XLV.	Jessop.	Sanguineous effusion.	1	—
XLVI.	Jessop.	,, ,,	1	—
XLVII.	Jessop.	Purulent ,,	2	—
XLVIII.	Raynaud.	Hydarthrosis.	1	—
XLIX.	Raynaud.	Blennorrhagic hydarthrosis.	3	—
L.	Le Bèle.	Sanguineous traumatic effusion.	2	—

Besides these cases, which have been published or communicated to me in detail, and which are quite in favour of aspiration, I have received documents and information attesting without reservation to the harmlessness of aspiratory puncture in effusions into the knee. M. De Kieter, professor of clinical surgery at St. Petersburg, has been kind enough to send me a report (dated Dec. 6th, 1872), on the results of aspiration in Russia. The following is a summary of that part which treats of articular effusions :—

At the military hospital Nicholas, at St. Petersburg, five cases of hydarthrosis have been cured by aspiration, without accident. At the civil hospital, St. Marie, Dr. Kadé, the chief physician, reports two cases ; at the hospital of Kieff, two cases ; at the great military hospital at Moscow, four cases ; Professor de Kieter, one case. Not a single accident imputed to aspiration is any where discussed.

In the journals of England and the United States, I find cases which bear witness to the harmlessness of aspiratory punctures in articular effusions.

Dr. Jessop * (of Leeds) reports four cases of hydarthrosis cured by aspiration ; and these, he says, he selected from a considerable number of cases which have been similarly treated. Dr. Laffan † (of Dublin) has treated many cases of hydarthrosis by aspiration, and always found it quite harmless. MM. Barbosa and May Figueira (of Lisbon) have obtained the same result. M. Rasmussen (of Copenhagen) has obtained analogous success. Dr. Mollière recently wrote me from Lyons, " Aspiration is here so well established for the treatment of articular effusions, that we do not even take notes of the cases."

These are the collected documents which plead in favour of the harmlessness of the aspiratory punctures.

SECOND CATEGORY.

Aspiratory Punctures which have caused Accidents.

In this category I find but one case,‡ which is the one which was reported by M. Dubreuil to the Société de Chirurgie, at the meeting of October 9th, 1872. It occurred in a patient who, in consequence of a fall from a great height, was taken into the Beaujon Hospital, with a transverse fracture of the patella. " The joint was distended by a considerable effusion, which separated the fragments and caused the patient sharp pain. Hoping to relieve him, I thought of evacuating the synovia, by the aid of Dieulafoy's ap-

---

* *Loco citato.*   † *Loco citato.*

‡ To this must be added a fatal case since recorded by Dr. Macdonnell of Dublin, *Irish Hospital Gazette,* January 1st, 1873.—TRANSLATOR.

paratus. A first puncture was made on the internal side of the patella, with the medium-sized trocar, but it gave issue to nothing at all. I withdrew the instrument, and punctured outside the patella ; this puncture was as useless as the first, not a drop of fluid was evacuated. The punctures were immediately covered with a collodion plaster. The lower limb was placed in a splint, and the knee covered by a large poultice."

The next day, intense fever ; the external wound was gaping, and under the influence of a slight pressure on the joint, a considerable quantity of a sanguineous fluid came out ; later on, pus escaped by the puncture ; the patient at first passed through a phase of improvement which lasted for some days, then new accidents occurred, and he succumbed.

This case raised a discussion in the Société de Chirurgie, in which many eminent surgeons refused to admit the harmlessness of aspiratory punctures, whilst other members of the society supported a different opinion.

" The accidents of arthritis which occurred with this patient," said M. Le Fort, " were not due for certain to the puncture, for a fracture of the patella, with a considerable effusion of blood into the joint, is a very serious thing."

As to ourselves, desiring to judge the question with the greatest impartiality, we think that the best means of doing so is to place the two categories of cases that we have compiled side by side ; on one side 150 successful cases, and on the other one unfortunate one.*

In the first group are collected 150 aspiratory punctures performed on the knee for effusions of different causes and kinds, occurring after traumatism, blennorrhagia, and rheumatism. The fluid was, according to the case, serous, sanguineous, or purulent ; the punctures were repeated five, eight, ten, and even fifteen times in a few days on the same joint, and nowhere is mention made of

* Two.—TRANSLATOR.

the slightest accident. The observers are unanimous in declaring the harmlessness of the aspiratory puncture; in no case is articular swelling, erysipelas, or arthritis mentioned.

In the second group we only find one unfortunate case. The operator had placed himself in the best possible conditions, the puncture was made with care and ability, but the patient, having fallen from a great height, had fractured the patella; he complained from the first of intense pain in the joint. This case was then serious enough by itself, and, as observed by M. Le Fort, there are no very strong grounds for referring its fatal termination to the aspiratory puncture. But if it could be, what would this accident prove? It compels us to use prudence in articular lesions, complicated by fractures, effusion, pain, &c.; but it has nothing in common with the effusions of the first category.*

Thus, after having fully considered this unfortunate case, and after having placed it, with regard to its serious articular lesions, in a special category, we have still 150 aspiratory punctures which have not caused the least accident, and they are cases of the most different natures;

---

* The following are the leading particulars of Dr. Macdonnell's case. We quote from the *London Medical Record* for January 22nd.—In an article translated in the *Irish Hospital Gazette* for January 1st, Dr. Valdemar Rasmussen, in some observations on the use of the aspirator, says:—"In arthritis of the knee, both chronic, which does not yield to ordinary treatment, and acute, which causes violent pain from the great distension, aspiration is also a useful remedy." In the same journal for January 15th, Dr. Robert Macdonnell records the case of a man who had no other ailment than that of chronic effusion into the knee-joint. With the aspirator, as much clear glairy synovia as twice filled the syringe was withdrawn, and the patient was carried back to bed. Severe pain, rigors, and suppurative arthritis set in, and the patient was dead within a week. Dr. Macdonnell adds, "I have never met within my practice any case which made a sadder or more profound impression on me."

examples particularly favourable to aspiration have not been chosen, for we find amongst the number eight traumatic effusions, with hematic fluid, hyper-acute hydarthroses, and collections becoming purulent, &c.

Are these numerous operations not sufficient to establish the harmlessness of the aspiratory puncture? Here are 150 aspirations that have only been followed once by failure, and then in an exceptional case, and ought we to hesitate to affirm the harmlessness of the operation? It seems to us that a process of operating which, put in force 150 times, has only once provoked accidents, is as anodyne as possible. If hesitation could be felt in recognizing it as such, one must needs be careful not to apply leeches for fear of hæmorrhage, not to bleed for fear of phlebitis, not to cup for fear of erysipelas.

Every kind of fluid contained in the knee-joint may, then, be aspirated without fear or danger; my conviction is not the result of a theory, it rests on 150 clinical facts. One single case may inspire us with doubts, that is when we have to deal with violent traumatism and fracture and consecutive accidents.·

Before leaving this question of harmlessness, it is good to point out a cause of accident which, for want of precautions, might be imputed to the operator. To take an example—I suppose a person suffering from hydarthrosis for whom aspiration has been decided on. The aspirator is armed, and needle No. 1 is thrust into the joint, but the fluid does not flow, and the operator, surprised, asks himself if the needle is not too fine, or if the fluid is not too thick; he assures himself by many to-and-fro movements that the instrument has well penetrated the joint, and thinking to help the issue of the fluid, he has resort to a deplorable manœuvre, and presses the joint between his hands. To be brief, he withdraws needle No. 1, which he replaces by needle No. 3, and this time the fluid is quickly extracted. But in the evening, the patient feels the preliminary pains of arthritis, which the next day increases in intensity, and the operator hastens, a little too quickly, from one isolated example, to condemn aspiration as a treatment for hydarthrosis. How can we explain, however, that which has taken place? The first cause of accidents is so insignificant in appearance, but it is not the less of great importance, and is worthy of our attention. At the time of using the needle, the operator is not always careful to assure himself of its permeability, and its canula is so fine that a few grains of rust or dust are sufficient to fill it up. It is not at all astonishing, therefore, that the fluid is stopped in its passage. Hence the manœuvres of which I have just spoken, pressure on the joint, the introduction of a more voluminous trocar, of which the irritation of the serous membrane and the consecutive arthritis are the results.

We will return at greater length to these practical questions when on the subject of the mode of operating; our aim for the present is to establish the harmlessness, which we declare to be complete if the operation is done well. We can, therefore, undertake the second part of our work, that is to say, the treatment of hydarthrosis, of traumatic and purulent effusion into the knee-joint, and see if aspiration is a real improvement on the processes used before it. Here, as elsewhere, we take clinical observation and analysis of facts as the basis of our work.

ARTICLE II.

Treatment of Hydarthrosis by Aspiration.

Whether hydarthrosis be acute or sub-acute, rheumatic or blennorrhagic in its origin, the treatment is always the same; the fluid must be steadily evacuated until there is no longer any tendency for it to reappear. The different serous membranes have a very varying tendency to pathological secretion; thus, while the fluid of simple pleurisy is very rarely reproduced, that of the knee-joint is, on the contrary, reformed with great facility. The tenacity of the fluid depends chiefly on its origin. It may be said that the more local and direct the change in the serous membrane, the less the tendency of the fluid to reproduction ; when, on the contrary, a general condition is concealed behind the apparently local cause, the fluid seems to form afresh with so much the more facility as its originating cause is the more hidden or the less easily grasped.

What is certain is, that the condition is aggravated as the effusion grows older, the presence of the exudation is capable of exercising an injurious influence on the nutrition of the synovial membrane ; the effect becomes a cause, the serous membrane is thickened, the ligaments lose their elasticity, and the cure becomes difficult in proportion as the treatment has been long deferred. There is, then, in our opinion, only one course to take, and in presence of hydarthrosis we must evacuate the fluid without concerning ourselves with the acuteness and the age of the malady.

CATEGORY I.

Cases of Hydarthrosis cured by Aspiration.

CASE I.—HYDARTHROSIS IN THE COURSE OF RHEUMATISM —THREE ASPIRATIONS—CURE IN NINE DAYS (DIEULAFOY). —A man, æt. 38, entered the Beaujon Hospital, and was under the care of M. Axenfeld. For ten days he had suffered from acute articular rheumatism ; he had been successively seized in the left knee, the left hand, and the right foot. Hydarthrosis had begun seven days back, it was seated in the left knee ; movement was very difficult but little painful ; the synovial membrane was so distended, that the impact of the patella on the condyles could not be felt ; the joint was deformed, and measured 39 centimetres

in circumference. The fluid was aspirated the day following the patient's admittance, Aug. 23rd, and 70 grammes
were drawn off; the fluid was thick, slightly turbid, and
by the microscope a very notable quantity of leucocytes
were found. The puncture was covered by a little square
of plaster dipped in collodion; M. Dussaussay, the house
surgeon, applied strong pressure to the joint and bandaged the leg to prevent œdema. The next day, the 24th,
the fluid was not reproduced; pressure was continued.

August 26th.—The fluid having partly reappeared, 45
grammes were aspirated; fewer leucocytes were found in
it under the microscope.

August 28th.—The third and last puncture was made,
and 80 grammes of fluid drawn off; the knee was compressed. The following days the effusion was not reproduced, and the patient left the hospital on the 31st, the
treatment having lasted nine days.

CASE II.—ACUTE HYDARTHROSIS — ASPIRATION—CURE
IN TWO DAYS (M. FAUCHER).—M. X——, æt. 50, was of
a good constitution and had no rheumatism. On April
2nd, 1870, in coming downstairs he slipped and missed
several steps at a time, stopping suddenly on the left leg,
and he felt at the same time a rather acute pain in the
left knee. From that moment M. X—— felt a sensation
of stiffness in the joint, to which swelling and discomfort
in moving were soon added. On Wednesday, April 6th,
the patient went to bed, applied a blister to his knee, but
did not send for his medical man till the next day.
Aspiration of the fluid was proposed, but it was thought
better to wait till the blister was healed. On Tuesday,
April 12th, the swelling was still greater than on the previous day. The knee measured 39 centimetres in circumference, the pain was acute. Needle No. 2 was
introduced on the outer side of the articulation, and 45
grammes of a yellowish and slightly turbid fluid were

x

drawn off. Pain immediately disappeared, and the knee resumed its normal shape; rather firm compression was applied to the articulation, and the patient kept at rest. The next day, April 13th, all trace of swelling had disappeared; the bandage was again applied as a precautionary measure, and the patient was able to walk away forty-eight hours after the puncture, completely cured.

Case III. (At the St. Charles Hospital, at Rochefort, under the care of Dr. Duplouy.)—Hydarthrosis of the Left Knee—The Failure of various. Means—Cure after One Aspiration. (Case reported by M. Lécuyer, assistant physician in the Navy.)—A man called Ernest Hurteau, æt. 20, a joiner, of a vigorous constitution, was admitted into the St. Charles Hospital, June 8th, 1870, for double hydarthrosis, without appreciable cause, and two months old. Though by reason of the intense pain that the patient had felt at the beginning, the hydarthrosis may be referred to acute pre-existing arthritis, there did not exist any inflammatory symptom on admission. The effusion, which was very slight in the right knee, was, on the contrary, very abundant in the left; the superior culs-de-sac of the synovial membrane were greatly distended, and the characteristic shock of the patella against the condyles left no doubt as to the presence of fluid in the joint. Iodine paintings had been frequently tried without result since Hurteau's admission into the hospital; a large flying blister had been applied to both knees, and in the right had produced a rapid improvement; but the effusion in the left knee continued stationary. It was found in the same condition after it had been kept immovable for a month by means of a compressive bandage.

July 18*th*.—Professor Duplouy decided to puncture the articulation by means of needle No. 2 of Dieulafoy's apparatus, thinking that this insignificant puncture would, owing to powerful aspiration, offer every possible guarantee of harmlessness and efficacy. The instrument was used in the Clinic for the first time.

After having driven the fluid into the culs-de-sac by compression, the operator thrust the needle obliquely into the external cul-de-sac under the triceps tendon, and allowing it to remain, he successively made two aspirations with the body of the pump; he drew off thus 76 grammes of a reddish-yellow fluid, viscous and homogeneous at the moment of extraction, but which on standing soon separated into two distinct layers; the upper was of a clear yellow colour, limpid and transparent; the lower coloured more strongly, glutinous, formed for the most part of water and an albuminous network, coloured by blood globules. The microscope revealed, besides, the presence of pus globules.

Exact compression was applied to the knee, and the limb was placed in Bonnet's large splint for twenty-five days.

The hydarthrosis was not reproduced, but the patient was kept in the hospital till September 15th, so as to be assured of the thoroughness of the cure.

CASE IV.—HYDARTHROSIS OF THE LEFT KNEE— ASPIRATION—IMMEDIATE FAVOURABLE RESULT—UNCERTAINTY OF THE CONSECUTIVE RESULTS.—(Case under M. Lécuyer, assistant physician in the Navy.)—Pierre Gaudin, a peasant, at Gentet, near Cognac, came to consult M. Duplouy. He had considerable hydarthrosis of the left knee, of traumatic origin. He had been treated for four months by the most various means. He was punctured May 5, 1872, by means of the aspiratory needle No. 3, and the knee was submitted to methodical compression, and kept immovable in a splint. At the same sitting 105 grammes were extracted of a fluid slightly

x 2

syrupy, perfectly homogeneous, and of a citron colour. The fluid was not reproduced six days after the puncture, but the impatience of the patient did not allow us to judge of the ulterior result; he left in a good condition, and we have never had any further information about him.

CASE V.—DOUBLE HYDARTHROSIS—THIRTY ASPIRATIONS—CURE (DIEULAFOY.)—A man, æt. 47, a restaurant-keeper by trade, was admitted October 26th, into the Beaujon Hospital, under the care of M. Axenfeld. He had double hydarthrosis; the knees were so distended that the patella could not be moved; the right knee measured 41½ centimetres, and the left 39½ centimetres. The pain had begun a fortnight back, without swelling of the joints, but in four days the effusion had made rapid progress, and the pain was very acute. The patient had neither blennorrhagia nor a cardiac affection. The other joints were quite free.

October 26th.—I performed. double aspiration, and drew off from the right knee 70 grammes, from the left 60 grammes. The pain disappeared immediately, but returned at midnight. The fluid was slightly purulent.

October 27th (morning).—The fluid had been reproduced in the night, and at ten o'clock in the morning I drew off 70 grammes from the right knee, 60 grammes from the left. After the evacuation of the fluid no pain, but it returned afresh at 3 o'clock.

October 27th (evening).—Double aspiration, right knee 65 grammes, left knee 65 grammes. Five hours' repose after the operation, then the suffering revived with intensity.

October 28th (morning).—Double aspiration, right knee 70 grammes, left knee 60 grammes. The fluid was still slightly purulent, and, placed in a test-tube, it was seen to separate into two parts, one almost transparent, the other rather solid, composed of fibrine and leucocytes.

October 29th (morning).—Aspiration; right knee 70 grammes, left knee 60 grammes. The patient had ice-water compresses applied to the knee. The pain discontinued during the day, but the effusion formed afresh.

October 29th (evening).—Aspiration; right knee 60 grammes, left knee 50 grammes. The application of ice-water continued; the patient began to move his legs without pain.

October 30th (morning).—Aspiration; right knee 60 grammes, left knee 50 grammes.

October 30th (evening).—Aspiration; right knee 50 grammes, left knee 40 grammes. No pain.

October 31st (morning).—Aspiration; right knee 50 grammes, left knee 40 grammes.

October 31st (evening).—Aspiration; right knee 50 grammes, left knee 35 grammes. The pain less acute, and the nights good.

November 1st (morning).—Aspiration; right knee 50 grammes, left knee 35 grammes.

November 2nd (morning).—The tumefaction of the knees was diminishing visibly, and the fluid withdrawn was less purulent.

November 4th (morning).—Aspiration; right knee 58 grammes, left knee 45 grammes. The night bad and the pain reappeared.

November 5th (morning).—Aspiration; right knee 60 grammes, left knee 50 grammes.

November 9th (morning).—Aspiration; right knee 25 grammes, left knee 20 grammes. The fluid was hardly purulent, and a few leucocytes could be discovered with difficulty by the microscope.

The improvement continued, the patient began to walk on the following days, and he left November 17th.

To recapitulate : here was double and slightly purulent

hydarthrosis, for which thirty punctures were performed. The treatment lasted almost three weeks ; the effusion was reproduced with such rapidity that in four-and-twenty hours each joint yielded 120 grammes of fluid ; the intense pain disappeared immediately after the puncture, but it reappeared with the effusion. The application of ice-water was efficacious. The serous membrane of the knee received no harm from these fifteen punctures which were made in a space not larger than a franc-piece.

CASE VI.—HYDARTHROSIS—TWO ASPIRATIONS—CURE (Extracted from the *Abeille Médicale*, July 10th, 1871, PHÉLIPPEAUX).—On the 8th of September, 1870, a patient named Daunas, a conscript of the Commune of Bord, presented himself at our consultation. This young man limped. The right knee was larger than the left. The part was hot without redness, the tissues thickened, and the instep swollen. The examination was not painful, but walking was impossible. Inside the knee there was a marked elasticity, and a deep fluctuation. For about six months he had noticed the mischief. No appreciable cause, except, perhaps, the fatigue resulting from agricultural work. I proposed aspiration of the supposed fluid. The previous vacuum was made in the body of the pump, and with the small No. 1 needle I made a puncture on the fluctuating spot, on the inner side of the knee, and I pressed the needle in about a centimetre. The aspiratory reservoir was immediately put into communication with the tube, and whilst the needle, by pressure and rotation, was slowly penetrating, a translucid fluid was suddenly seen to rise and spurt into the body of the pump. I drew off 35 grammes. The knee diminished in size, and movement became easy. I did not, however, content myself with this. On the inner side I made a fresh exploratory puncture ; but it gave issue to no fluid.

It was the same with two other punctures made on the external side of the knee, and to a great depth, so as to touch the bone. The instrument aspirating nothing, I dismissed the patient, who walked home, a distance of ten kilometres.

On the 20th of September, Daunas presented himself again with the same affection. He had walked and worked much since the operation. The punctures had not caused the least pain. Fatigue alone, he said, was the cause of this relapse. Aspiration was performed on the inner side of the knee by one puncture. 40 grammes of fluid were drawn off and filled the body of the aspirator. Local applications of alcohol were prescribed and used. Daunas, whom I saw some time afterwards, was quite cured. From that time he had no relapse.

To recapitulate : slight chronic hydarthrosis cured by the aspiration of 75 grammes of fluid. The extracted fluid became, after a time, of a clear grey colour, slightly clouded. A white, pulverulent, albuminous precipitate was thrown down in the phial, which contains it still.

CASE VII.—HYDARTHROSIS—TWO ASPIRATIONS—CURE (Case reported from the Hospital St. Antoine, under the care of M. LABBÉ, by M. Hubert, house surgeon).— *January 8th*, 1871.—François X——, artilleryman, æt. 26, was admitted into the St. Antoine Hospital under the care of M. Labbé. This man, who was very tall and strong, had had typhoid fever four years previously. No actual blennorrhagia, nor previous attacks of rheumatism. Two days previously, after a night passed in the trenches, he felt pain in the joints of the wrist and knee on both sides, at the same time that rather violent fever showed itself. He had, besides, in the left tendon Achilles, a wound made by the pressure of his boot, for which wound he was admitted to the surgical ward. The day following his entrance into the ward, it was observed at the morning visit that the fever had increased. The pulse was higher, and the skin hotter. The articular pain had, more-over, become more intense, especially in the right knee. Nothing the matter with the heart. Under the influence of rest and poultices, the wound was already better. The knees and wrists were sprinkled with laudanum, and wrapped up in thick folds of cotton-wool. Bicarbonate of soda, 4 grammes.

January 10th.—The pain had not decreased in inten-sity, and it prevented the patient from moving at all. Same treatment as the day before.

January 11th.—In spite of the administration of an opium pill, his sufferings were so acute that he could not sleep. The cotton-wool was removed, and the wrists were found tumefied and red. The swelling was much larger on the knees, especially on the left ; but at this spot the skin had, however, almost entirely kept its normal colour. A subcutaneous injection of morphia was made into part of each knee. Vapour baths. The bicarbonate of soda con-tinued.

January 12th.—The injection of the preceding day had done little to allay the pain ; it was done afresh, without more success.

January 13th.—The right knee being very large, and the fluctuation very manifest, M. Labbé allowed me to make a puncture with the aspirator. The vacuum having been made previously, needle No. 2 was thrust into the superior and internal part of the synovial cul-de-sac. The stopcock was opened immediately after the skin was pierced. About 120 grammes were obtained of a trans-parent fluid, amber-coloured, without clots, entirely re-calling by its external characters the synovia which flows from a recent articular wound. As a dressing, compression with cotton-wool.

January 14th.—The patient felt himself so much re-lieved that, by his request, a fresh puncture was made on the other knee, and which produced as good a result. The wrists were not very painful, but the skin was rather red. The bicarbonate of soda continued.

On the 15th, 16th, and 17th the febrile symptoms and pain decreased. On the 18th the bicarbonate of soda was discontinued and 4 grammes of *extrait mou de quinquina* were given in its place, the patient being very anæmic. The cotton-wool was taken off to examine the knees, which no longer contained any fluid. On the 22nd he left the hospital to finish his convalescence in a private ambulance.

Case VIII. — Blennorrhagic Arthritis — Three Aspirations—Cure (Le Bêle of Mans).—Joly, of the 12th Cuirassiers, was admitted into the Hôtel Dieu October 10th, 1871, with an enormous swelling of the right knee, extending from the thigh to the leg, and causing apprehensions of extensive phlegmonous erysipelas. I performed three aspirations in succession with No. 2 needle, the effusion gradually disappeared, movement returned into the joint, and the patient left cured on February 20th, 1872.

Case IX.—Simple Hydarthrosis—Two Aspirations (Le Bêle).—François G—— was admitted into the Hôtel Dieu February 6th. He had an effusion in the left knee, not very painful, but very extensive. Two aspirations were performed at some days' interval, and he left cured on March 6th.

Case X.—Hydarthrosis—The Ordinary Treatment Insufficient—Two Aspirations—Cure (By Dr. Vergely of Bordeaux).—M. B——, æt. 25, showed unmistakable signs of scrofula. In April, 1871, after having given himself up with ardour to the pleasures of the chase, he felt some pain in the left knee. To this pain was joined a noticeable swelling of the articulation. A medical man prescribed three blisters in succession, and the pain, as well as the swelling, disappeared.

M. B—— returned to his occupations, but after five or six days the same symptoms reappeared in the left knee. Fresh blisters were applied, and friction with iodine was prescribed; the patient took a complete rest, and twenty-five days of treatment made the joint its normal size again. But M. B—— had hardly begun to walk than the articular swelling reappeared afresh. He then applied to me, praying me to cure him as quickly as possible, as he was anxious to return to his occupations, which he had left for three months.

Then, in November, 1871, the diseased knee measured 2 centimetres more than the healthy knee; the lateral and superior culs-de-sac were distended by fluid, the patella was floating; the patient did not complain of pain in any one spot, but he could not walk without immediately feeling extreme fatigue, and without fear of falling.

I prescribed friction with mercurial and belladonna ointment, paintings with tincture of iodine, and I recommended absolute repose. I then applied silicated bandages, after having surrounded the joint with bands of cotton-wool, as in Burgrave's apparatus. After ten days the apparatus becoming loosened, I removed it and replaced it by a second, after having ascertained a diminution of half a centimetre in the joint. The second apparatus was kept on for twenty-five days, and the patient declaring that he could tolerate it no longer, I removed it and found no improvement in the state of the knee.

I then proposed aspiration, which I performed with the assistance of Dr. Demons. After having applied the ether spray at the level of the superior and external cul-de-sac of the synovial, I made a puncture with Dieulafoy's needle No. 2, and drew off 66 grammes of a limpid serous fluid. I applied cold-water compresses to the knee, and the patient was kept quiet. Six days later the fluid was slightly reproduced. The difference between the two knees was not more than a centimetre in favour of the diseased joint. Eight days later I performed a second aspiration, and drew off 30 grammes of a fluid yellower than the first. After eight days' rest in bed, the swelling not having reappeared, the patient got up and occupied himself in his business. The cure has been perfectly maintained for eight months.

To recapitulate : this hydarthrosis, after having resisted ordinary processes, such as blisters, iodine frictions, repose, and compressions, was cured in twenty days by means of two aspirations.

CASE XI.—HYDARTHROSIS OF THE RIGHT KNEE IN THE COURSE OF ACUTE ARTICULAR RHEUMATISM—ASPIRATION—CURE WITHOUT RELAPSE (DR. DOUAUD, OF BORDEAUX).—In the *Bordeaux Médicale*, for November 10th, 1872, M. Demons, à propos of a communication made to the Société de Chirurgie of Paris, by M. Dubreuil (at the meeting of Oct. 9, 1872), appealing to all physicians who had performed aspiratory punctures, requested that they would publish the happy or unfortunate results observed by them, so that we might establish with certainty " the indications and contra-indications of aspiratory punctures in the different cavities of the body, and according to the nature of the effusion, so as to encourage the timid, or to moderate the enthusiastic."

I replied to his appeal, and I hope I was not the only one to take part in the inquiry.

Case.—Mlle. P——, æt. 18, healthy, though rather pale, menstruated regularly, and who had not consulted me before, except for sebacious acne, which covered her face and the scapular region ; this slight affection troubled her much.

Aug. 13th, 1872, she was seized with acute articular

rheumatism, which affected the right knee, and the left shoulder and wrist. The pain was sharp in the knee, and the swelling increased rapidly; in the other affected joints the pain was less severe and the swelling less. Intermittent fever of the tertian type complicated the disease.

The rheumatism and intermittent fever yielded gradually to an appropriate treatment, but the fluid accumulated in the knee was not absorbed. A blister having produced no effect, and the patient refusing to have others applied, I proposed to her aspiration with Dieulafoy's apparatus. This instrument had just then rendered me great services in enabling me to empty without accident a large purulent collection, which had developed under the great pectoral muscle of a child eighteen months old, and also to extract, in a case of intestinal obstruction, a quantity of gas and from 150 to 160 grammes of fluid fæcal matter, without the occurrence of the least sign of inflammation of the peritoneum.

September 4th.—After having pushed the fluid into the superior culs-de-sac of the articular synovial, and arming the aspirator, I thrust needle No. 2 into the outer culde-sac and drew off above 60 grammes of a viscous fluid of a clear chocolate colour. I withdrew the needle, and after placing a piece of sticking-plaster on the puncture, I bandaged the foot, leg, knee, and part of the thigh, taking care to exert rather firm compression at the level of the knee-joint.

September 5th.—Mlle. P—— did not suffer, and asked to be allowed to walk. But though the fluid had not been reproduced, and the patient felt no pain in the knee, I forbade her to get up and applied the bandage again.

The next day, the 6th, I found Mlle. P—— walking in her room. A few days afterwards, on the 14th, the rheumatic pains returned, and till the end of the month they affected various joints, but the cure was maintained in the right knee. At the commencement of October, I had reason to consider the illness over. I prescribed a general appropriate treatment, and discontinued my visits.

On October 23, I was called in again by Mlle. P——, who told me that for a week the pains had returned, but more particularly in the left knee, where the affection had followed the same course as in the right knee, without the same acuteness. She had not called me in sooner, for fear I should apply blisters; but now, as there was nothing more than water in the articulation, she asked for it to be punctured. The quantity of fluid seemed to me to be much less than there had been in the other knee; I resorted to medical means, and, the patient refusing to have blisters, I prescribed painting with iodine, compression, rest, and diuretics. Mlle. P——, who was very anæmic, was submitted for some time to tonic treatment (syrup iod. ferri, vin de quinquina).

October 28th.—There was much improvement, but it was not till November 10 that the hydarthrosis completely disappeared.

Reflections.— The effusion into the right knee was considerable, and not amenable to blisters; treated by aspiration, it was cured in twenty-four hours. The effusion into the left knee was much more insignificant, but treated by paintings with tincture of iodine, compression, and rest, was not cured for seventeen days. These different results speak too strongly in favour of capillary aspiration for it to be necessary for me to insist longer on its usefulness.

Not only this fact, but others that came under my observation, those published by M. Dieulafoy, or communicated by him to the Société de Chirurgie (nineteen cases of effusions into the knee-joint, treated by sixty-five aspiratory punctures, none of which was followed by an accident), have convinced me that capillary aspiration, performed with every possible precaution, in the articular and other serous membranes, induces none of the dangers attributed to it, either in the Société de Chirurgie or in the Académie de Médicine. As to employing it to the exclusion of all other treatment, my conduct in the case which I have just related shows that that is not my way of viewing it. As to sanguineous effusions, though I have often seen Jarjavay, when I was his assistant, puncture with the lancet not only large sanguineous effusions consecutive to contusions, and which he malaxated to squeeze out the clots, but even hemo-hydarthroses; but I think it is more prudent not to puncture them, even with the aspirator.*

Extracted from the *Bordeaux Médicale*, Jan. 12th, 1873.

PARAGRAPH II.—DURATION OF THE TREATMENT—VALUE AND EXAMINATION OF THE METHOD.—I could add a large number of cases to those I have already reported, but it would be simply an useless repetition. All the patients of whom we have spoken have recovered after having been operated on by simple aspiration, without any consecutive injection.

The duration of the treatment was variable, and the interesting point is to establish with precision how long the treatment was continued. We want to know if aspiration cures hydarthrosis more certainly and quickly than blisters, alternating with pressure and paintings, expedients which are generally prolonged for several weeks. We will include three categories, based on the duration of treatment by aspiration.

In the first group may be placed the hydarthroses which have given way under one, two, or three aspirations, that is to say after a treatment of from three to eight days. Instances are not rare; we have brought forward a dozen

---

* Farther on it will be seen what opinions may be formed of these hematic effusions.

such cases in our table. These very rapid cures are more usually observed when the hydarthrosis is of traumatic origin, or when it comes on acutely, with violent pain and immediate swelling. It is true that hydarthroses are occasionally seen which are cured spontaneously and without any interference. These cases, although exceptional, are met with, as for instance, in articular rheumatism; it is well to point them out, and we shall bear them in mind.

The fluid extracted from the articulation in hydarthroses of the first category is very thick, thready, and fibrinous, of a greenish colour, containing a comparatively large quantity of leucocytes.

In the second group we shall rank the hydarthroses in which it is necessary to perform four, five, or six aspirations, and of which the treatment lasts from a week to a fortnight; this is the largest category.

These hydarthroses develope themselves without apparent cause, after great fatigue; they are as insidious as in the blennorrhagic form, described by M. A. Fournier.[*] They generally appear slowly, almost without the knowledge of the patient, following in that respect the usual course of effusions of the serous membranes, which seem to develope themselves the more according as they are latent. The fluid of these hydarthroses contains a large quantity of leucocytes, in much greater number than in the fluids of the preceding group.[†]

---

[*] Article BLENNORRHAGIE in the Dictionnaire de Médecine et de Chirurgie.

[†] In a communication made to the Académie de Médicine, at the meeting of the 16th of July, 1872, M. Laboulbène thus gives a summary of the composition of the blennorrhagic fluid taken away from the knee by aspiration:—

1. The fluid contained in the articulation of the knee during the period of the blennorrhagic rheumatic state is of a deep yellow; it is composed of viscous, alkaline, thick, and purulent serosities.

Finally, a third group takes in hydarthroses of old standing, or certain recent effusions which, from a cause we cannot detect, reproduce themselves with astonishing facility. We cite Case V. as an example of this, where two aspirations were necessary in the same day. The pain disappeared only on that condition, but the serous membrane secreted as much as 60 grammes of fluid between the morning and the evening. In general these hydarthroses give way in the course of the third week; if they persist then comes the moment for considering the question of irritant injections.

The questions we must set before us are, is the treatment of hydarthrosis by aspiration superior to other methods? what are its advantages? and what are its drawbacks? I believe I can affirm that the plan of operation, as I have described it, is entirely harmless; I have seen performed, or I have myself performed, more than a hundred and fifty aspirations on the knee-joint, and I have never remarked the least accident in hydarthrosis. The pain is *nil*, especially if the precaution be taken to locally anæsthetize the part. The operation is as simple as a puncture performed by means of Pravaz's syringe, and the introduction of air into the cavity is impossible, since everything goes on between the articular cavity and a receptacle in which the previous vacuum has been created.

I do not, therefore, see any objections to using aspiration; it remains to be ascertained if there are any advantages in so doing. In hydarthrosis of a painful type, such as those which supervene very rapidly after a chill, or in acute articular rheumatism, the pain, sometimes extremely sharp,

It does not contain mucine, and holds globules of pus and fibrino-albuminous matters.

2. It differs from articular synovia.

3. It resembles arthritic fluid.

4. Aspiratory puncture may be performed with advantage to remove this fluid, and it deserves to come into ordinary practice.

ceases immediately the fluid is evacuated, and the movements of the joint, which were difficult, are then effected with scarcely any annoyance. We are far from obtaining similar results by painting with iodine or blistering. As to the duration of the treatment, it varies according to the causes which have given rise to the hydarthrosis, and according to the individuals who are suffering from it. We are now stumbling against a question which is but little elucidated ; and it is scarcely possible to say, at least up to the present day, by the examination of a pathological fluid extracted from a serous membrane, whether the effusion is likely to have a greater or less tendency to reproduce itself. It matters little whether the fluid be poor in coagulable substances, like that found in ascites or hydrocephalus ; whether it be very fibrinous, like that of hydarthrosis ; whether it be more or less rich in leucocytes ; there are conditions in the reproduction and in the transformation of pathological fluids which elude us, and we believe that it is preferable to be silent, rather than to hazard a classification which would rest on bases as yet too uncertain.

The notions we possess respecting the obstinacy of the effusion are somewhat of an indefinite character, and if we have included three groups in the varying duration of hydarthroses, it is only to establish facts, without pretending to seek to interpret them. It would be possible, it is true, by taking an average, to see what is the advantage of aspiration over other treatments as regards duration ; but this method, strict in the exact sciences, appears to us to be little applicable to medicine, for we should be obliged to associate together cases too dissimilar in character. Experience has demonstrated that a certain number of large painful hydarthroses, of some days' standing, give way rapidly after one or two aspirations followed by compression. In other circumstances, the treatment lasts twelve or fifteen days, and in rare instances attains to three weeks.

In Case XI. (Vergely) a hydarthrosis which had resisted compression by iodine plasters and three blisters, was cured by two aspirations. In a case we owe to Dr. Ménard, two aspirations did more in eight days than four blisters in six weeks.

In Case XIII. (Douaud) both the knee-joints were attacked at the same time by rheumatic hydarthrosis; one was cured in twenty-four hours by one aspiration, and the other in seventeen days by treatment with blisters and painting with iodine. These different comparisons plead strongly in favour of aspiration, and when we ask a patient who has already experienced the good effects of aspiratory puncture, to choose between a blister or a puncture, he quickly decides in favour of the latter.

We therefore think that, unless special circumstances are present, we ought to give up the different medications for the treatment of hydarthrosis, none of which, it is true, are in very great repute. They are:—1. Calomel, given to salivation, extolled by O'Beirne, of Dublin, a fruitful source of stomatitis, and one barren of good results. 2. Emetics in large doses, recommended by M. Gimelle, who began by administering 20 centigrammes in the twenty-four hours, and increased 10 centigrammes a day until he attained to 90 centigrammes, a dosing which was also often only a prelude, since the authors of the Compendium think that it is frequently necessary to associate with it, or follow it up by other means. 3. Painting with tincture of iodine, blisters renewed several times or kept open during several weeks, regarding which we have already expressed our opinion. These various treatments ought to make way for aspiration, which to us appears to be the rational treatment of hydarthrosis.

ARTICLE III.

Sanguineous Effusions.—Treatment of Hemarthrosis of the
Knee by Aspiration.

Until quite lately it was regarded as very bold to touch
the sanguineous effusions of the cellular tissue and of
closed cavities, for experience had shown that operations
performed in the sanguineous foci were often followed by
penetration of air into the cavity, by the inflammation of
the walls of the focus, by abundant suppuration, and by
accidents of a sufficiently serious nature to cause the death
of the patient.

These fears appeared still more legitimate when a sanguineous articular effusion was in question, and the joint
was a *noli me tangere*, on which we were satisfied to act by
remote and but slightly efficacious means. It appears to
us that there is no longer room for having the same fore-
bodings now that we have aspiration at our command ; we
are in possession of a certain number of cases of sanguineous effusions into the cellular tissue and the joints,
which have been treated by the aspiratory needle, and the
operation has never been followed by any accidents. It is,
however, to be remarked that this kind of fluid collection
is cured more completely and quickly than serous and
purulent effusions.

Thus, with regard to the affections of the knee-joint,
while a simple hydarthrosis sometimes resists five, six—
nay, ten aspirations, it is not uncommon for a hematic
effusion to give way to the first or second aspiratory
puncture. The ten cases I have collected, and which I
am about to report in detail, will afford confirmation of
what I advance, and it will be seen that the cure of these
hematic effusions has been rapidly obtained, without
there being the slightest question of troublesome complications.

And indeed, if the aspiration be well performed, whence should accidents arise? The puncture made by No. 2 needle is insignificant, introduction of air into the joint is not possible, since everything takes place in a closed cavity and an instrument in which the previous vacuum has been created; if accidents supervene it seems to us that they must be imputed to the manipulatory part of the operation. The operator commits an error if he makes use of too large a needle or trocar; he is wrong if he squeezes the joint between his hands on the pretext of favouring the issue of the fluid, or if he allows his patient to get up and walk directly after the operation. It does not indeed suffice to have a needle and an aspirator in our hand—we must also know how to manage the vacuum, to suit the size of the needle to the particular case, and conform to the rules which experience has enabled us to establish. Under these conditions, I do not fear to affirm that aspiration is completely harmless.

We have already said that the sanguineous effusions of the knee are cured by aspiration with great rapidity; here indeed the morbid cause is entirely local. This cause, which is, according to circumstances, a bruise, a contusion, a false step, exhausts its hurtful action at the first blow, and then disappears. It only leaves as a trace of its passage the pathological condition of the serous membrane, of which the principal manifestation is a sanguineous exudation. If this exudation were left to itself it would be slowly reabsorbed—it would play the part of a foreign body, and might, under certain circumstances, become a cause after having been an effect, and by its presence bring on the developement of an articular disease. If, on the contrary, the effusion is repressed, the serous membranes are placed in the best conditions for cure; after each fresh aspiration, the fluid, if it reproduce itself, is less hematic and less abundant, and I have never in any of the ten cases seen its purulent transformation pointed out. It thence results that an affection which was justly regarded as being somewhat serious, and which one approached in fear and trembling, may be easily combatted by our present methods. In the Cases II. and III. (Aubry), V. and VI. (Jessop), a single aspiration sufficed to produce a cure. Dr. Jessop owns that he felt some uneasiness before undertaking the operation, but he declared it to be completely innocent after he had observed its good results.

Case I.—Traumatic Effusion of the Knee—Hematic Fluid—Three Aspirations—Cure in Eight Days (Dieulafoy). — A man 37 years old entered M. Axenfeld's wards at the Beaujon Hospital. This patient was attacked by scarlet fever of medium intensity, but he complained particularly of a severe pain in the right knee, which had come on about four days previously, after a fall. The joint was rather large; it measured 41 centimetres in circumference. The knee was out of shape, the tissues were strained, the concussion of the patella against the condyles was very slightly manifest, pain was unceasing, day and night, and was exasperated by the least movement. A fixed position, poultices, and other means, not improving matters in any way, we made a puncture in the joint with the needle No. 2, and we drew off by aspiration 70 grammes of fluid, deeply coloured with blood.

The relief was immediate, motion became easy, and the knee soon resumed its normal form. This aspiration was performed eight days after the patient went into the hospital; at that time there was no further trace of scarlatinous eruption. After the evacuation of the fluid, compression was made over the joint, and the night passed without pain.

The next day, the knee again contained a certain quantity of fluid, 20 grammes were extracted, and the joint was compressed by means of a roller.

Two days after, a fresh and last aspiration, and issue of 20 grammes of pinkish fluid. Five days afterwards, the patient walked and left the hospital, completely cured of his eruptive fever and his articular effusion.

CASE II.—TRAUMATIC EFFUSION OF THE KNEE—HEMATIC FLUID — ONE ASPIRATION — CURE (AUBRY).— Julien Bacherey, 46 years of age, a working mason, fell on the 7th of November, 1871, at half-past four in the afternoon, from a height of nearly 1½ metre, whilst descending a ladder, carrying a chest of tools. He wished to recover himself, missed the step, turned round on the ladder, and fell on his knees in the midst of a heap of rubbish. When he got up, he believed he had only suffered in the right knee and the right hand; his elbows, however, were somewhat severely bruised. The right knee became extremely painful, and he was taken to his home. I could not find either luxation or fracture, and I only prescribed cold compresses, applied *loco dolenti.*

On the morning of the next day, the 8th of November, the right knee was enormously swollen, measuring 40 centimetres, the patella was raised up, and fluctuation in the joint manifest. The knee was surrounded by a compressive bandage to facilitate the flow of the fluid. Puncture was made with Dieulafoy's No. 2 needle; aspiration produced 100 grammes of a black, uncoagulated fluid; the patient said he felt great relief. I covered the puncture with collodion, the knee was surrounded with a slight layer of wadding and some sheets of pasteboard, and I then used compression by means of a flannel bandage. On the 9th of November, the effusion was not renewed, I replaced the apparatus, by way of precaution, and ordered the patient not to get up until I had given him permission to do so.

On the 10th of November the patient disappeared, and as he only lived temporarily in the street where his work took him, I could not obtain his address. Ten days afterwards, I met him in another part of the city, engaged in whitewashing a wall; he was perfectly well, and only suffered some inconvenience from his elbows. The wounds were suppurating.

CASE III.—HEMATIC EFFUSION—ONE ASPIRATION—CURE (AUBRY).—Emile Thomas, aged 29, formerly a soldier, of good constitution, received suddenly on his knee a basket of plaster which he was lowering by a pulley from a third story. The next morning the knee was 45 centimetres round, the patella fixed by the fluid. Aspiration was made; 120 grammes of a viscous fluid, mixed with blood, but in smaller proportion than in Case II. Compression was made, and a cure effected in two days. I have since then seen the invalid; he has not felt anything more in the knee.*

CASE IV.—HEMATIC EFFUSION OF THE KNEE—THREE ASPIRATIONS—CURE (DIEULAFOY).—A man 35 years old came into the Hôtel Dieu, on the 16th of December, 1872, under the care of M. Tardieu, whose place was supplied at the time by M. Martineau. The patient related how, some days before, in coming downstairs he made a false step, and experienced a somewhat acute pain in the right knee.

Sharp pains came on in the evening, and the joint swelled. When he went into the hospital, his knee was painful and large, measuring 44 centimetres in circumference, that is to say 5 centimetres more than the

* These two last cases are extracted from the thesis of M. Aubry, *loc. citat.*

healthy knee. Walking and articular movements became, so to speak, impossible, the external and internal *culs-de-sac* of the synovial cavity stood out in strong relief, but neither ecchymosis nor change of colour were found in the skin. I performed the aspiration of the fluid by means of No. 2 needle and the rack aspirator, and withdrew 85 grammes of a sanguineous and almost black fluid.

The relief was instantaneous, the joint resumed its normal form, and the patient could accomplish movements of flexion and extension without pain. Compression was performed on the joint and the leg by M. Massigas, the dresser on duty.

Two days afterwards, the fluid had partly formed again ; a fresh aspiration was made, 45 grammes were withdrawn, and it was observed that the effusion was less sanguineous than the first time. Compression was employed. Three days later, the fluid having re-collected, I took away 30 grammes of it of a rather deep colour. The patient recovered completely.

CASE V.—HEMATIC EFFUSION OF THE KNEE—ONE ASPIRATION—CURE (DR. JESSOP OF LEEDS).—A young man of 21 had a fall, and felt a rather violent pain in the left knee. I administered purgatives, prescribed rest, ordered lotions, but after a month of this treatment, there was no appreciable change in the joint distended by fluid.

On the 6th of August I performed aspiration with the smallest needle, and I brought away 7 ounces of fluid, almost entirely composed of blood. This was the first occasion on which I found myself in presence of a case of this kind, and I experienced some uneasiness as to the issue of the treatment. But the fluid did not reappear, and on the 9th of August I allowed the patient to rise, after having surrounded his knee with a plaster bandage.

Six weeks afterwards, the bandage was removed, and the young man only retained a little weakness in the joint.

CASE VI.—HEMATIC EFFUSION OF THE KNEE—ONE ASPIRATION—CURE (DR. JESSOP).—A man of 40 years of age, while trying to climb over a high wall, fell on his left knee. He returned home on foot, though suffering great pain. His knee also swelled, yet he still continued his work for three days. After several days' rest, tincture of iodine was applied, and the patient was admitted into Leeds infirmary.

On the 18th of September, I aspirated three ounces of fluid tinged with blood. The leg was bandaged until the 28th September, and then placed in a plaster bandage.

On the 14th of October, the apparatus was removed, and the patient left, completely cured, and able to resume his occupations.

CASE VII.—SANGUINEOUS EFFUSION OF THE KNEE— ONE ASPIRATION—CURE (LE BÊLE, OF MANS).—Auguste Glade, a soldier, came into the hospital at Mans under the care of M. Le Bêle. This man had never suffered from any disease previously, except blennorrhagia. He entered the hospital for an effusion into the knee, which came on under the following circumstances. Wishing to mount a horse without using the stirrup, he fell back on his right foot, then on the right knee, and felt a violent pain in the knee. He kept his bed for a week in the barrack infirmary, and as the pain increased, he asked to be allowed to go to the hospital. On examination, his knee showed a somewhat considerable effusion, and during ten days the joint was fomented with camphorated brandy. The tumour remained in the same state, and the patient complained of the same pain.

On the 18th aspiration was performed with No. 2

needle of M. Dieulafoy's aspirator, and the tumour disappeared completely. The patient did not experience any uneasiness or feverishness during that nor the following days. On the 22nd he began to get up, on the 28th he walked in the garden without any fatigue, and on the 15th of January, the cure being complete, he left the hospital. These few cases prove that hematic effusions are cured by aspiration, without any accidents, and with great rapidity. Two hospital surgeons, MM. Horteloup and Tillaux, have had two cases of this kind in their practice. One of the joints contained 120 grammes of black uncoagulated blood. In both instances, a single aspiration sufficed to produce cure. Professor Axenfeld has had an analogous case, in which two aspirations and six days' treatment were sufficient to produce a cure.

ARTICLE IV.

Treatment of Purulent Effusions of the Knee by Aspiration.

The degree of purulence of a fluid is very variable, from that specimen which scarcely looks turbid, to a decidedly purulent fluid; and as we find more or less leucocytes in all effusions of the knee without exception, it would be difficult to say exactly where purulence begins. However, in a clinical sense it is easy to understand where purulence begins, and we know perfectly well what is meant when a purulent fluid is designated. It is probable that effusions of this kind may sometimes claim the intervention of modifying injections; but I have never yet had occasion to employ them, and I do not see them mentioned in the cases—but few, it is true—that I have collected on this subject. Aspirations, repeated a certain number of times, have sufficed to exhaust the source of the purulent fluid.

CASE I.—HYDARTHROSIS WITH PURULENT FLUID—SEVEN ASPIRATIONS—CURE (DIEULAFOY).—A young woman, aged 24, entered the Beaujon Hospital, under M. Axenfeld's care on the 5th of November, 1870. For a week previously the patient had felt rheumatic pains in the right arm and the left knee ; the pain in the arm had disappeared, but that in the knee increased ; at the same time the joint swelled, until it measured 38½ centimetres in diameter.

On the 6th of November 40 grammes of deep-coloured fluid were aspirated, in which a quantity of globules of blood and pus were found by the aid of the microscope ; the patient applied iced water to her knee. On the 7th the fluid reappeared, the joint was painful, the same quantity of fluid was withdrawn. The applications of iced water were continued. On the 8th the condition was the same ; aspiration was made of 35 grammes of fluid of similar appearance. A moderate pressure of the knee was performed. On the 9th the pressure was well supported, the quantity of fluid taken away was rather less than 30 grammes. On the 10th aspiration of 25 grammes ; pressure. On the 11th the pain had disappeared, the swelling had diminished, 20 grammes of fluid were aspirated, presenting a similar purulent appearance. On the 14th there was no longer any swelling, the patient extended the leg without pain. Moderate pressure was continued.

On the 20th the patient walked with ease ; the shock of the patella was perceptible, without the presence of any fluid in the articulation. The above case was an example of painful, purulent, rheumatic hydarthrosis, for which seven aspirations were necessary. The whole treatment only lasted fifteen days.

CASE II.—PURULENT EFFUSION OF THE KNEE—TWO ASPIRATIONS—CURE (MÉNARD, OF VITRY-LE-FRANÇAIS).— I have performed aspirations on two different occasions on the wife of a colleague, attacked by spontaneous arthritis with considerable effusion into the knee-joint. The patient had been treated in the first instance for a fortnight by repeated blisters, and by frequent application of leeches.

The first aspiration gave issue to a milky fluid, and the pain, which had until then been intolerable, was quieted immediately. The second aspiration was performed eight days after the first, and removed a reddish fluid of a very fibrinous and coagulable character. Pressure was made immediately, and the knee was surrounded by a wadded and starched bandage. Fifteen days later, the patient, though still feeling a little stiffness in the joint, could walk with ease.

CASE III.—PURULENT EFFUSION OF THE KNEE—ASPIRATION—CURE (DR. JESSOP OF LEEDS).—A young man aged 21 came into the Leeds General Infirmary on the 19th of September, 1871, with acute periostitis of the right humerus; the pus was removed by means of incisions. On the 14th of October fever declared itself, and the left knee-joint became painful. On the 27th of October, the left knee swelled and became the seat of violent pain, Aspiration was performed in the knee on the 1st of November, and two ounces of a limpid fluid were removed. But the general condition of the patient continued equally unsatisfactory, the joint swelled afresh, and on the 10th of December, nine drachms of thick pus were removed. The operation had marvellous results; the pain disappeared immediately, the health improved rapidly, and on the 12th of January, 1872, the patient left the hospital.

ARTICLE V.

.Method of Operation in Serous, Hematic and Purulent Effusions
of the Knee.

When aspiration of a fluid contained in the knee-joint
is to be made, the diseased leg ought to be placed in a
position of extension, for in that position the articular
surfaces of the femur and the tibia are brought one over
the other to a considerable extent, and the fluid being
driven forward makes the patella and the triceps project.
It is advisable to encompass the joint with an india-rubber
bandage, which has an advantage over the linen bandage
in exercising an uniform and continuous pressure during
the flow of the liquid. However, in default of an india-
rubber bandage, an ordinary linen bandage can be used,
taking care, as a matter of course, to leave bare the point
in which the puncture should take effect. This point
varies according to the wish of the operator; we should by
preference indicate the outer synovial *cul-de-sac* at the
level of the upper extremity of the patella and at about
2 centimetres outside that bone.

To perform the puncture, either No. 1 or No. 2 needle
is used, but never No. 3, the too great diameter of which
may bring on accidents. For still stronger reasons the
use of the trocar must be proscribed. No. 1 needle, of
which the diameter only measures half a millimetre,
appears to us a little too fine. Though it has often
been used with advantage, we prefer No. 2 needle, which
fulfils all conditions, and which has never given rise to the
smallest pathological phenomenon. The aspirator being
set—that is to say, the previous vacuum being created—
the needle is placed in communication with the body of
the pump by means of an india-rubber tube; it is then
introduced into the tissues at the level of the spot designated for the puncture. The corresponding tap of the

aspirator is then opened, and this needle, which carries the vacuum with it, is slowly pushed forward, until a jet of fluid crossing the crystal index, or appearing in the body of the pump, indicates that we have penetrated into the articular cavity.

The fluid is aspirated to the last drop; it is useless to press the joint or malaxate it, for this manipulation would only have the inconvenience of irritating the serous membrane, by multiplying its points of contact with the needle.

As soon as the fluid is evacuated the needle is withdrawn, and we apply over the puncture (although this is not absolutely necessary) a small square of goldbeater's skin and a few drops of collodion. We must then occupy ourselves with the pressure, and we ought to use special care in this part of the treatment, for it is one of the essential elements of success. The knee is encircled with a thin layer of wadding, a somewhat energetic pressure is made by means of linen, or, better still, flannel bandages. But this is not all, it is necessary to surround the foot and leg with a roller bandage, so as to avoid œdema, which would not be slow in making its appearance, and it is well to place the leg in such a position that the foot should be the most elevated part.

Twenty-four hours after the operation, the dressing should be removed, and note taken of what has occurred. Two circumstances may occur—in the one case, the fluid is not reproduced, or at least but a very small quantity is formed. A fresh aspiration is therefore not necessary, but it is needful to apply compression afresh without delay. If, on the contrary, the effusion has assumed rather large proportions, aspiration is performed, and pressure exercised as on the previous day. The next day the same process is repeated, and so on during several days, still searching for the fluid and aspirating it as it accumulates, until cure is achieved. The introduction of the needle produces scarcely any appreciable pain, and that may be obviated (an attention for which the patients are always very grateful) by locally anæsthetizing the spot where the puncture is to be performed by means of Richardson's apparatus, or by the help of a mixture of salt and ice.

The treatment I have just described is equally applicable to serous, hematic, or purulent effusions of the knee. Before introducing the needle, we cannot be too careful to assure ourselves of its cleanliness and its permeability. It is from neglect of these details that we sometimes expose ourselves to the risk of accidents. By introducing a closed-up needle, we do not see the fluid make its appearance, and we then ask ourselves if we have penetrated thoroughly into the joint; we impart to-and-fro movements to the needle, which irritate the serous membrane; we try a larger needle, and, in short, we resort to manipulations which result in bringing on symptoms of arthritis.

Aspiration, or repeated aspirations, followed by pressure, appears to us to be the rational treatment for serous, hematic, or purulent effusions of the knee. We have already made a formal declaration of our opinion on this subject. When a fluid, whatever may be its nature, accumulates in a serous cavity, and when this cavity is accessible to our means of investigation without danger to the patient, our first care ought to be to remove the fluid. If it reforms, to withdraw it again, and so on even for several times, if it be necessary to do so, so as to exhaust the serous membrane by a mechanical and perfectly harmless method, before thinking of modifying its secretion by irritant and sometimes dangerous agents. But if aspiration within the limits we have indicated do not suffice, we believe that we must, without any intermediate means, have recourse to irritant injections; the mode of operating is of the most simple kind. Thanks to the aspiratory-injectors, it is possible to regulate the quantity of the injection to within a gramme; either to leave it *in situ*, or to remove it to the last drop without having to dread the introduction of air, for the needle which has served to extract the pathological fluid also serves to introduce the modifying fluid.

HYDARTHROSIS OF THE RIGHT KNEE—MULTIPLE ASPIRATIONS — ONE INJECTION — CURE (CHARIOU).— M. ——— had suffered five years from hydarthrosis of the right knee, but the pain was so bearable and the quantity of fluid so small, that M. ——— could walk without difficulty, and follow his occupations.   One day, after excessive fatigue, he felt acute pain in the right knee, and the joint soon swelled to enormous proportions.   I endeavoured to give the patient some relief by means of poultices and morphia injections, but seeing that I did not arrive at any satisfactory result, I decided on performing aspiration of the fluid.

On the 12th of November, 1871, I took away 100 grammes of a yellowish fluid by means of Dieulafoy's No. 2 needle.   The relief was immediate, but the collection speedily reformed.

On the 15th, aspiration of 80 grammes of fluid was performed.

On the 22nd, fresh aspiration; then seeing that the fluid reformed with such obstinacy, and in so short a time, I decided on injecting 10 grammes of alcohol. The improvement was progressive, and the patient might be considered as cured on the 15th of December.   Since that time I have had occasion to see M. ———, and the cure has proved radical.

CHAPTER IV.

The analogy existing between effusions of the serous bursæ and of the synovial cavities, would give rise to the supposition that the treatment of these differing diseases would be identical. I possess but few data on this subject, therefore I shall not allow myself to make any comments, but shall content myself with relating the cases.

Case I.—Hygroma of the Right Knee—Six Aspirations and Four Injections — Cure (Dieulafoy). —A woman, 43 years of age, went into M. Axenfeld's wards in the Beaujon Hospital, for a hygroma of the right knee, on the 7th of April, 1870. Its origin was unknown. The tumour was as large as a small apple; walking was painful and difficult, and flexion of the leg impossible. Several aspirations were performed at intervals of a few days, and somewhat energetic pressure was made after the aspiration. The fluid removed, of a pale yellow colour, soon became of a pinkish hue. Seeing that the fluid accumulated again without intermission, after the seventh aspiration, I injected a mixture composed of three-fourths of water and one-fourth of alcohol, and I left 15 grammes of fluid in the serous bursa. No accident supervened, the fluid did not appear again after the fourth injection, and the patient left the hospital with only a slight halt in her walk.

z

CASE II.—SYNOVIAL CYST OF THE INSTEP—TWO ASPIRATIONS—CURE (MARKHEIM).—A lady had a tumour on her instep, the size of a large almond; there was no pain, no change in the colour of the skin, but the mere situation of the tumour rendered locomotion very troublesome. A first aspiration was made with Dieulafoy's No. 2 needle, and gave issue to a thick, thready fluid of a reddish colour. A moderate pressure followed this operation, but the fluid reappeared. A new aspiration was performed, and a fluid of the same nature, but less abundant in quantity, was taken away. This second aspiration was followed by recovery.

CASE III.—HYGROMA OF THE CUBITUS—ASPIRATION—CURE.—In the report of M. de Kieter, of St. Petersburg, I find the two following cases briefly pointed out. A hygroma of the cubitus was, after several aspirations, cured in a fortnight; and Dr. Yanovitch-Tshaïnsky also relates a case of dropsy of a serous bursa cured by one aspiration.

CHAPTER V.

THE cases which I have collected on the treatment of
hydrocele are neither sufficiently numerous nor sufficiently
detailed to enable me to establish the value of aspiration
in the treatment of that disease. The question is whether
the fluid of hydrocele may be exhausted by successive
aspirations without injections. I believe it to be so, but
I could not affirm the fact, not having a sufficient number
of cases in my possession to enable me to formulate that
proposition.

In Professor de Kieter's report, mention is made of
four cases of hydrocele cured by aspiration; one at the
military hospital of Moscow; the three others at the
St. Nicholas Hospital, in St. Petersburg.

To these cases we add the five following, in which
hydrocele was cured by successive aspirations without
injection.

CASE I. — HYDROCELE — TWO ASPIRATIONS — CURE
(DIEULAFOY).—Alexander D—— had a large hydrocele
of the left side, which had come on a year previously
without any appreciable cause. I performed aspiration by
means of No. 1 needle, and I removed 220 grammes of
limpid fluid. The effusion was tardy in reappearing. I
performed a second aspiration a month later, and the
fluid did not accumulate again.

z 2

CASE II. — HYDROCELE — FOUR ASPIRATIONS — CURE (DIEULAFOY).—M. X—— was struck by a spent ball at the fight at Buzenval, in the inguino-scrotal region. Some months afterwards a hydrocele showed itself. I made a first aspiration, which gave issue to 240 grammes of very clear fluid. However, in a fortnight the effusion was reproduced. Fresh aspiration. This time the fluid reappeared, but much more slowly, and the third aspiration allowed me to take away only 60 grammes. After the fourth aspiration M. X—— was completely cured.

CASE III.—HYDROCELE — THREE ASPIRATIONS—CURE (LIBERMANN).—D——, a soldier, went into the hospital at Courcelles, on the 8th of February, 1872. This man had a hydrocele of the left side, which had attained to a considerable size. The testicle appeared larger than that on the healthy side, and the hydrocele had developed itself without appreciable cause.

I performed aspiration with No. 2 needle of Dieulafoy's apparatus, and drew off 120 grammes of fluid. On the 12th, the fluid having collected again, I made a fresh aspiration, which gave issue to the same quantity. The bursæ were enveloped with compresses steeped in alcohol. The fluid reappeared, but this time more slowly, and I then performed a third aspiration, and drew off 80 grammes.

On the 22nd the effusion appeared again, but in very small quantity, and a fourth aspiration gave issue to about 25 grammes of fluid. From that time the source of the fluid was completely dried up, and the patient was able to leave the hospital the following week.

CASE IV. — HYDROCELE — ONE ASPIRATION — CURE (CRAMOISY).—A coachman, 37 years of age, had a hydrocele of the tunica vaginalis on the right side. The tumour was of medium size, transparent, and had never been operated on.

On the 16th of November, 1872, I performed aspiration with Dieulafoy's No. 2 needle, and drew off 150 grammes of pale yellow fluid.

The fluid did not re-accumulate.

CASE V.—LEFT HYDROCELE—ONE ASPIRATION—CURE (CRAMOISY).—A man of 52, a cabinet-maker by trade, came to consult me for a large hydrocele which had made its appearance four months previously, without any apparent cause, and which, during the last two months, had been complicated with acute pain.

On the 17th of December, 1872, I performed puncture by means of No. 2 needle of Dieulafoy's aspirator, and drew off 200 grammes of clear and transparent fluid. The pain disappeared immediately, and the fluid did not again accumulate.

CHAPTER VI.

ASCITES.

EFFUSIONS into the peritoneum—ascites in particular—are of very little interest in reference to the aspiratory treatment; in fact the fluid is so abundant, issues forth with so much facility, and the accidents consecutive on the operation are so rare, that the ordinary trocar fulfils all the conditions requisite when it is desirable to give vent to an effusion in the great peritoneal cavity.

Nevertheless, cases do occur in which the plan of operation may be modified with advantage; for instance, individuals whose abdominal walls are indurated, thickened, or œdematous, and patients in whom the fluid is reproduced with great rapidity. In these cases, if paracentesis abdominalis be performed with a large trocar, we run the risk of seeing the opening become fistulous, a circumstance which might cause the most serious accidents to the peritoneum. These two conditions, œdema of the abdominal walls, and rapid formation of fluid, are most generally combined in persons attacked by a double hepatic and cardiac lesion; in them, the tissues of the abdomen, but slightly supple and elastic, are powerless to obturate the orifice left by the trocar, and the fluid, finding an easy issue, flows through the lips of the wounds, and a fistula is established.

Under these circumstances it is preferable to replace the large trocar by a small one, and to favour the issue of the fluid by means of aspiration. It is not necessary for the aspiration to possess its full power, it is sufficient to change the aspirator into a syphon, and the abdominal effusion flows with ease through an aperture so minute, that the fistulous course and its consecutive accidents need not be dreaded.*

* This subject has been treated by Dr. Festy, in his inaugural thesis:—Des complications de la paracentèse abdominale et des moyens d'y remédier. Paris, 1873.

PART IV.

THE TREATMENT BY ASPIRATION OF EFFUSIONS INTO THE CELLULAR TISSUE.

THE deep or superficial cellular tissue of the limbs, and of the splanchnic cavities, may become the seat of effusions of different kinds, cystic, hematic, or purulent, which do not escape the action of the laws regulating the formation and transformation of fluids in the organs and in the serous membranes, and which consequently ought to be accessible to the same mode of treatment.

Cystic accumulations, so common in certain organs, such as the liver, are very rare in the cellular tissues, and scarcely deserve to arrest our attention.

Hematic effusions, tumours, and sanguineous swellings show themselves under widely differing conditions, according as they are the consequence of a serious general condition, such as purpura, scorbutus, or variola, or the result of traumatism, such as a wound, fracture, or contusion.

As to purulent collections, their frequency in the cellular tissue is very natural, since this tissue is the agent in their formation ; but their genesis and method of developement assume, according to circumstances, different modes of progression, having a great influence over the therapeutic method. There is a great difference between the progress of an acute abscess, which forms in a few days, and the slow progress of a metastatic abscess, which will be months and years developing itself; and again, what a difference between a phlegmon, of which the pus remains for a long time in the interstices of the cellular tissue, and an abscess, in which the rapidly-accumulated pus immediately strives to make a path for itself, and to make its appearance outwardly. These distinctions in the formation and in the developement of suppurations of the cellular tissue, show us that the same treatment is not applicable to all cases; it is by generalizing a method unduly, that its efficacy is compromised. We must discriminate; an anthrax, certain abscesses, or certain phlegmons being given, no kind of medication can take the place of incisions and large openings, while in the case of a metastatic abscess, of a collection in the iliac fossa, or of a suppurating bubo, aspiration appears to be the best treatment to employ. Here, as elsewhere, aspiration is at once an element of diagnosis and of treatment. Whether the purulent state be set up rapidly in the acute stage, or slowly in the chronic stage, the diagnosis is sometimes surrounded by such difficulties that the discovery of the fluid is the only means of certainty. The diagnosis is the more difficult according as the tumour is more deeply seated; its form and its precise situation may be masked or changed in character by the surrounding tissues, and it often happens that it simulates a solid tumour and leads us into error. If the progress of the purulence be acute, the rapidly-accumulated pus will make a passage for itself, at the expense of the neighbouring organs or serous membranes, grave accidents will startle us, and we shall repent not having sooner made sure of the diagnosis, and not having acted in due time.

When we only possessed the services of the exploratory

trocar, improperly termed capillary, a deceptive and unreliable instrument, at once too large and too small, it is comprehensible that hesitation was felt in confirming the diagnosis, by puncturing in search of the purulent accumulation situated in the depths of delicate regions like the abdomen. Consecutive peritonitis was justly dreaded, and the only controlling power which could give certain indications of the existence and the situation of the fluid tumour was abandoned. But at the present time what reason have we for apprehension or for delay? We are in possession of instruments exercising a strong aspiratory power, and allowing the densest fluids to pass through the finest needles; the aspiratory needle does not present either the uncertainty or the danger of the exploratory trocar, and the numerous punctures made without accident in all regions and in all organs, give us complete security, and allow us, when we think the opportune moment has arrived, to acquire an absolute certainty as to the presence and the nature of the fluid effusion.

Exploration ought to be made with No. 2 needle, or with No. 1 if the region to be operated on is particularly delicate; the needle, armed with the previous vacuum, is introduced into the tissues, and is guided slowly in search of the fluid, which rushes into the aspirator as soon as the needle has met it. By this method, we can search without danger for deep-seated accumulations, such as perinephritic abscesses, iliac phlegmons, tumours of the pelvis, &c.

The treatment of hematic and purulent effusions into the cellular tissue, is in accordance with the rules we have already set forth for other cases. When a fluid has accumulated in any situation, our first care ought to be to aspirate it; if it form anew, to evacuate it again, and so on several times in succession if necessary; so as to exhaust the source by purely mechanical means, before thinking of modifying the secretion by irritant and sometimes dangerous agents. These successive and frequently repeated aspirations, without consecutive injections, which have afforded such good results in the treatment of hydatid cysts of the liver, in hydarthrosis, in purulent pleurisy, &c.,.are equally applicable to the different accumulations of the cellular tissue.

The harmlessness of the aspiratory punctures allows of their being frequently repeated without the least inconvenience and successfully ; and thus we shall find suppurating buboes treated during several weeks end by yielding to the twelfth or fifteenth aspiration. We shall report cases of chronic and metastatic abscesses, reproducing their fluid as quickly as it is withdrawn, and at last disappearing after the eighth or tenth aspiration. It is, as we have already said, a sort of struggle between the fluid which is secreted and the operator who excretes it, and, in the great majority of cases, it ends by the exhaustion of the fluid.

When the accumulation has a great tendency to reproduction, we must not wait till it has attained its original volume before we again evacuate it ; if the tumour contained, let us say, 200 grammes of fluid, we should perform aspiration as soon as 100 grammes are reproduced, then recommence as soon as the tumour contains 50 grammes, and so on until complete exhaustion has been secured. If the fluid resist this purely mechanical treatment, we then make use of injections frequently repeated and given in small doses, after the process which I have described at length in the treatment of purulent pleurisy and in hydatid cysts of the liver. The application of a trocar like the hepatic and thoracic trocars might, in such a case, render us the greatest services.

CHAPTER I.

THE accidents which were frequently consequent on operations performed in hematic effusions, the inflammation of the walls of the focus, the suppuration of the sac, the accesses of purulence, and the symptoms of infection, had induced surgeons to use the greatest caution in the treatment of these effusions. However, M. Voillemier had demonstrated the harmlessness of puncturing these sanguineous foci, provided that the puncture was performed by the help of fine needles and subcutaneously. Aspiration unites all the conditions of success, since it places at our service on the one hand extremely fine needles producing a trifling puncture, and on the other a powerful aspiratory force, attracting the effused fluid, and opposing itself to the introduction of the least globule of air into the interior of the sac. If the fluid accumulates a second and a third time, it is again aspirated, and pursued by this purely mechanical method until it is exhausted, without the necessity of performing injections. At each fresh aspiration the fluid loses its hematic character, and forms again in smaller quantity, especially if care be taken to exercise a gradual and methodical pressure on the affected part after aspiration has been performed.

CASE I.—SANGUINEOUS TUMOUR OF THE THIGH—ONE ASPIRATION—CURE (DIEULAFOY).—A woman 43 years of age entered the Beaujon Hospital in M. Dolbeau's service, after a violent bruise of the left thigh. This woman had been thrown down the day before by an omnibus, and one of the wheels of the carriage had bruised her buttock and hip on the left side. There was no fracture, but motion was painful and scarcely practicable; the skin presented a large extent of ecchymosis, and palpation showed a fluctuation extending from the great trochanter to the median portion of the thigh. In consequence of the extent of this effusion, I performed aspiration with No. 2 needle, and drew off 500 grammes of a blackish sanguineous fluid, inodorous and free from coagula.

Immediate relief followed the operation, and the puncture made in the skin was so insignificant that it was scarcely possible to find it again after the tissue had retracted.

The affected part was surrounded by wadding and bandages, rolled so as to exercise a rather powerful pressure. No accident supervened on this aspiration, the fluid did not form again, the patient soon began to walk, and ten days after left the hospital completely cured of the effects of the accident.

CASE II.—SANGUINEOUS TUMOUR OF THE LUMBAR REGION—ONE ASPIRATION—CURE (LIBERMANN).—M. H——, 38 years of age, fell from a horse on the 5th of October, 1872; he became unconscious, and was obliged to be taken home in a carriage. The next day, being called in to see the patient, I discovered a violent contusion of the whole dorsal region, which everywhere showed purple marks, indicating great sanguineous extravasation. At the lower part of the lumbar region, a little towards the right, there was a sanguineous swelling as large as the head of an infant, the pain was acute in the sacro-lumbar region, radiating into the right thigh, and the patient was unable to make the slightest movement.

I could not discover any fracture. I ordered applications of cold water and arnica, and rest in bed; but the pain continued, the swelling retained the same dimensions. Ten days after the accident, therefore, I decided on making an aspiration by means of Dieulafoy's instrument.

The puncture was made with No. 2 needle, and gave issue to 450 grammes of a blackish inodorous fluid. The patient was relieved immediately, and was able to go out the next day and follow his ordinary occupations, which were very fatiguing, for he was an engineer on one of our railways, and his duties imposed very long journeys on him. The puncture was scarcely ended before the prick closed up without leaving any trace.

In order to induce the complete resolution of the tumour, in which there only remained slight induration, we prescribed some Russian baths, and on the 10th of October the patient was completely cured.

CASE III.——HEMATIC TUMOUR OF THE RIGHT ILIAC FOSSA—ONE ASPIRATION—CURE (CHAIROU).——A woman, 30 years of age, a sister in the Asylum at Vesinet, consulted us in the month of January, 1871, for a very painful tumour situated in the right iliac fossa. The patient dated the commencement of her affection four years back, but the pain, which had been bearable during that period, had during the last six weeks become so intense that all work had become impossible, and the patient was obliged to keep her bed. It must be remarked in this case, that this woman suffered at the same time from very pronounced hysterical troubles, as vertigo, loss of memory, anomalous sensations, insensibility of the epiglottis, and irregularly disseminated cutaneous anæsthesia.

When I examined her I found a considerable tumefaction, without fluctuation, in the right iliac fossa. The belly was very painful and increased in size ; menstruation was very irregular, and during the last fortnight shiverings, sweats, and in fact slight febrile attacks of an irregular intermittent character, had come on.

I diagnosed a phlegmon in the right iliac fossa, and I performed aspiration by means of Dieulafoy's No. 2 needle. I obtained 650 grammes of a fluid which proved to me that I had no phlegmon to deal with, but an old sanguineous focus. Its aspect and its nature appeared to me so singular, that I had it examined by M. Méhu, the chief chemist of the Necker Hospital. The result of the analysis was as follows :—

This very fluid liquid, the colour of Malaga wine, or infusion of burnt coffee, coagulated very incompletely when it was warmed to boiling point, on account of its alkalinity. On the contrary, when it was freely acidulated by acetic acid, all the albuminous matter which it contained coagulated completely. Its density was 1·020.

A kilogramme of this fluid submitted to evaporation gave a well-dried residue weighing 58 grammes, of which 9 grammes consisted of anhydrous mineral matters, and 49 grammes of organic matters. The ashes of this liquid were ferruginous, its colour indicated the presence of blood, of which the colouring matter had undergone the transformations it habitually undergoes in old effusions.

This fluid was not precipitated by acetic acid, whence absence of pus, likewise there were no leucocytes. It was abundantly precipitated by four volumes of a saturated solution of sulphate of magnesia, as occurs with the serum of blood and dropsies, such as ascites and pleurisy.

In fine, this fluid had no character which made me particularly recognize the anatomical situation whence it proceeded, but I am rather disposed to believe that it came from an encysted, serous, sanguinolent tumour of long standing.

It was not necessary to perform fresh aspirations, the fluid did not form afresh, and the patient was cured by means of this simple puncture.

CASE IV.—HEMATIC TUMOUR OF THE AXILLA—ASPI-
RATION—CURE (M. DE KIETER, OF ST. PETERSBURG).—A
patient had an enormous cystic tumour in the left axilla,
the pulsations of which at first suggested the presence of
an aneurism. An aspiratory puncture was made with
Dieulafoy's No. 1 needle, and gave issue to a sero-sanguineous fluid, which was completely evacuated.

The operation over, a compressive bandage and application of ice were made. The patient was cured by this
single aspiration.

CHAPTER II.

We have collected fifteen cases of metastatic and chronic abscesses treated by aspiration, through the kindness of M. A. Bergeron, house surgeon in Paris. These abscesses were treated by means of successive aspirations, and in two cases only was any use made of injections.

The operators almost always employed No. 3 needle, the diameter of which, though only a millimetre and a half, is large enough to allow the passage of the very thick pus of these purulent collections. No accidents have been recorded in any case, none of the patients were attacked with fever, shiverings, or symptoms of infection. The source of purulence was dried up at the first, fifth, or twelfth aspiration, according to circumstances, and during this local treatment the patients were placed under a general treatment, of which cod-liver oil, quinine, and phosphate of lime formed the basis. These fifteen cases were all either cured or improved, and although these statistics are prepared from a small number of cases, they suffice to give us the measure of the value of aspiration in this class of affection. These cases are summarized in the following table :—

* *Abscès par congestion* is here translated *metastatic abscess*, as being the nearest English expression. French pathologists distinguish three kinds of abscess : acute, chronic, and "*par congestion.*" The last-mentioned are "abscesses arising by purulent absorption or infiltration, and formed at a distance from the lesion which gives rise to them."

METASTATIC AND CHRONIC ABSCESSES TREATED BY ASPIRATION.

Cases.	Operators.	Nature of the Disease.	Number of Aspirations.	Result.
I.	Dolbeau.	Metastatic abscess of the iliac fossa.	4	Cure.
II.	Dieulafoy.	Chronic abscess of the thigh.	5	—
III.	Broca.	Abscess surrounding a coxalgia.	—	—
IV.	Jessop.	Metastatic abscess.	2	—
V.	Dolbeau.	Metastatic abscess in the right hypochondrium.	—	—
VI.	Dieulafoy.	Metastatic abscess in the crural region.	7	—
VII.	Dolbeau.	Metastatic abscess at the level of the great trochanter.	1	Improvement.
VIII.	Dolbeau.	Metastatic abscess in the ileo-inguinal region.	4	—
IX.	Dubreuil.	Metastatic abscess in the lumbar region.	1	Cure.
X.	Dubreuil.	Metastatic abscess on the serratus anticus.	—	—
XI.		Metastatic abscess below the pectoralis major.	—	—
XII.	Dubreuil.	Metastatic abscess of the inguino-crural region.	—	Improvement.
XIII.	Dubreuil.	Metastatic abscess above the inguinal fold.	2	—
XIV.	Polaillon.	Metastatic abscess of the left wrist.	1	—
XV.	Polaillon.	Chronic abscess of the pectoral region.	2 and injection.	Cure.

CASE I.—POTT'S ABSCESS—METASTATIC ABSCESS SITU-
ATED IN THE LEFT ILIAC FOSSA—FOUR PUNCTURES WITH
No. 3 NEEDLE—SIX MONTHS' TREATMENT—CURE (DOL-
BEAU. Case reported by M. Bergeron, house surgeon.)
—Jean Gaudey, an official on the Eastern Railway, entered
the Beaujon Hospital on the 9th of June, 1871, in
M. Dolbeau's ward. He had a large painful tumour in the
left inguino-crural region, which interfered with his power
of walking. Questioned as to his antecedents, he declared
that he had never had either syphilis or any serious
disorder; he remembered that he was subject to glandular
engorgement, and to affections of the eyelids, in his childhood. Three years ago, after having gone through a very
laborious winter, he felt pain in the dorsal region, which,
at first slight and fugitive, finally obliged him to leave off
work. Three weeks' rest enabled him to resume his
occupation.

Eight months ago he again felt the same pain, which
radiated as far as the left leg; locomotion became difficult,
and two months since, he became aware of the existence
of a tumour, which reached almost to the upper third of
the left thigh. At the time of entering the hospital this
tumour was indolent, the skin was of normal appearance,
with the exception of numerous networks of veins, which
showed themselves on its surface. To palpation the
tumour was distinctly fluctuating, and the left hand applied
to the iliac fossa felt an evident sensation of fluctuation
when the fluid in the crural region was compressed.
The presence of these facts proved that a fluid collection
occupied the left iliac fossa, extending as far as the thigh.
Where, then, did this tumour originate? Exploration of
the pelvis afforded no indication, but at the level of the
twelfth dorsal vertebra and the first lumbar vertebra a
deformity was found. This point was very painful to
pressure. We were therefore in presence of a metastatic

abscess, originating in the vertebræ above indicated, which had probably travelled along the psoas muscle, and had passed below the crural arch so as to form in the thigh in front, and to the inner side of the femoral vessels.

July 15*th.*—The tumour situated above the crural arch had considerably increased in size. The skin had become slightly red, and the leg was decidedly flexed, and rotated inwards. M. Dolbeau then, whilst continuing a general treatment of cod-liver oil and quinine, decided on surgical intervention.

July 20*th.*—A first aspiration was performed by the help of M. Dieulafoy's No. 3 needle. The puncture was made at 2 centimetres above the Fallopean arch, and at 3 centimetres inside the anterior superior iliac spine : 250 grammes of thin inodorous pus were removed. The patient was considerably relieved, and no accident nor febrile reaction supervened.

August 4*th.*—A fresh puncture was made, and 180 grammes of pus removed.

August 6*th.*—The patient complained of nausea. He had no appetite, the pulse 100, a red patch appeared on the skin, and the enlargement of the neighbouring glands clearly indicated the existence of erysipelas. This attack of erysipelas was easily explained by the vicinity of a patient, who having come into the hospital some days previously with an erysipelatous wound of the head, had already communicated the erysipelas to two of his neighbours.

An emetic, much diluted, was administered for three days, the symptoms diminished, and the patient became convalescent. Though the tumour had attained some size, M. Dolbeau only decided on making a third puncture on the 18th of September, when 200 grammes of pus were taken away.

November 10*th.*—A fourth aspiration, giving issue to 80 grammes of fluid, was made.

The tumour, after that time, did not reappear, movement became easy, pain diminished so much that walking became possible, and the patient left on the 20th of December, 1871, after six months' treatment, to resume his work on the Eastern Railway.

CASE II.—COLD ABSCESS OF THE THIGH—FIVE ASPIRATIONS—CURE (DIEULAFOY).—On the 25th of January, 1871, I was consulted by a patient who had an enormous abscess situated on the upper part of the left thigh. The sensation of fluctuation was most distinct, and the tumour, ascending to the buttock, descending to the two lower thirds of the thigh, and passing round the limb in its upper portion, made me suspect the presence of about a litre of fluid. The skin was tense and marked with a bluish network, but it did not appear anywhere attenuated, nor inclined to ulcerate.

Madame ———— told me that her disease had made its appearance six years previously, and the prescriptions of several practitioners attested that the fluid had been forming for at least three years. At the present time the pain was acute, and the left leg was flexed, and rotated inwards.

I performed a first aspiration, and after having taken away 400 grammes of pus, I arrested the flow so as not to leave too large a cavity, and then exercised a moderate compression over the entire limb.

The patient experienced some relief from this operation, and a week afterwards I performed a second aspiration by means of No. 2 needle, and I stopped the issue after 300 grammes of fluid had escaped. This pus was healthy and homogeneous, without odour or red tinge.

On the 12th of February the improvement was considerable, and locomotion became easier; the fluid reformed apparently only in very small quantity. I performed a third aspiration, and took away 120 grammes of pus, a moderate compression being made as usual.

On the 25th of February a fresh aspiration was made, and 80 grammes of pus taken away; and on the 10th of March a fifth and last aspiration with No. 2 needle, 40 grammes of pus being withdrawn. During this treatment, the patient was under a regimen of cod-liver oil and bark, which she continued for some months. The fluid did not accumulate again, and the patient only suffered from slight lameness.

CASE III. — ABSCESS ROUND A COXALGIA OF TEN MONTHS' DURATION — FIVE ASPIRATIONS—CURE (BROCA. Case communicated by M. Bergeron, house surgeon.)— On the 10th of April, 1871, Marie Guyonner, five years old, was brought by her parents for consultation to M. Broca, at the Clinical Hospital. Ten months previously this child had coxalgia on the right side, and nine months after an abscess made its appearance on the upper third of the thigh, towards the external region. The abscess soon became as large as one's fist.

M. Broca saw the child on the 10th of April. He emptied the sac by means of Dieulafoy's aspirator, using No. 3 needle. The aspiration gave issue to 250 grammes of thin pus. The little patient was put on vin de quinquina and cod-liver oil.

On the 25th of April her parents brought her again, and a second aspiration was performed, giving issue to 150 grammes of pus. On the 14th of May another was performed, 85 grammes of pus being removed.

For more than two months the parents brought the child for advice at different intervals; the abscess did not increase in size. However, an access supervened, which determined M. Polaillon, who at that time replaced M. Broca, to make a fourth puncture with No. 3 needle, and 150 grammes of pus were withdrawn. On the 30th of

November a last puncture was made, and only 50 to 60 grammes of pus were found. During the course of this treatment no accident occurred, and the general health of the child was not deranged for an instant.

Case IV.—Metastatic Abscess—Two Aspirations— Cure (Dr. Jessop, of Leeds).—M. T———, 40 years of age, came to consult me in May, 1871, for a violent pain situated in the lumbar region and in the course of the spine, from which he had suffered for nearly six years. There was a slight deviation of the vertebræ, at the point of junction of the dorsal and lumbar regions, accompanied by a psoas abscess, which was about the size of an orange when the patient stood up.

On the 10th of June I withdrew, by aspiration, six ounces and a half of pus, emptying the abscess as completely as possible. The fluid formed again, and on the 28th of June I performed a fresh aspiration, removing three ounces and a half of pus. From that moment the abscess might be considered as cured, for although I introduced the needle on the 7th of January, in case the fluid had reformed, I could not discover any.

There was then no difference between the two sides, and the patient was free from all pain. The deviation of the vertebræ still, however, continued, and as a measure of extreme precaution, I recommended great care in motion, and prescribed frequent recourse to the recumbent posture.

Case V.—Metastatic Abscess situated in the Right Hypochondrium — Two Aspirations — Compression — Cure (Dolbeau. Case reported by M. Bergeron.)—Petit Cyrille, 85 years of age, came into M. Dolbeau's wards at the Beaujon Hospital on the 21st July, 1871.

This man was of a scrofulous diathesis, and had con-

tracted syphilis eight years previously, but had not experienced any effects from it since that time. For the last
seven months he had suffered from a soft, indolent fluctuating tumour in the right hypochondrium, which had
not produced any change in the colour of the skin. The
tumour was subcutaneous, and when first noticed was
a small lump, about the size of a walnut, at the level
of the last rib. The tumour soon increased in size, and
in doing so, it had a tendency to descend and extend
superficially, without increasing in depth.

When the patient came into the hospital it was the size
of the head of a fœtus, and without being painful, was
sufficiently distressing to the patient to oblige him to seek
surgical aid. He was at first placed on a tonic and
restorative treatment, and on the 1st of August a puncture
was made with No. 3 needle, which gave issue to 240
grammes of serous pus.

On the 3rd of August a fresh aspiration was performed,
removing 300 grammes of similar fluid. These two
punctures were not followed by any accident, the abscess
did not form again, and the patient was able to leave on
the 19th of August for Vincennes.

CASE VI.—METASTATIC ABSCESS—SEVEN ASPIRATIONS
—CURE (DIEULAFOY).—On the 10th of March, 1870,
Dr. Marchal de Calvi asked me to see, in consultation, a
patient, who was suffering from a metastatic abscess, situated in the right inguino-crural region. This abscess was
about the size of a large orange, and partly disappeared
under strong pressure, ascending almost into the abdomen, where it was also possible to detect fluctuation, by
pressing on the iliac fossa with the hand.

Although there was no visible deformity of the vertebral column, the patient complained of having suffered
from a somewhat acute and strictly limited pain at the
level of the last dorsal vertebræ. The tumour was only

slightly painful, but the skin was attenuated, and locomotion was very difficult. I performed a first aspiration
with No. 3 needle, and removed 80 grammes of very
thick, yellowish pus.

On the 17th of March a second aspiration was made,
and 60 grammes of pus removed, and on the 23rd of
March a third, when 50 grammes of pus were withdrawn.
The patient was considerably relieved, the tumour had
almost entirely disappeared, and walking became easier.

On the 15th of April, fluctuation having again made its
appearance, I performed one aspiration, and removed 80
grammes of pus. The patient having fatigued himself
greatly on the following days, the opening became fistulous,
and the pus escaped drop by drop. After three weeks this
opening closed up, and the patient was thought to be
cured; but the purulent sac again made its appearance.
On the 20th of May a puncture gave issue to 55 grammes
of healthy pus. The general condition of the patient was
good, and the pain situated at the level of the last dorsal
vertebræ had almost completely disappeared. Two other
aspirations were performed at intervals of some days, and
since that time the fluid has not reformed, and the patient
might be considered cured.

CASE VII.—METASTATIC ABSCESS AT THE BASE AND ON
THE OUTER SIDE OF THE RIGHT TROCHANTER MAJOR
—PUNCTURE—IMPROVEMENT (DOLBEAU).—Julien Charles
Rodier, 17 years old, weak, ill-developed, and bearing
all the appearance of a scrofulous diathesis, came into
M. Dolbeau's wards at the Beaujon Hospital on the 28th
of July.

He said that he had fallen on his right side about a year
previously, that he had kept his bed for three weeks, and
that soon after a tumour appeared on the upper part of the
thigh, on the outside and rather towards the back. This

tumour had been constantly increasing in size ever since, and at the time of his admission into hospital was of the size of a large orange. It was situated at the level of the trochanter major, and was almost spherical in form. It was soft, fluctuating, and indolent, without any change in the colour of the skin.

The movements of the thigh on the pelvis were difficult and painful. The patient was placed on a regimen of cod-liver oil and bark. On the 18th of August the tumour became larger, the skin became red, hot, and tense, and an aspiration was performed with M. Dieulafoy's No. 3 needle, and 300 grammes of thin sanious pus were withdrawn. A wadded compressive bandage was applied over the great trochanter, and rest in bed enjoined. The abscess had not formed again after the lapse of a fortnight, but there still remained some difficulty in moving the thigh. The patient was placed on an expectant plan of treatment, and the fluid not having reappeared, the man was able to leave the hospital on the 30th of September.

CASE VIII.—METASTATIC ABSCESS IN THE RIGHT ILEO-INGUINAL REGION — FOUR ASPIRATIONS — COMPRESSION—IMPROVEMENT (DOLBEAU. Case reported by M. Bergeron, house surgeon.)—On the 5th of April, 1872, Caubet Pascal was admitted into the Beaujon Hospital under the care of M. Dolbeau.

This patient displayed all the attributes of the scrofulous diathesis; his complexion was pallid, and the glands were enlarged. He bore on the anterior portion of the left tibia a depressed, corrugated cicatrice, adhering to the bone, indicating former osseous lesion. He said that an abscess which had formed at that point had given passage to two bony fragments. There was no history of syphilis. Four years previously, a violent contusion in the dorsal region had been caused by a fall; the patient kept his bed for six weeks, and could only resume his work after the lapse of seven months. At the commencement of the preceding March a tumour made its appearance, without any apparent cause, in the fold of the groin on the right side. This tumour was about the size of one's thumb, then it gradually increased, until it became the size of a large orange. Its precise situation was on the anterior and superior portion of Scarpa's triangle. It was soft, indolent, fluctuating, and could be reduced without any audible gurgling. When the abdominal wall at the level of the right iliac fossa was strongly depressed with the left hand, another tumour communicating with the first could be felt at that point, and the fluïd could be made to pass from the one to the other.

The vertebral column was not deformed, but a fixed pain, increased by pressure, existed at the level of the last dorsal vertebra.

On the 7th a first puncture, performed with No. 3 needle, gave issue to 280 grammes of thin pus. On the 13th a fresh aspiration of 150 grammes of fluid was made, and on the 19th a third of 90 grammes. On the 24th a fourth puncture was necessary, which produced 50 grammes of pus. None of these punctures gave rise to febrile reaction ; a compressive bandage was always applied over the groin. The patient retained his usual appetite during treatment. On the 7th of September he left for Vincennes, without a trace of the tumour.

CASE IX.—METASTATIC ABSCESS OF THE LEFT LUMBAR REGION — ONE ASPIRATION — COMPRESSION — CURE (DU-BREUIL. Case reported by M. Rémond, house surgeon.) —A man, 38 years of age, was admitted into the Beaujon Hospital on the 10th of June. He had suffered for four years from an abscess which had gradually become immensely large, and which was situated in the left lumbar region. The tumour was subcutaneous and indolent, with fluctuation plainly perceptible.

On the 11th of June an aspiration was made with Dieulafoy's No. 3 needle; 220 grammes of pus were removed, and a compressive bandage immediately applied.

The patient did not suffer from any results of the puncture, the fluid did not reform, and on the 28th of June the man left the hospital.

CASE X.—METASTATIC ABSCESS ON THE POSTERIOR SURFACE OF THE SERRATUS ANTICUS, CONSEQUENT ON CARIES OF THE TWO LAST RIBS—ONE ASPIRATION— CURE (DUBREUIL).—A man named Bonhomy, 40 years of age, entered the Beaujon Hospital on the 8th of July, for a painful, fluctuating tumour, situated on the posterior surface of the serratus anticus. A puncture was performed on the 12th of July with No. 3 needle. The fluid did not reaccumulate, and the patient, without having suffered from any accident, left the hospital on the 22nd of July.

CASE XI.—METASTATIC ABSCESS BELOW THE RIGHT PECTORALIS MAJOR, CONSECUTIVE ON CARIES OF THE THIRD RIB — ONE ASPIRATION — CURE (DUBREUIL).— Margaret Méguin, 63· years old, went into hospital on the 17th of July, 1872.

Above the right breast, about three fingers' breadth below the clavicle, was a fluctuating tumour, insensible to pressure and the size of a large orange. It first showed itself about two years previously, and had developed rapidly during the last three months only. During the last eight days the skin had begun to redden and to grow thinner. A puncture was made with No. 3 needle. It gave issue to 80 grammes of thin pus, without any bony fragments. At the same time an injection, composed of equal parts of water and tincture of iodine, was used. On the 19th of August, the fluid not having reaccumulated, the patient left the hospital.

Case XII.—Metastatic Abscess of the Left Inguino-Crural Region—Pott's Disease—One Aspiration—Improvement (Dubreuil).—Héloïse Vauler, 15 years old, was admitted into hospital on the 1st of September, 1872. She had, below the left inguinal fold, a tumour, bearing all the appearance of a purulent focus. A small hump, very painful on pressure, was discovered at the lower part of the dorsal region of the vertebral column. The disease had commenced about three years previously.

On the 12th of September a puncture, with No. 3 needle, was made, giving issue to 250 grammes of inodorous serosanguineous pus. A woollen compressive bandage was applied. On the 3rd of October, as the pain had diminished, and the tumour had not reformed, the patient was able to leave the hospital.

Case XIII.—Metastatic Abscess situated above the Right Inguinal Fold—Pott's Disease—Two Aspirations—Improvement (Dubreuil. Case reported by M. Rémond, house surgeon.)—On the 7th of May, 1871, a patient, who for two years had been suffering from curvature and prominence of the three first lumbar vertebræ, entered the Beaujon Hospital. The man complained of a rather painful fluctuating tumour, which had appeared about six months before, above the right inguino-crural fold. An aspiration was performed with No. 3 needle on the 12th of May, and gave issue to 300 grammes of pus : this operation did not cause any accident. After three weeks the swelling appeared again, but smaller, and 150 grammes of fluid were again evacuated. Compression was exercised after each operation. The pain disappeared, walking became easy, and on the 5th of July the patient left the hospital free from any trace of the tumour.

CASE XIV.—METASTATIC ABSCESS OF THE LEFT WRIST —ONE ASPIRATION—IMPROVEMENT (POLAILLON).—A man, 48 years of age, was admitted into the Clinical Hospital on the 16th of December. Three years previously the two radio-carpal joints were affected by fungoid arthritis. During his stay in M. Richer's ward he was treated by the actual cautery, and by drainage of the right side. At the time of his admission into the hospital an abscess was discovered at the level of the dorsal surface of the left wrist, the size of an egg, covering the radio-carpal joint, and ascending on the forearm. An aspiration, with Dieulafoy's No. 3 needle, was made on the 23rd of September, and 40 grammes of thin pus were extracted. Up to the 8th of January the pus had not formed again.

CASE XV.—COLD ABSCESS OF THE LEFT PECTORAL REGION—TWO ASPIRATIONS—INJECTIONS OF TINCTURE OF IODINE — CURE (POLAILLON. Case reported by M. Bergeron, house surgeon.)—A man, 27 years of age, was admitted into the Clinical Hospital, on the 31st of August, 1872. The patient had a soft, fluctuating, indolent tumour below the left clavicle ; it was as large as one's fist, and covered by the fibres of the pectoralis major. Its origin dated five months back. The patient had shown numerous symptoms of a scrofulous diathesis in his childhood, but he had never contracted syphilis. On the 2nd of September, M. Polaillon made a puncture with a No. 3 needle, which allowed the evacuation of 160 grammes of thin pus. Tincture of iodine and iodide of potassium were then injected. The patient left the hospital on the 11th of September, but his tumour having reappeared, he returned on the 30th of September. A second aspiration was made, and followed up by a second injection, and the patient was able to leave, cured, on the 4th of October. We have not seen him since that time, and the cure may be considered certain.

CHAPTER III.

TREATMENT OF ACUTE ABSCESS BY ASPIRATION.

Summary.—Abscess of the Pectoralis Major.—Iliac Phlegmon.—
Perinephritic Phlegmon. — Phlegmonous Angina. — Peri-
œsophageal Phlegmon.

CASE I.—ENORMOUS PHLEGMON FORMED BELOW THE
PECTORALIS MAJOR OF A CHILD EIGHTEEN MONTHS OLD—
TWO ASPIRATIONS—CURE (DOUAUD, OF BORDEAUX).—Some
months ago, Madame C—— sent for me to see her child,
of eighteen months old, who had been suffering acute
pain for some days. She told me that the little invalid
shrieked and cried, could not move the right arm, and had
a swelling on the right side of the chest. I found, on
examination, that the whole of the right antero-superior
part of the chest was swollen and puffy, the skin was
tense and hot, but not very red. Pressure on the tumour
and attempted movements of the arm made the child
scream violently. On examining the affected region I
found distinct but deep fluctuation; these different
symptoms, added to the fever, made me think of a phlegmon formed under the pectoralis major muscle. The
cause of the phlegmon was no doubt a fall which the child
had had some days previously. Not thinking it prudent
to give issue to so considerable an effusion by an incision,
more especially as the patient was of so tender an age, I
resolved to perform aspiration. The fluctuation being yet
more apparent the next day, I made a puncture in the
most projecting portion of the tumour with M. Dieulafoy's

B B

No. 2 needle.   I pricked the skin, and made it slip over
the needle, so as to avoid the introduction of air ; then I
traversed the pectoralis major and reached the cavity.
Twenty grammes of tenacious pus rushed instantly into
the aspirator ; but a sudden movement of the child
having displaced the needle, I put off the conclusion of
the operation to the next day, and placed a piece of
sticking-plaster over the puncture.   Two days afterwards
the swelling was considerable, the pain had returned,
and the fever was high.   I performed another aspiratory
puncture, which gave issue to 60 grammes of healthy
pus.   Compression was made, and the arm was fixed.
The next day the child was well, the compression was
removed, and from that time he has enjoyed perfect
health.

CASE II.—ILIAC PHLEGMON—TWO ASPIRATIONS—CURE
(LE BÊLE).—Madame Lemonnier, 32 years of age,
having already had several children, had a good confinement at the Lying-in Hospital of Mans, on the 2nd of
November, 1870.   There was head presentation.   She
left the hospital on the 12th of November.
    On the 19th of December she came back into my ward,
suffering from violent fever, and complaining of pain in
the left iliac fossa.   Exploration per vagina and abdominal examination gave no indications, but a manifest fluctuation soon became apparent in the left iliac
fossa.   Two aspirations were performed in that region at
intervals of some days, giving issue to a somewhat considerable amount of pus.   The patient was greatly
relieved, and the fever disappeared.   The last opening
was fistulous for some time.   The patient left the hospital in good health, on the 19th of January.

CASE III.—ILIAC PHLEGMON AFTER DELIVERY—TWO
ASPIRATIONS—CURE (LE BÊLE).—Madame G——, 23

years of age, primipara, had a natural confinement on the 20th of October, 1871. Recovery, however, was slow, and she was attacked by an interminable intermittent fever, which was quite beyond the influence of quinine. Pain, at first vague, but afterwards more strongly marked, became developed in the right iliac fossa. This region was puffy and swollen, and very soon fluctuation became distinct. On the 5th of January, 1871, nearly three months after the confinement, the purulent collection was completely formed. I performed aspiration with Dieulafoy's No. 2 needle, and removed 200 grammes of pus, giving great relief to the patient.

On the 6th, I made a fresh aspiration with the same result. The resolution of the tumour went on gradually, without the necessity of making another aspiration, and without any fistulous opening. Madame G——'s health was completely restored in a few weeks.

Case IV.— Non-Puerperal Iliac Phlegmon — One Aspiration—Fistula—Cure (Le Bêle).—I was called in in January, 1871, to take charge of Madame ————, aged 32 years. She had had pain for a long time in the left lumbar region, and in the iliac fossa on the same side. A swelling gradually appeared in the iliac fossa, and fluctuation soon became apparent. I performed aspiration with No. 2 needle, and removed a certain quantity of pus. The opening continuing to be fistulous, I used iodized injections, and the patient was cured after some weeks' treatment.

Remarks.—These three iliac phlegmons were treated and cured by aspiration. There are, however, some peculiarities in their treatment worthy of remark. In Case I. the second puncture became fistulous, but the fistulous passage soon closed. In Case III. iodized injections were employed; and the patient in Case II.

recovered without the employment of injections or the occurrence of any fistula.

CASE V.—PERINEPHRITIC PHLEGMON—ASPIRATIONS AND INJECTIONS—CURE (CHAILLOU, OF TOURNY).—M. P——, lawyer's clerk, 30 years of age, who had never been ill, fell down a stone staircase some weeks back.   The following days he said that he did not feel any inconvenience from the accident, but towards the end of September, 1870, he came to consult me for an acute pain situated below the last rib of the left side.   He likewise complained of general discomfort, his appetite was bad, and from time to time irregular accesses of fever came on. Although the respiration was not affected, I expected to see the developement of pleurisy, and I prescribed a blister.   Two days afterwards I saw the patient again, the pain continued, the uneasiness and fever increased, and as the respiration continued to be normal, I gave up the idea of pleurisy.   On the same evening and the following days, M. P—— was taken with a strongly-marked attack of fever, with its three periods : percussion of the spleen showed no increase in its size.   I prescribed sulphate of quinine.   These intermittent accesses continued, notwithstanding my treatment, and the lumbar pain became very acute : on the 6th of October two cupping glasses were applied.   This pain, accompanied by increase of fever, made me think of the formation of a perinephritic abscess. To combat the continual constipation, I gave small doses of rhubarb.   On the 10th of October I discovered a puffiness, accompanied by deep-seated pulsations in the left lumbar region, but I did not perceive a deep fluctuation until the 24th, when I made an exploratory puncture with the hypodermic syringe, which produced one drop of pus.

October 26th.—I performed aspiration with the largest trocar of Dieulafoy's apparatus, on the external edge of the lumbar square, and I aspirated 300 grammes of healthy phlegmonous pus. This operation was followed by immediate relief.

October 28th.—I performed a fresh aspiration, which produced the same quantity of purulent fluid; I kept the orifice open by means of a thick thread folded backwards and forwards, and twisted into the shape of a screw. The following days I employed injections of water and carbolic acid by means of the aspirator, and later on iodized injections. In consequence of the penetration of air into the cavity, the pus altered in character, and symptoms of putrescence showed themselves immediately. The fever, which had disappeared after the first puncture, then reappeared, the skin was burning, but washing out the cavity, by means of a female catheter deeply inserted, removed these symptoms immediately. Appetite returned, the patient became stronger, suppuration diminished considerably, and the iodized injections were continued with regularity. Some weeks later he was completely cured.

CASE VI.—PHLEGMONOUS ANGINA—ONE ASPIRATION—CURE—(GAURIER).—A young woman named Martha, 18 years of age, came into the Hôtel Dieu, in M. Tardieu's wards, on the 27th of November, suffering from an intense pain in the head, caused by the sudden cessation of the menses, which had stopped abruptly from the effects of a chill. On the fifth day the patient felt a violent constriction of the throat, and deglutition became painful and difficult to the last degree. When making my rounds on the 28th, all the symptoms of a phlegmonous angina in the suppurative stage were discovered. The right side of the velum of the palate was displaced forwards, and the isthmus of the throat was almost entirely closed. Two glasses of seidlitz water and an astringent gargle were prescribed. There was no amelioration the next day, so M. Gaurier performed aspiration by means of No. 3 needle of Dieulafoy's aspirator, and took away 30 grammes of pus. The relief was immediate, deglutition became easy, and the patient left the hospital on the 2nd of December, perfectly cured.

CASE VII.—PERI-ŒSOPHAGEAL PHLEGMON—TWO ASPIRATIONS—CURE (LE BÊLE).—A young man named Guiton, 19 years of age, was admitted into the hospital on the 17th August, 1870. I found an œdematous swelling of the neck, accompanied by very serious symptoms and impending suffocation. The countenance was purple, the head thrown back, and the man labouring under the greatest distress. I diagnosed a deep phlegmon of the neck, and I introduced No. 2 needle of the aspirator between the edge of the sterno-cleido mastoid and the thyroid region. I aspirated about 50 grammes of pus, and relief was immediate.

On the 18th of August, the patient had a fresh attack of dyspnœa, but less violent than the preceding one. I performed a fresh aspiration, and again removed 40 grammes of pus. The small opening became fistulous, but the cavity closed quickly, and on the 12th of September the patient left, cured.

CHAPTER IV.

TREATMENT OF ADENITIS AND SUPPURATING BUBOES BY ASPIRATION.

SUPPURATING glands may be treated with advantage by aspiratory punctures ; the pus generally forms again with great rapidity, but we can aspirate it as quickly as it is reproduced, and, if necessary, perform two or three aspirations a week until complete exhaustion is secured. The absence of a cicatrix is not the least of the advantages of this treatment; we have seen scrofulous cervical adenitis cured by a certain number of aspirations, without its being possible to discover the point where the punctures were made. The same method has been applied with advantage to the treatment of suppurating buboes.

M. Libermann, surgeon to the military hospital of Gros-Caillou, has been good enough to communicate to us a summary of his as yet unpublished work on the treatment of inguinal, suppurating glands, and it is to him that the honour is due of having first applied aspiration to the treatment of buboes. The following case will afford an exact account of the method employed, and the result obtained :—

A soldier was admitted into the hospital at Courcelles on the 3rd of October, 1871. The man had been ill for three weeks; he had three soft chancres on the prepuce, going on to cicatrisation, and a bubo as large as a hen's egg in the left groin. Palpation of the tumour showed a slight fluctuation, and the skin retained its normal aspect. On the 4th of October a puncture was made with No. 1 needle of Dieulafoy's aspirator, and gave issue to 30 grammes of pus mixed with a little blood. One drop of this pus was inoculated into the thigh, and four days after reproduced a soft chancre, which was rapidly cured by cauterisations with nitrate of silver. Immediately after the aspiration of the bubo, compression was applied by means of a woollen spica bandage. On the 6th of February a fresh aspiration was made, 35 grammes of pus taken away, and compression applied. On the 7th the pus had formed again ; 30 grammes were withdrawn, and a fresh aspiration performed every day. After the ninth puncture, the pus became serous, and after the eleventh, the fluid was not reproduced. Some days later, the resolution of the tumour was complete. The punctures left no trace, and the patient left the hospital on the 25th of October.

M. Libermann applied aspiration to thirty-six cases of inguinal adenitis ; of which nine were virulent, and twenty-seven sympathetic.

In the nine virulent cases of adenitis, the aspiratory method completely succeeded in five cases, and failed in four. In the five successful cases, the average length of treatment was twenty-two days, and the average number of aspirations, ten. In the four unsuccessful cases, the punctures became ulcerated, and formed a cutaneous chancre which required the usual time to cicatrise.

If the cause of the want of success in the cases last mentioned be sought for, we may refer it to the time when the aspiration was made, success being so much the more likely if we do not wait for the skin to be red, attenuated, and detached. The twenty-seven cases of sympathetic buboes are thus divided : sympathetic buboes resulting from soft chancres, ten ; sympathetic buboes resulting from hard chancres, fourteen; sympathetic buboes of undetermined origin, three.

In the category of buboes which have not supervened after soft chancres, we find four cures obtained in the space of from four to eight days, and six cures in an average of a fortnight to three weeks. In the category of buboes supervening on indurated chancres we find nine cures in an average of a fortnight, and five cures in a space of from three weeks to a month. As to the buboes of undetermined origin, two were cured at the end of a week, and one in a month. Although these statistics are limited in number, they prove that aspiration applied to the treatment of buboes may be of great value. According to M. Libermann, it shortens the duration of the treatment of a long and painful disease, and in the greater number of cases it prevents the skin from becoming ulcerated and detached from the subjacent tissues, and also prevents the indelible scars and the phagædenic affections which are so much to be dreaded.

Dr. Schonfeld, surgeon to the military hospital at Kieff, who has employed aspiration in the treatment of seventy-six suppurating buboes, has arrived at analogous conclusions, and thus formulates them :—

1. It is possible by the use of the aspirator to evacuate the pus of buboes at a period when the integuments are still in a normal condition, and without fearing the introduction of air into the cavity.

2. This operation prevents subcutaneous infiltrations, cure is effected with sufficient rapidity, the cicatrix is almost invisible; repeated aspirations therefore constitute the most rational treatment for suppurating buboes.

PART V.

ASPIRATORS.

ARTICLE I.

History.—General Idea of the Aspirator.

WHAT is an aspirator ? An aspirator is a pneumatic machine of varying shape and size, which is intended, by means of fine hollow needles introduced into the tissues, to remove the morbid fluids effused into and collected in the organs, the serous cavities, and the different regions of the economy.

The historical aspect of this question, the birth and origin of the aspirator, have been touched on and discussed in the early part of this work * at sufficient length, to render it useless to descant further on it. We should have wished to have banished all personal elements from the study of this subject, but we have been forcibly brought on this ground by the somewhat sharp attacks to which we have been exposed, and we then undertook a scientific inquiry on the question of priority, which has enabled us to affirm that before our presentation to the Academy of Medicine, at the meeting of the 2nd of November, 1869, neither aspirator nor method of aspira-

* *See* page 3 and *sequitur.*

tion existed.   If the problem has not been solved before,
it is not for want of searching for the solution ; for, since
the time of Galen, who seems to have invented the first
pyulcon, until our days, dozens of instruments, of which I
omit a particular enumeration, have been invented for the
purpose of extracting morbid fluids.

But the inventors moved perpetually in the same circle;
they contented themselves with modifying pyulca and
syringes, instruments with a subsequent and imperfect
vacuum, without perceiving that changes which only affected the form or the name of the apparatus were no real
advance in the therapeutics of morbid fluids.

It is easy to see the reason. of this inferiority.   The
vacuum obtained by these instruments was a subsequent
and very imperfect vacuum.*

Aspirating morbid fluids only with great difficulty, it
resulted, as a matter of course, that the trocars intended
to give passage to these fluids were necessarily of a
relatively large size, which would make them inappropriate
for introduction into delicate organs.

Thus, a large trocar and very imperfect aspiration, one
producing the other, was the hereditary defect of the
instruments which had been applied for generations to the
extraction of fluids ;   from   the   pyulcon of Galen   to
Laugier's ball syringe ; from M. Van den Corput's trocar
to M. Guérin's syringe.

These are the reasons why these instruments and all
resembling them (their name is legion) were not aspirators, that is why, possessing the same defects and
offering neither the harmlessness of puncture, nor the
requisite conditions for aspiration, they fell successively
into   well   merited   oblivion,   and   surgery possessed
no   instrument   which   could   be   used efficaciously for
the   extraction   of   morbid   fluids   at   the   time when we

---

* *See* the remarks on the subsequent vacuum, the previous
vacuum, page 12 *et seq.*

introduced the first aspiratory apparatus. If other proofs were wanting, the written testimony of such men as M. Trousseau and M. Nélaton would suffice to attest what I advance : Trousseau had just performed paracentesis in a case of pericarditis ; the fluid flowed badly, in driblets, as is usual in this operation ; the idea then occurred to him to introduce a sound for the purpose of assisting the outflow of the fluid, and to apply a syringe at the end of the sound, hoping by these means to arrive at a better result. But this proceeding was so insufficient, and these attempts were so unsuccessful at this time as well as at others, that Trousseau hastened to add : " It is useless to try the different expedients which have been recommended to hasten the evacuation of the fluids, the use of aspiratory pumps not being of any assistance, and complicating the instruments used in operating in a very tiresome manner." *

This quotation sufficiently enlightens us as to the state of aspiration some years ago ; where, then, were the so-called aspiratory instruments ? If they had been in existence, as has been stated, would Trousseau have misrepresented or overlooked them ; he, a man of progress, always ready to bring scientific innovations into notice ? M. Nélaton, in his pathological treatise, discussing the treatment of strangulated hernia, and speaking of the frequently repeated attempts which had been made to puncture the intestine in order to disembarrass it of its fluids and gases, condemns this method of operation in the following terms : " Of two things one," he says ; " either the opening of the intestine will be very small, and nothing will come out, or it will be larger, and we shall be exposed, after reduction has been effected, to an effusion into the abdominal cavity." Now, if the aspirator had been in existence, and if aspiration had been known for several years at the time that these lines were written, can it be

* Clinique Médicale de l'Hôtel Dieu. Paracentèse du Pericarde, 186. T. II., p. 26.

supposed that M. Nélaton would not have made use of a method which soon after was destined to give such brilliant results in the treatment of strangulated hernia.　It is useless to accumulate a greater number of proofs in favour of the established origin of the aspirators.　That the idea of aspirating morbid fluids existed for many centuries, is a fact ; trite from its very truth, we constantly meet with this idea in the history of medicine, but it had remained, without form and void, in the theoretical stage, because it had not assumed a practical form ; and it has only become a medico-chirurgical method since the day the aspirator was invented.

At the present time, the diagnosis and treatment of morbid fluids have entered on an entirely new phase. The aspirator was based on principles which made it entirely different from the instruments which had preceded it.　Aspiratory power, so imperfect in the pyulca and syringes, was here replaced by the much more powerful force of the pneumatic machine; large trocars, unfit for exploration, were succeeded by hollow needles of extreme delicacy, and a most essential matter, the previous vacuum, took the place of the subsequent vacuum.　The power of aspiration allowed the thickest fluids to pass through the finest needles, the smallness of the needles guaranteed the harmlessness of the punctures, the previous vacuum put an aspiratory needle carrying the vacuum within it at our service, and it allowed us to explore, vacuum in hand, the depths of the most delicate organs.

This new idea appeared so seductive, it was so various in its applications, so quickly adopted everywhere, that, to respond to its needs, seventeen aspirators were invented in France and other countries.　From the list of aspiratory instruments I will mention the following :—

Dieulafoy's notched aspirator ;
Dieulafoy's rack aspirator ;
Hamon's aspirator ;

Potain's aspirator ;
Smith's aspirator (London) ;
Rasmussen's aspirator (Copenhagen) ;
Myrop's aspirator (Copenhagen) ;
Weiss's aspirator (London) ;
Weiss's superposed aspirator ;
Castiaux's aspirator ;
Regnard's aspirator ;
Leiter's aspirator (Vienna) ;
Thénot's aspirator ;
Fleuret's steam aspirator ;
Dieulafoy's double aspirator.

All these aspirators may be arranged in two classes, which I shall proceed to examine in the following article.

ARTICLE II.

Summary. — The Parts composing an Aspirator. — The Working Barrel.—Aspirators with an unvarying Vacuum.—Aspirators with a varying Vacuum.—Aspirators with unvarying Vacuum are Aspiratory Injectors.—Needles and Trocars.

An aspirator is made up of essential parts and accessory parts. The latter may be modified, but the essential parts are unvarying, for they of themselves constitute the principle on which aspiration is based. An aspirator, of any description whatsoever, must be made up of, first, the body of the pump, in which the previous vacuum is made ; secondly, fine and hollow needles, intended to be introduced into the tissues in search of fluids.

The size and shape of the apparatus may be varied infinitely, but the principle on which the aspirator rests cannot be modified ; therefore, the instrument must, from the outset, attain an unsurpassable degree of perfection. In fact, however perfect may be the vacuum obtained by an aspiratory apparatus, its power of aspiration cannot be superior to that of one atmosphere ; and however fine the aspiratory needles may be, it is still necessary that they should be of sufficient calibre to allow the passage of hematic and purulent fluids.

Thus, both the perfection of the vacuum and the fineness of the needles have their limits in an aspiratory apparatus, beyond which it is impossible to go. This is the reason why the numerous aspirators which have been constructed during the last three years, as well as those which are brought out every day, are of necessity based on the same plan as the original model. They only differ from each other in quite secondary points of detail ; they cannot depart from the established type, and they cannot pass the limits which are inexorably imposed on them. All the difference is involved in the working of a tap, in the form of the instrument, or in the manner of producing the vacuum. These differences we will proceed to examine.

The first aspirator, the instrument which was laid before the Academy of Medicine, was the notched aspirator, in which the vacuum is created by a single stroke of the piston, and the piston retained at the top of the pump by a notch, transforming the instrument into a true pneumatic machine. This extremely simple method of creating the previous vacuum in the barrel of a pump which holds 50 cubic grammes, would become fatiguing and impracticable if the receiver were larger. Thus, in the 150 gramme aspirator, we replaced the notch by a rack, and the vacuum is equally well made in the barrel of the pump by a single stroke of the piston. To sum the matter up, the action of the notched aspirator, of the rack aspirator, and of the double aspirator, which are based on the same principle, consists in a piston working in the barrel of a pump of fixed dimensions. I call these instruments

" aspirators with an unvarying vacuum," because the capacity of the graduated receiver in which the piston moves cannot vary, the aspiratory power in it is always the same, and produced by the first stroke of the piston.

In another class of aspirators, instead of the vacuum being made by a single stroke, it is obtained by means of an indefinite number of strokes of the piston, the number depending on the capacity of the receiver, in which the air is progressively rarefied. This receiver, in which the vacuum is made, is infinitely variable, resembling, according to circumstances, a hollow ball, a bottle, or a flask with two tubular openings. MM. Potain and Castiaux's French aspirators, M. Myrop's Danish, and M. Weiss's English instruments, are constructed on this principle. I shall call these instruments " aspirators with a varying vacuum," because the amount of vacuum placed at the service of the operator varies according to the capacity of the receiver, and according to the number of piston strokes necessary for the rarefication of the air contained in this receiver. Such are the two chief classes of aspirators ; as for the other aspirators which create a vacuum by more or less complicated chymical methods, I only refer to them from memory, and without describing them, so unpractical do I consider them. We will make a comparative examination of aspirators with the varying and unvarying vacuum. The aspirators with the varying vacuum offer as an advantage the power of being able to accommodate the dimensions of the receiver in which the vacuum is created, to the capacity of the cavity containing the morbid fluid. They simplify the operation, since it suffices to make a vacuum in a bottle holding about a litre, instead of doing it several times in a 150 gramme aspirator. These aspirators are good when the emptying of a large collection, such as an effusion into the pleura, is in question, but that is their only advantage, and for other purposes they are less useful than aspirators with an unvarying vacuum.

In fact, they are not instruments of precision like the latter, possessing the power of adapting themselves according to necessity both to the previous and subsequent vacuums. They are ill adapted to the delicate processes of washing out and injecting, which we have described at length in the treatment of hydatid cysts of the liver and of purulent pleurisy. The aspirators with a varying vacuum are only intended for simple aspiration, whilst the aspirators with an unvarying vacuum are also aspiratory injectors; their mathematically graduated receiver affording means of ascertaining the amount of aspirated or injected fluid set in motion. This apparatus likewise gives us information as to the dimensions and the capacity of the morbid cavities. It allows us to follow day by day the gradual contraction of these cavities, and by the aid of the piston working in the barrel of the pump, it is easy for the operator to impart to the fluid injected the force required to wash out a morbid cavity in its most hidden parts and anfractuosities. The action of thoracic and hepatic trocars is based on the mechanism of the aspiratory injectors, as are likewise the processes of successive washings out and graduated injections.

THE NEEDLES.—It would be an advantage if the needles of all the aspirators were constructed by unvarying standards; which will be easily understood when a puncture made with No. 1 or No. 2 needle is in question. The diameter of the needle is, in fact, the most essential condition of the harmlessness of the aspiratory punctures. When, for example, it is necessary to puncture a hernial intestinal loop, or a bladder distended with urine, it is not a matter of indifference whether we make use of a needle one millimetre, two millimetres, or two millimetres and a half in diameter.

No. 1 is the finest needle; its diameter is only half a millimetre. Instruments of greater delicacy might be constructed, but, for practical purposes, it is not possible to pass this limit, or continual obliteration of the passage would be the consequence. This No. 1 needle is but rarely employed; for our part, we reserve it for very delicate explorations, or for the extraction of fluids similar to that found in hydrocephalus.

No. 3 needle, which is a millimetre and a half in diameter, is only useful in cases where a purulent fluid is very thick, and may hold in suspension detritus of false membranes. No. 2 needle is the most generally employed; it is a millimetre in diameter, and is the needle to be used in thoracentesis, hydarthrosis, cysts of the liver, retention of urine, strangulated hernia, &c.

Diameter of the needles :—

No. 1 needle (long and short), half a millimetre.
No. 2 needle (long and short), one millimetre.
No. 3 needle, one millimetre and a half.
No. 4 needle, two millimetres.

THE TROCARS.—In some exceptional cases, we can replace the needle by a trocar (for instance, for the puncture of ascites), but we must not confound the needle and the trocar, and take good care not to use No. 2 trocar when the No. 2 needle is indicated. It seems to me useless to recur to the description of the thoracic and hepatic trocars, on which I have dilated in the treatment of purulent pleurisy and cysts of the liver. I therefore refer the reader in quest of further details to those chapters.

The diameters of these trocars are as follows :—

Simple trocar, No. 1, one and a half millimetre.
—   —   No. 2, two millimetres.

Curved thoracic trocar,   No. 1, one millimetre and a half.
—   —   No. 2, two millimetres.
Right hepatic trocar,   No. 1, a millimetre and a half.
—   —   No. 2, two millimetres.
—   —   No. 3, three millimetres.

DIEULAFOY'S RACK ASPIRATOR.

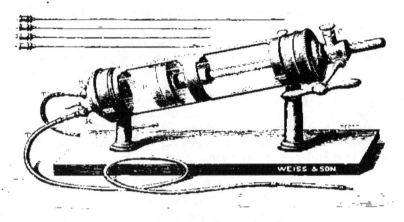

The Aspirator with an Unvarying Vacuum.

The rack aspirator is an aspiratory injector, with an unvarying vacuum. It holds a larger quantity of fluid than the notched aspirator, since it holds 150 grammes, while the other can only receive 45. Its manipulation is easier, as the operator keeps both his hands free at the moment of aspiration; the length of the india-rubber tube allows the apparatus to be placed at some distance from the patient, and the action of the rack allows a piston, of which the surface measures 35 millimetres in diameter, to be drawn up without fatigue, a proceeding which was impossible by the simple movement of the notched aspirator.

EXPLANATORY NOTE.

P   Piston.
C   Spring intended either to hold or to disengage the rack.
RR' Taps.
T   Aspiratory tube; a glass index, intended to allow the fluid to be seen as soon as it has been met by the needle, may be observed towards its anterior extremity.

T' Discharging tube, which is at the same time the injection tube by which the fluid to be injected through the tube T into the morbid cavity is introduced into the aspirator.

Plan of Operation.—The vacuum is created in the aspirator as follows :—

1. The taps RR' are closed by placing them at right angles, that is to say perpendicularly to the jet of fluid.

2. The piston is drawn up to the top of the barrel by means of a rack, and from that moment a vacuum is created in the aspirator.

3. The needle to be used is applied to the india-rubber tube T, which is placed in connection with the aspirator by the tap R.

4. As soon as the needle is introduced into the tissues to be explored, the corresponding tap of the aspirator R is opened, and a vacuum is consequently produced in the needle ; this needle is then driven slowly into the tissues in search of the fluid. As soon as the needle meets the fluid, the latter rushes into the aspirator, and at once reveals its presence by traversing the glass tube situated in the course of the india-rubber tube.

5. When it is desired to drive out the fluid contained in the aspirator, the tap R is closed, and the tap R' is opened, and the rack is disengaged by drawing the catch C out of its notch ; it is retained in this position by a slight rotatory movement, and the fluid is driven out by means of the piston which is sent down the barrel of the pump. To drive out the fluid more easily, an india-rubber tube, which dips into a basin, is fitted to the tap.

6. If it be desired to inject a medicated fluid, or to wash out the morbid cavity just emptied, a plan directly inverse to that which we have just described is adopted. The fluid to be injected is aspirated through the india-rubber tube fitted to the tap R' ; then this tap R' is closed, the tap R is opened, and the injection is driven into the cavity. The aspirator being graduated, we know with great exactness, to within a few grammes, what is the quantity of fluid set in motion. We can ascertain the capacity of the morbid cavity into which the injection is thrown, and follow the retrocession of this cavity and its progress towards cure. Thanks to the play of the piston, we have under control a force powerful enough to send the modifying fluid into all the anfractuosities and windings of the morbid cavity.

This apparatus is thoroughly adapted to the washings and injections performed with the hepatic and thoracic trocars we have described in detail in the course of this work. If it be desired to make the injecting operation still more convenient, it suffices to have an aspirator with three taps and three tubes ; the first for aspiration, the second for injection, and the third for the expulsion of the fluid which has been used for washing out the cavity.

There are two conditions essential to the regular manipulation of the aspirator.

1. Before operating it is necessary to make sure of the permeability of the needle, and this needle, replaced in the box, ought always to have a wire passed and left in it.

2. If the aspirator be but seldom used, the piston is liable to become dry ; we must therefore take the precaution, at the proper time, to aspirate a little water and allow it to remain in contact with the piston for some moments, so as to soften the lower layer, which ensures the creation of the vacuum in an almost complete manner.

It is very easy to transform the aspirator into a syphon : the fluid being first drawn into the barrel of the pump, the tube T must be placed in a depending position, the piston pushed down, driving back the fluid, the two taps R and R' left open, and the syphon is established. We very rarely advise this plan, as the aspiratory power with a syphon of this description is six times less than the power obtained by means of the aspirator.

ASPIRATORS WITH A VARYING VACUUM.

The woodcut on the opposite page shows the Pneumatic Aspirator which has been contrived and is manufactured by Messrs. WEISS & SON, of the Strand.

The Aspirator consists of—

1. A Glass Bottle or Reservoir, A, mounted with a two-way stop-cock, B, and having an opening at the bottom for the insertion of the tube, C.
2. An exhausting syringe, D, with elastic connecting tube, H.
3. A tubular needle, E, to be attached to the reservoir by an india-rubber tube, F.

A syringe and stop-cock for injecting astringents or other fluids is supplied if desired. The stop-cock is in such cases fixed to the tube F at its juncture with stop-cock B. Thus the tube can be detached from the Aspirator without any chance of air entering the cyst.*

DIRECTIONS FOR USE.

Adjust the Aspirator as figured in the diagram with the stop-cock B turned vertically, that is, open to the bottle; close the stop-cock in the tube C, and form a vacuum by a few upward and downward movements of the piston of the exhausting syringe D.

Insert one of the needles beyond the two eyes, attach tube F to it, turn the stop-cock B towards the needle, namely, horizontally, and continue the insertion of the needle until fluid is seen to flow through the short glass tube G into the reservoir.

To empty the latter turn stop-cock B vertically, detach the syringe tube, and open the stop-cock in tube C.

The presence of fluid having been established by the use of one of the fine needles, it is recommended for more quickly emptying the cyst to use one of the larger needles or trocars.

The introduction of the needle into the tissues requires some pre-

---

* Messrs. WEISS & SON inform me that their apparatus possesses certain advantages: such as simplicity of construction, facility for keeping it in order, the possibility of creating a complete vacuum, and the non-liability of the piston of the syringe being injured, as the fluid does not come into contact with it.

ATIONS.

SURGERY AND
CORMAC, F.R.C.S., Senior
Post 8vo.

PHYSIOLOGY. By
of Physiology, King's College

ICAL AND **PATHOLOGICAL**

MEDICINE, in its Legal,
By W. H. MICHAEL, F.C.S., Bar-
M.A., M.D., Oxon.; and J. A.
Post 8vo.

guidance of Medical Officers of Health
in the performance of their duties,
and others interested in questions of
diseases by the application of Sanitary

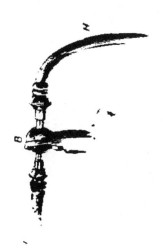

IA MEDICA AND THERA-
the Physiological Action, and the
By T. LAUDER BRUNTON, M.D., D.Sc.,
Therapeutics at St. Bartholomew's Hos-

PRACTICE OF MEDICINE.
D., F.R.C.P., Physician and Joint Lecturer
Hospital. Crown 8vo.

MANUAL. Being a Guide to
Obstetrical Society of London. By J. H.
to the Chelsea Hospital for Women, Hon.
Society of London. Post 8vo.

ACY: A Vade-Mecum relating to the
of the Insane in Public and Private Asylums.
NSLOW, M.B., M.L., Cantab.; D.C.L. Oxon.;
Post 8vo.

OLUTIONS OF THE BRAIN. By Pro-
Translated by JOHN C. GALTON, M.A., M.R.C.S., F.L.S.,
n Comparative Anatomy at Charing Cross Hospital.

cautions.   In place of endeavouring to penetrate by pressure as with an ordinary trocar, it is preferable to combine pressure with rotation, by taking the needle in the forefinger and thumb, and rolling it between them.   Such a manœuvre is rendered necessary by the extreme fineness of the needle, which would be liable to bend or twist if driven in by direct pressure.   Before using a needle it is well to be assured of its permeability.

LONDON : PRINTED BY
SPOTTISWOODE AND CO., NEW-STREET SQUARE
AND PARLIAMENT STREET

SMITH, ELDER & CO.'S

MEDICAL PUBLICATIONS.

IN THE PRESS.

A MANUAL OF PRACTICAL SURGERY AND SURGICAL ANATOMY. By WILLIAM MAC CORMAC, F.R.C.S., Senior Assistant Surgeon, St. Thomas's Hospital. Post 8vo.

TEXT-BOOK OF PRACTICAL PHYSIOLOGY. By WILLIAM RUTHERFORD, M.D., Professor of Physiology, King's College and Royal Institution. Fcp. 8vo.

PART 1.—PRACTICAL HISTOLOGY.
PART 2.—EXPERIMENTAL PHYSIOLOGY.
PART 3.—PRACTICAL PHYSIOLOGICAL AND PATHOLOGICAL CHEMISTRY.

A MANUAL OF PUBLIC MEDICINE, in its Legal, Medical, and Chemical Relations. By W. H. MICHAEL, F.C.S., Barrister-at-Law ; W. H. CORFIELD, M.A., M.D., Oxon. ; and J. A. WANKLYN. Edited by ERNEST HART. Post 8vo.

, This Manual is intended for the guidance of Medical Officers of Health and Members of Local Sanitary Boards in the performance of their duties, and for the information of medical men and others interested in questions of public health and the prevention of diseases by the application of Sanitary Science.

A MANUAL OF MATERIA MEDICA AND THERAPEUTICS ; including the Pharmacy, the Physiological Action, and the Therapeutical Uses of Drugs. By T. LAUDER BRUNTON, M.D., D.Sc., Lecturer on Materia Medica and Therapeutics at St. Bartholomew's Hospital. Post 8vo.

A MANUAL OF THE PRACTICE OF MEDICINE. By JOHN SYER BRISTOWE, M.D., F.R.C.P., Physician and Joint Lecturer on Medicine, St. Thomas's Hospital. Crown 8vo.

THE MIDWIVES' MANUAL. Being a Guide to the Examination of the Obstetrical Society of London. By J. H. AVELING, M.D., Physician to the Chelsea Hospital for Women, Hon. Sec. to the Obstetrical Society of London. Post 8vo.

MANUAL OF LUNACY : A Vade-Mecum relating to the Legal Care and Custody of the Insane in Public and Private Asylums. By LYTTLETON WINSLOW, M.B., M.L., Cantab. ; D.C.L. Oxon. ; M.R.C.P. London. Post 8vo.

ON THE CONVOLUTIONS OF THE BRAIN. By Professor ECKER. Translated by JOHN C. GALTON, M.A., M.R.C.S., F.L.S., late Lecturer on Comparative Anatomy at Charing Cross Hospital.

READY.

A SYSTEM OF SURGERY : PATHOLOGICAL, DIAG-
NOSTIC, THERAPEUTIC, AND OPERATIVE. By Samuel D.
Gross, M.D., LL.D., D.C.L., Oxon. ; Professor of Surgery in the
Jefferson Medical College of Philadelphia, &c. Fifth Edition, greatly
enlarged and thoroughly revised, with upwards of 1,400 Illustrations.
2 vols. 8vo. 3*l.* 10*s.*

A TREATISE ON HUMAN PHYSIOLOGY; designed for
the Use of Students and Practitioners of Medicine. By John C.
Dalton, M.D., Professor of Physiology and Hygiene in the College of
Physicians and Surgeons, New York, &c. Fifth Edition, revised and
enlarged, with 284 Illustrations. 8vo. 28*s.*

A PRACTICAL TREATISE ON FRACTURES AND DIS-
LOCATIONS. By Frank Hastings Hamilton, A.M., M.D., LL.D.,
Professor of the Practice of Surgery with Operations, in Bellevue
Hospital Medical College, New York, &c. Fourth Edition, revised
and improved. With 322 Illustrations. 8vo. 28*s.*

SURGICAL DISEASES OF INFANTS AND CHILDREN.
By M. P. Guersant, Honorary Surgeon to the Hôpital des Enfants
Malades, Paris, &c. Translated from the French by R. J. Dunglison,
M.D. 8vo. 12*s.* 6*d.*

ESSENTIALS OF THE PRINCIPLES AND PRACTICE
OF MEDICINE. A Handbook for Students and Practitioners. By
Henry Hartshorne, A.M., M.D., Professor of Hygiene in the University
of Pennsylvania. Third Edition, thoroughly revised. Post 8vo. 12*s.*

A PRACTICAL TREATISE ON URINARY AND RENAL
DISEASES, INCLUDING URINARY DEPOSITS. Illustrated by nu-
merous Cases and Engravings. By William Roberts, M.D. Second
Edition, revised and considerably enlarged. Small 8vo. 12*s.* 6*d.*

A PRACTICAL TREATISE ON DISEASES OF THE
LUNGS : including the Principles of Physical Diagnosis and Notes on
Climate. By Walter Hayle Walshe, M.D. Fourth Edition, revised
and much enlarged. Demy 8vo. 16*s.*

A PRACTICAL TREATISE ON THE DISEASES OF THE HEART AND GREAT VESSELS ; including the Principles of their Physical Diagnosis. By WALTER HAYLE WALSHE, M.D. Fourth Edition, thoroughly Revised and greatly Enlarged. Demy 8vo. 16s.

AN INTRODUCTION TO THE STUDY OF CLINICAL MEDICINE: Being a Guide to the Investigation of Disease, for the Use of Students. By OCTAVIUS STURGES, M.D. (Cantab.), F.R.C.P., Assistant Physician to Westminster Hospital, and formerly Registrar of Medical Cases at St. George's Hospital. Crown 8vo. 4s. 6d.

AUSCULTATION AND PERCUSSION, together with the other Methods of Physical Examination of the Chest. By SAMUEL GEE, M.D. With Illustrations. Fcp. 8vo. 5s. 6d.

DEMONSTRATIONS OF ANATOMY. Being a Guide to the Knowledge of the Human Body by Dissection. By GEORGE VINER ELLIS, Professor of Anatomy in University College, London. Sixth Edition. With 146 Engravings on Wood. Small 8vo. 12s. 6d.

ON EXERCISE AND TRAINING, AND THEIR EFFECT UPON HEALTH. By R. J. LEE, M.A., M.D. (Cantab.). Lecturer on Pathology at Westminster Hospital, &c. 1s.

SYPHILIS AND LOCAL CONTAGIOUS DISORDERS. By BERKELEY HILL, M.B., Lond., F.R.C.S. Demy 8vo. 16s.

THE ESSENTIALS OF BANDAGING : Including the Management of Fractures and Dislocations, with Directions for using other Surgical Apparatus. With 122 Engravings. By BERKELEY HILL, M.B., Lond., F.R.C.S. Second Edition, revised and enlarged. Fcp. 8vo. 3s. 6d.

HOUSEHOLD MEDICINE : Containing a Familiar Description of Diseases, their Nature, Causes, and Symptoms, the most approved Methods of Treatment, the Properties and Uses of Remedies, &c., and Rules for the Management of the Sick Room. Expressly adapted for Family Use. By JOHN GARDNER, M.D. Seventh Edition, revised and enlarged, with Numerous Illustrations. Demy 8vo. 12s.

SMITH, ELDER & CO., 15, WATERLOO PLACE.

NAME	DATE DUE

Check Out More Titles From HardPress Classics Series In this collection we are offering thousands of classic and hard to find books. This series spans a vast array of subjects – so you are bound to find something of interest to enjoy reading and learning about.

Subjects:
Architecture
Art
Biography & Autobiography
Body, Mind &Spirit
Children & Young Adult
Dramas
Education
Fiction
History
Language Arts & Disciplines
Law
Literary Collections
Music
Poetry
Psychology
Science
…and many more.

Visit us at www.hardpress.net

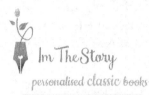
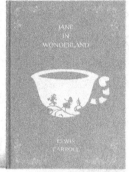

CPSIA information can be obtained
at www.ICGtesting.com
Printed in the USA
BVHW092246270819

556849BV00015B/2268/P